1r46   2306/10   16.14   2.95

The End of Innocence

THE END OF INNOCENCE
Britain in the Time of AIDS

SIMON GARFIELD

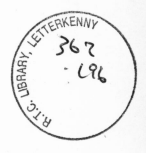

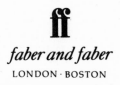

faber and faber

LONDON · BOSTON

For Diane

First published in 1994
by Faber and Faber Limited
3 Queen Square London WC1N 3AU

Photoset by Intype Ltd, London
Printed in England by Clays Ltd, St Ives plc

© Simon Garfield, 1994

Simon Garfield is hereby identified as author of this work in accordance
with Section 77 of the Copyright, Designs and Patents Act 1988

A CIP record of this book is available from the British Library

ISBN 0-571-15353-4

10 9 8 7 6 5 4 3 2 1

Contents

List of Illustrations

Author's Note

Shortly after I began researching this book, I was struck with fear. What if people decided not to talk? What if people believed that no one who was not touched intimately by AIDS could write a fair account of it? What if they failed to share my enthusiasms that this story had almost everything – sex, blood, death, science, religion, scandal, filmstars?

Whenever I asked anyone for an interview, I gave a little speech. I said that I wanted to write a history of Britain over the last ten years with AIDS at its core; an account that would tell you some interesting things about a lot of institutions and systems (health, politics, education, charities, democracy, medical research), not by addressing these topics directly, but by examining how they coped when faced with what everyone was calling the biggest health crisis since the Second World War. It was like they say in those corny true-crime straight-to-video films: from a detailed examination of one terrible thing, we may emerge with a greater truth. This is what I told them; it was true and I hope it is true now. But when I told people this, especially gay people and haemophiliacs and others who have been most affected by AIDS in this country, I usually felt that I was selling them short. Ultimately, however you cut it, AIDS is about dying, or fighting not to die. And I suppose I felt guilty about not attending enough AIDS funerals.

Actually, this didn't bother people too much. When I asked for their opinions, or for access to their notebooks or minutes, no one told me that I was unqualified to write this history (although they may have believed it and may believe it still), and for that I was grateful. What a lot of people wanted to know was: 1) who else had I talked to, 2) why did I want to do it, and 3) did it have a title.

Other than the fact that HIV and AIDS had always fascinated me, because it seemed to affect us all dramatically, yet few intimately, I explained that when I had written a magazine article about the drug AZT, I had scrambled around for something that would put it all in perspective, but could find little apart from medical journals or cuttings of other articles. When I thought deeper I also reasoned that having a brother who died in his twenties (not of an AIDS-related ill-ness) may have had something to do with it too.

This book has no claims to be a definitive history of AIDS in Britain; that would take 30 volumes, and most likely be unbearable to write and read. Besides, the history is far from over. But it is, I believe, a full and accurate account, and one that reflects the main events, and some of the lives, that have shaped its course thus far. As I hope will become clear from the text, it seemed like a good time to take stock and look around.

The bulk of the book is in chronologically themed form, but the last chunk is a year-long journal kept while researching and writing, a structural conceit intended to tie up some loose ends, spear some absurdities and throw light on the future. Not all the text for this last chapter was written at the time of the action it records.

As all but one of the main events described occurred in the last 13 years, I have leant heavily on first-hand accounts. With the exception of 'Steve' in Chapter 11, all the names are real. I owe a large debt to many people who have helped me, either by agreeing to talk on the record, or by supplying valuable background information and docu-mentation.

In particular I am grateful to: Derek Jarman, Dr Ray Brettle, Dr Laurence Gruer, Prof Tony Pinching, Prof Michael Adler, Prof Ian Weller, Dr Jane Cope, Dr Alan Stone, Dr David Ho, Dr John Leonard, Dr Trevor Stretton, Dr Peter Jones, Dr George Williams, Prof Trevor Jones, Dr Jerome Horwitz, Christopher Spence, Nick Partridge, Stephen Fry, Holly Johnson, Tom Hanks, Angela Serota, Geoff Crawford, Sir Norman Fowler, Baroness Cumberlege, Lord Kilmarnock, Chris Smith, Sir Donald Acheson, Kate Grieves, Lindsay Neil, Claire Baron, Lyndall Stein, Jimmy Glass, Tony Whitehead, Simon Taylor, Rupert Haselden, Tim Clark, John Campbell, Joy Barlow, Ben Croall, Paul Trainer, Alastair Hume, Peter Stransky, Adam Sampson, Hugh Dufficy, Michael Cottrell, Karl Burge, Michael Scott, Ceri Hutton, Les Rudd, Linda Semple, Zoe Schramm-Evans, Andrew Butterfield, Robert Key, Edward King, Simon Watney, Esmee Seargent, Steve Mayes, Aamir Ahmed, Martin Harrington, Sammy Harari, Malcolm Johnson, Will Huxter, Peter Scott, Caroline Guinness, Philippa Easterbrook, Neville Hodgkinson, Margaret Jay, David Mellor, Edwina Currie, Jerry Hayes, the Revd Martin Smyth, Dawn Primarolo, David Morgan, Margaret Johnson, Jimmy

Somerville, Jonathan Grimshaw, Patrick O'Connell, John White, Sheila Dutch, Naomi Wayne, Richard Salmon.

A few passages from this book have appeared, in a slightly different form, in the *Independent* and *Independent on Sunday*, and I am grateful to several editors who demonstrated their skills and offered support: David Robson, Liz Jobey, Richard Williams and Ian Parker. The staff of the *Independent* library were always knowledgeable and helpful. Thanks also for invaluable guidance to my agent, Pat Kavanagh, and to everyone who has supported this book at Faber, particularly my editor, Julian Loose.

Della Hirons, the librarian at the Terrence Higgins Trust was dazzlingly efficient. Nicky Wilson, Anne Moir and George Carey of Barraclough Carey provided some useful contacts and material, as did Tim Hulse at *Esquire* and Mig Lumley at *Horizon*. Lucy Thorpe at the Health Education Authority was extremely helpful, as was Sara Mosely at the London Lighthouse, Graham Barker at the Haemophilia Society and Ian Poitier, Keith Winestein, Julian Meldrum and Steve Coote at the National AIDS Trust. Neil McKenna provided encouragement and many contacts. My old friends Andrew Bud and Matthew Kalman read the typescript and offered many useful suggestions. For services too diverse to mention thanks also to Sue Terry, Liz Lynch, Richard Maude, Geoff Woad, Tehmina Boman, Pamela Esterson, Peter Tatchell, Richard Tomlinson, Roger Tredre, BJ, JC, and FD.

PART I

Chapter 1: Thirty-Five Years

'What is the black spot, captain?'
'That's a summons, mate.'
Robert Louis Stevenson, *Treasure Island*

Manchester, 1959

'Mr Carr, we'd like to keep you in for observation overnight.'

On 8 April 1959, David Carr was admitted to Manchester Royal Infirmary looking wasted, feeling feverish. He had managed to walk into outpatients, but the consultant on duty was certain that Carr would not be going home that night. A while later the consultant realized that Carr would never see his home again.

His blood pressure was normal and his lungs were clear, but the 25-year-old patient had many strange symptoms: he had an inflamed nostril and gums, an anal ulcer and some scaly brownish lesions on his back and shoulders. In the past five months he had experienced night sweats, breathlessness, loss of weight, tiredness and a high temperature.

Carr was placed on an open ward and was examined most days by either Dr John Leonard, the senior registrar, or Dr Trevor Stretton, the senior house officer. Unexplained cases were not uncommon on their wards, but neither of them had seen a case like this. The doctors ran tests and offered treatments, but the tests were all inconclusive and the treatments mostly inefficacious. The initial diagnosis was tuberculosis. Hodgkin's disease was also suspected, as was Wegener's granulomatosis, a rare condition of unknown cause. But when the tests came back from the labs they were all negative.

So they were stumped, though they couldn't admit this to their patient. Carr's immune system appeared to be simply shot to pieces. He became increasingly subdued, in great discomfort from his symptoms and weary from the examinations; every few days they took more samples, more swabs, more blood, more scrapes, and yet he continued to waste away, surrounded mostly by older men with established conditions.

His parents visited at the appointed hours, as did his girlfriend;

3

they were engaged to be married next year. They couldn't imagine what had caused such a sudden transformation. David was their strapping lad, a robust footballer at school, a keen apprentice printer on a local newspaper. He'd never experienced serious disease before and he had remained healthy throughout his stint of national service in the Royal Navy.

And now here he was, a medical mystery. All the experts came, the chest men, the skin men, the bacteriologists. He even attracted Professor Robert Platt, the consultant who later became President of the Royal College of Physicians. In the case notes Platt wondered whether, now that bacterial infection was in retreat from antibiotics, it wasn't possible that 'the viruses are going to come and plague us'.

In the last month of his life, Carr developed fresh ulcers and broncho-pneumonia. He died on 31 August 1959, 20 weeks after admission. His cause of death was entered officially as Wegener's granulomatosis. But the autopsy revealed something else.

Dr George Williams, a pathologist at the hospital, had also never seen anything like the body of David Carr. It was severely emaciated and covered in small lesions and fissures. One of his lungs was partially collapsed and his spleen and liver were enlarged. The samples Williams cut from his lungs revealed cysts in a honeycomb formation, suggesting a form of pneumonia, *Pneumocystis carinii*. The lungs also contained swollen infected cells typical of cytomegalic inclusion disease, a virus belonging to the herpes group. Considered separately, these factors were rare and seen most often in babies or small children. Considered together they were practically unheard of.

The doctors could offer no clue as to how their patient might have contracted such diseases, or how these diseases conspired to kill him so swiftly. They wrote the case up for the *Lancet*, but when their report appeared, more than a year after David Carr's death, they received no correspondence; no one else appeared to have any ideas either.

At the end of his autopsy, Dr Williams stored some tissue samples, the way he always did. These were tiny sections, perhaps a centimetre square, sliced from all the organs. Williams took more samples than normal, about 40, fitting, he believed, for such a perplexing case. He 'fixed' them in a formaldehyde solution for 24 hours, treated them with alcohol, embedded them in paraffin wax and stored them between pieces of stiff paper. This was standard and reliable practice and remains so today.

4

With many cases, the tissue samples are disposed of after a few years; others become untraceable or mislaid. David Carr's tissues were not destroyed or lost and survived two departmental moves. And that would have been the end of the story, another unexplained case in a regional teaching hospital many moons ago. But then, about 20 years later, young men began falling sick in New York and Los Angeles and San Francisco.

At the beginning of the 1980s, none of the Manchester doctors had forgotten their patient from 1959, such was the rarity of his condition. But their memory of the details was patchy. They had not seen a comparable case since. They had flourished in their respective careers, both in Britain and abroad. When news of 'the gay cancer' or Gay Compromise Syndrome or Gay Related Immune Deficiency (GRID) first came from America in 1981, the young doctors who had treated David Carr were in their fifties and had seen thousands of patients.

Dr Leonard clipped any articles that caught his eye in the *Lancet* and *British Medical Journal*, but the relevance of these early reports of Acquired Immunodeficiency Syndrome (AIDS) to David Carr's case was not immediately apparent. In the summer of 1983, when the reports of the syndrome began appearing in the national British press, he was working at Manchester's Withington Hospital. He called Dr Stretton at the Royal Infirmary. 'Do you remember that chap we saw with Pneumocystis? Do you know what I think he had?'

Stretton said he did. 'If he came in today I know which test I'd run first.'

Leonard called George Williams too and composed a brief letter to the *Lancet*. 'Could [our patient] have had AIDS?' the letter asked. 'He had previously been well. While in the navy (1955–57) he had travelled abroad. He was not married and we know nothing of his sexual orientation.'

There was little response, but the Centers for Disease Control (CDC) in Atlanta, Georgia, the organization that was tracking the epidemic in the United States, called Stretton to ask for some serum. There was none. Tests on tissue samples, if any could be found, would not be sophisticated enough to prove anything. The CDC asked Stretton to find out what he could about the man's past, but when he called David Carr's former GP in Stockport he was told that both his parents had died and his fiancée had moved to Australia. There was an elderly aunt in the area, but Stretton was advised that

5

she was frail and unlikely to welcome an inquiry of this nature. And so the matter came to rest again.

In the next few years, the case came to assume even greater potential significance. As research scientists studied the evolution of the virus, several wild theories about the origin of AIDS began appearing; the panic and prejudice AIDS engendered completely destroyed logical patterns of reasoning. Post-cholera, post-typhoid, post-polio, modern Western medicine could no longer be shocked by new epidemics. AIDS was no doubt man-made. Blame was the thing – who was *guilty*? The CIA or KGB released a virus as a form of germ warfare and/or to rid the world of homosexuals; it was the will of God and divine retribution; it came from outer space, the virus from another planet; it came from recreational drug use; it came from a polio vaccine programme; it came from telephone cables.

In fact, it is widely believed that Human Immunodeficiency Virus (HIV), the virus that leads to AIDS, originated in Africa, a mutation of a strain of virus prevalent in monkeys for many decades. But in the two or three years after the virus was isolated in 1983 there was so little natural history, so little convincing aetiology, that it was no wonder the crank theories took hold. The case of David Carr had the potential to lay at least some of them to rest, but his case appeared not to be unique. Also in 1959, an anonymous person from Kinshasa, Zaire, had serum drawn and stored which was shown many years later to be HIV antibody positive. In the same year, a 48-year-old New York clerk fell ill and developed symptoms similar to David Carr's: night sweats, fever, weight loss. The man had moved to Manhattan from Haiti three decades earlier. The autopsy revealed no underlying disease, but again detected Pneumocystis carinii pneumonia. When Dr Gordon Hennigar, the pathologist, was asked subsequently whether he thought the man had AIDS, he said, 'You bet.'

HIV infection before 1970 has also been detected in a Norwegian family. The father, a sailor who had travelled to African ports and contracted sexually transmitted diseases at least twice, fell ill in 1966 with recurrent respiratory infections and generalized lymphadenopathy (enlargement of the lymph nodes, a common trait in people with AIDS). His condition did not worsen until 1975, when he deteriorated rapidly and died the following year. His wife had health problems from 1967, including respiratory infections and candida, a fungal infection that affects the mouth and vulva. She also died in 1976, after severe weight loss, leukaemia and dementia. The youngest of three

6

daughters died at the age of eight with a lymphocyte depletion shared with her parents. Frozen serum samples all proved HIV positive. Sexual transmission was suspected in the case of the parents, while the daughter was believed to have been infected in the womb, or through breast feeding; she was thought to be the earliest recorded case of paediatric AIDS, certainly in Europe. The other two daughters were both healthy.

There were other cases too, including a 15-year-old boy from St Louis, Chicago, who died in 1969 and whose autopsy revealed a purplish lesion on his thigh and similar internal lesions. These are believed to have been malignant tumours called Kaposi's sarcoma, then almost unheard of in young men.

As news of these cases began to trickle out in the mid-1980s, the Manchester doctors realized that their patient might hold the earliest clues as to the origin of what had by then become a modern pandemic. George Williams had managed to locate the tissue samples in November 1987, although it was by no means clear how to proceed. He contacted Professor Maurice Longson, the consultant virologist, with a view to identifying a possible HIV protein on the tissue cells. The standard immunological methods were still primitive and no such virus was located. The following year, Williams got in touch with Dr Gerald Corbitt, another virologist at the hospital. Corbitt had recently become aware of a new American process of DNA amplification called the Polymerase Chain Reaction (PCR) that might prove suitable in the case of these tissues.

It was still an elaborate and time-consuming process which demanded rigid procedures. Sections were sliced from the wax blocks containing tissues from the brain, the liver, a kidney, throat, bone marrow and spleen. A control patient of a similar age to David Carr was located, a man who had also died in 1959, in this case from a road traffic accident. All the samples were coded by Williams before examination began and they remained blinded until the procedures were complete. The entire process – dewaxing, centrifuging, drying, resuspension with a range of chemicals, amplification – took several days. Of the 12 tissue samples examined, four were HIV positive. Decoding showed that all four came from David Carr. These samples were from the kidney, bone marrow, spleen and throat. Tissues from the brain and liver were negative, as were all six samples from the control. The conclusion was obvious and devastating: Carr had been infected with HIV.

7

There was much interest when the results of the tests were published in the *Lancet*, but for the results to have value many more questions had to be answered. Where exactly did Carr go on his travels? Was he gay or bisexual? Had he infected his fiancée? Had any of his shipmates shown similar symptoms?

The investigations continue today. His fiancée is well and lives in Australia. She believes her fiancé never had a homosexual relationship. In 1990 John Leonard wrote to the Admiralty for further details of his patient's ship movements and learnt that for much of his national service Carr was in Great Britain, at Chatham and Devonport, only travelling to Gibraltar and Tangier in February 1957, towards the end of his stint. Leonard's correspondent, a medical officer, noted that 'Tangier was (and still is) a hotbed of vice, where anything is available and discreetly catered for.' Leonard believes his patient was probably infected by a prostitute, either in Tangier or further south in sub-Saharan Africa, if indeed he had travelled that far. It is not known whether he sailed independently of the Royal Navy prior to his call up, perhaps as a merchant seaman; if he was infected in Tangier, the incubation period of the virus and his progression from infection to death – some two years – appear to be unusually short. When he was discharged from the navy in November 1957, his medical records showed no record of any illness.

The death of David Carr has further resonance. In 1992, Dr David Ho was working as the founding director of the Aaron Diamond Centre for AIDS research in downtown Manhattan when he heard of a new and initially attractive theory about the origin of HIV. This theory, reported at length in *Rolling Stone* magazine and subsequently in the national press, suggested that the large vaccination for polio virus in 1957 in the Congo may have initiated the AIDS epidemic by the introduction of simian (monkey) immunodeficiency viruses (SIVs). It was thought that the polio virus vaccine might have been grown in simian kidney cells. These monkey cells may have harboured SIV, which entered humans through vaccination and then evolved into HIV.

Dr Ho had been working in the AIDS field for eleven years. As a young clinician in Los Angeles in the early 1980s he had seen several of the first patients who presented with many of the unusual opportunistic diseases we now associate with AIDS. He had previously done work on other syndromes that also lacked an aetiology and it was a natural progression for him to make HIV his speciality.

It didn't take him long to distrust this new Congo theory; all his work had suggested that the virus dated back much much further. The problem was, there seemed to be no way of dismissing it absolutely. He was appointed to a special committee to look into the Congo evidence and it was then he remembered the Manchester case. From what we know of his travels and from what we understand about the incubation period, David Carr became infected before the vaccination programme began. But much more could be learnt from his tissue samples.

Ho wrote to Gerald Corbitt at the Royal Infirmary about the possibility of acquiring some of the samples; Ho was surprised that although the HIV testing had been done, no one had looked at the viral sequencing of the DNA. This was crucial to the understanding of how the virus has evolved over the years.

Corbitt consulted with George Williams, checked Ho's credentials and sent him a small piece of embedded kidney tissue. Ho and his researchers worked on this through much of 1993. He extracted the DNA from the section and, using the same PCR technique, amplified the entire virus in several chunks. These pieces were then cloned, and their nucleotide sequence determined. This sequence was then compared with current sequences from all over the world, in particular from North America and Europe. They were also compared to other sequences from monkeys and HIV-2 (a less virulent strain of HIV located in West Africa and still mostly confined to that area).

What Ho found in preliminary inquiries was that the virus from the 1950s was not very different from the one we see today, which suggests that these viruses have been going around for many decades and permits some rudimentary calculations. Ho believes that the divergence points from the chimpanzee virus must have occurred between 80 to 100 years ago and the divergence from HIV-2 and other monkey viruses must have been several hundred years ago. These are minimum estimates.

Dr Leonard, Dr Stretton and Dr Williams are semi-retired now and live within a few miles of each other in Cheshire. John Leonard is 67. His wife was a GP, their two sons are doctors. He has told his sons that the young man he saw in 1959 'is the only patient that I've ever seen that will live in history. I shan't live in history, but the patient will.'

He says he feels rather pleased about it, but what gives him most satisfaction is the fact that they wrote up the case in 1960. 'If we had just shrugged our shoulders and said, oh, too bad, and done nothing about it, then I think it would have been forgotten. That's our only claim to fame, and then twenty-four years later to have realized that it was AIDS, I think that was good too. I don't think we had ever really forgotten him.'

George Williams is also 67. He still writes and does a little work at Manchester University. He says he wasn't at all surprised that the tissues tested HIV positive, 'because it fitted so beautifully. But then the impact that it was the first authenticated case of AIDS in the Western world – that was exciting and interesting. There was also an element of relief and pleasure that the saga had been finally solved.'

He has had several requests for tissue samples since Dr Ho began his work, including one from the UK, but he has turned them down, aware that any new research would squander material on the sort of initial investigations Ho has already conducted. But in February 1994 he did send more samples to Ho. 'I'm keeping a strict eye on this,' he says. 'I don't want to lose it all. Having looked after the tissues very carefully so far, I have a pretty shrewd idea as to how much I can release for further investigation.'

David Ho's privately funded centre employs almost 70 staff engaged in a wide variety of scientific AIDS research. Situated across the street from the turmoil of Bellevue Hospital, it is a serene, plush place, elegantly furnished, immaculately appointed. Ho is a rising star of the field and has published several important papers in the international journals; highly specialized areas, minute but critical advances. For Ho, as with most sober AIDS scientists, the prospect of a sudden breakthrough (a much-loathed layman's concept) is unrealistic. A cure? Forget it. A vaccine? Many years away. There is some hope, of course, but there is much caution too, the result of too many false dawns. This is the long haul: every year Ho's people learn that they have so much more to know.

Of the Manchester case, Ho says: 'It's one of the fun things to do in science. It's somewhat different from the other projects we do, and this one has a nice twist to it. We think the sequence we've found here is real important.'

He says he's surprised at how slowly things have happened with the analysis:

If a case like this had happened in the United States, the Centers For Disease Control would have everything. It would have spent an enormous effort trying to find out more about this case. Nothing has been instituted by the Communicable Disease Surveillance Centre [the north London body that has monitored the spread of AIDS since 1982] until I wrote them, saying we have all this information. I do consider myself fortunate that when we asked we got the tissues.

Trevor Stretton is 62. He retired two years ago, disturbed by what he'd seen of the NHS reforms. Though he was never an AIDS specialist, he saw a lot of AIDS patients in his time as a respiratory expert. He, too, says he will never forget his first; an age away, an age away.

He was on our ward for months and we weren't hesitant at doing tests, mainly blood tests, biopsies of tissue as well. An open ward, and we were concerned of course in those days about cross-infection, but we didn't have disposable equipment: a syringe was reused, a glass syringe was a precious commodity and they were used until they got broken and the needles were reused until they became blunt and had to be thrown away.
   Needles were rinsed, washed and put in boiling water. We had a little boiler, a sterilizer sitting in the centre of every ward and we would put the needles and the syringes in there and reboil them and it was usually left to the most junior person. Very often medical students had the task of taking the blood; if ever there was a risk or an opportunity for a needle puncture or injury to another person, my goodness it was there.

Stretton remembers another patient of his, a middle-aged man he'd known for years, suddenly falling very sick in the mid-1980s. He'd had an operation in 1982 and picked up some contaminated blood.

Of course by that time we knew. He had a wife, had a loving, supportive family who went bananas when they knew what I thought he'd got, they were offended, distressed. About that time I was beginning to see haemophiliac patients, simply because the regional haemophilia centre is based in the Royal Infirmary.

One saw the occasional person who was homosexual, but we also saw people from Africa who were over here for academic reasons, post-graduate students at the university and whose disease was probably acquired heterosexually. All this distance away from their families and we'd got to counsel them and help them as best we could.

London, 1994

I'm a farm boy from Sussex. My dad was a farmer. My parents divorced when I was eight. I have a brother and a sister. I was sent away to boarding school which I neither liked nor hated and then I realized: I lay in bed at school when I was thirteen and said to myself, 'Rupert, you're homosexual.' I remember being rather pleased. I remember thinking this was going to be a key to meeting all sorts of people in a strange underground world. Far from being horrified, frightened, I remember thinking it was going to be the most fantastic adventure.

Rupert Haselden, 36, is sitting on a large sofa in his house in Balham, south London. It is early February 1994, clear and crisp, and the room is stifling, made airless by a wheezing fan heater. He's wearing two sweaters and heavy jogging pants. He is thin and pale but quite dashing, a little like the English comic actor Jeremy Lloyd, a big Roman nose and thin oaty hair. He has a rich voice, almost plummy. The room is elegant, packed with a traveller's treasures, framed by large paintings, giving way to a wild garden visited, this particular afternoon, by an inquisitive heron. By his side there are tea and digestives, and remote controls. By the controls a large black metal box containing his pills. Sam the dog has a noisy nightmare on the sofa opposite.

I was fourteen when I first got picked up by a man in London. In order to get to and from school I had to go to London on the train and change, and on one of these train changes I had gone to the toilet on Waterloo and got picked up by some bloke. I was somewhere between fourteen and fifteen when I went into Piccadilly Circus toilet one day and followed a chap out who seemed quite nice and he turned round to me and said, 'Are you rent?' I thought it must be some sort of slang for 'Are you queer?', so I said yes. He said, 'Well so am I, so there's no way then is there?'

He realized that I was naïve and took me off to coffee at Swan and Edgar's and told me that he was a rent boy and explained what all that meant and I was transfixed. He lived in Earl's Court he told me, and that sounded terribly exotic. But I went with him to Earl's Court and he lived in this terrible hole of a flat with about eight other rent boys.

But it became, this flat which was one of the most dreadful places I've ever seen, became like a second home to me really. During school holidays for the next few years and with the other kids – we were all teenagers – I used to sort of do rent, as they say.

It was wonderfully naïve and childish. It was basically wanking off old men in the staff bathrooms at the Regent's Palace Hotel. You got a tenner for it and then you went off to the James Bond movie in the evening. The rent boys got into the few nightclubs that there were for free. This is about 1972–3. I certainly didn't feel like a prostitute, not that I would have cared if somebody had said I was.

I finished my schooling and my mother split up with this second husband and I wanted very much to live in London.

I had a year between school and university, but I didn't want to continue doing the rent. I wanted to make it a bit more legit and so I wrote four letters: to the Tate, to the Royal Academy, the zoo and to Buckingham Palace asking for work. I said anything would do, and they all wrote back and said no, all except for Buckingham Palace which wrote back and said: 'Well we might have something, come and talk to us.'

And I got a job as a sort of glorified office boy, working under the master of the household, and I had a year that I could never have imagined, it was just fantastic. Wherever She went I went, and I met her every day and sort of glammed around and had absolutely nothing to do all day except putting a couple of things in a file. I was just a clerk, but I had an office of status which always amused me and I just swanned around. I mean there I was in Buckingham Palace ... I used to do things like going and organizing the private little details of the royal family's life, so I'd go off to Harrods in one of the cars with a driver and be shown up to the VIP suite. I'd choose binoculars or something ridiculous and take them back to the Palace and get the OK or not.

We would shoot off to Windsor for the weekend and then we

would go off to Sandringham for a few weeks and maybe Balmoral and then be on the yacht and nobody actually seemed to have anything to do. There must have been a few people working terribly hard but nobody else did, and we all spent the time being drunk, jumping in and out of bed with each other.

It's quite rare to meet somebody who isn't gay at the Palace. Office staff tended not to be quite as gay as the footmen and under butlers and kitchen people. I remember the very first night I spent with the royal household, it was in August 1976 and we travelled up on the train, the whole royal entourage to Balmoral. The weekend before I had thought, 'Oh my goodness, going to the deepest, darkest Scottish highlands for twelve weeks, there won't be any sex at all, ghastly.' So I'd had a bit of a binge that weekend in London. I arrived at King's Cross to meet the train, that was when I really met all the staff for the first time. Two hundred and fifty of us travelling north, and I just looked and it was like some sort of huge gay convention. By the time the train left the station I realized I was in for a ball.

So I had a wonderful year with them, and then they asked me if I'd like to stay on a second year because it was her Jubilee, and I thought it would be great and it was. But during that year I realized something. I had sort of been going to do medicine as a career, and I'd realized I wasn't a scientist. The whole medicine thing was one of those childhood things where whenever anybody asked it was, 'Oh Rupert's going to be a doctor.' So I didn't go to medical school, instead I decided I'd better go to New York, get out of it because I didn't have a clue what to do.

His partner, a BBC film maker, comes into the room. They've been together for 13 years. He's off to South Africa on a business trip. He says: 'I've made a will, Rupert, very rough, just in case anything happens to me. It's been so long since I made my last one. It's really about what happens to the house. Here.' He hands him a handwritten sheet of A4, both sides covered. 'I'll leave it on my desk upstairs.' A little later his taxi comes. They kiss goodbye. 'See you soon,' Rupert says. 'Do phone.'

I arrived in New York in 1978 with no money. I think I had a couple of hundred quid at the most for the summer. I had one telephone number of somebody I didn't know at all, a friend of a friend of a friend. I spent the first night in this dreadful dump. On the second night I phoned this telephone number and this chap was extremely

nice and helpful and he said, 'Oh I'll show you the Village tonight.'
During that evening we bumped into some friends of his and we went
back to one of them. He was called Bob, and it was clear that Bob was
a very, very successful young designer and had this spectacular loft
apartment. The next day Bob contacted me and invited me to dinner
and there and then said he was going off, away for the summer, and
did I want his apartment? Well of course I said yes, but then it turned
out to be much more than his apartment.

He also had a wonderful house on Fire Island in the Pines [a fabled
gay resort in Long Island, New York]. He used to fly me out each
weekend, and he and I became terribly close, non-sexually actually.
He was round about forty, twenty years older than me. He had come
from nothing and had made a huge amount of money and he just
quite obviously loved spoiling me. He loved doing things like, he'd
phone up and, it's all so ridiculous, he'd phone up and say, 'Look out
the window,' and there'd be a limo. He'd say, 'Get in it,' and then it
would take me off to the sea plane. He would introduce me to all
sorts of other famous designers that were around on the Island at that
time. I had a summer like I couldn't believe. Like everybody else, I
fucked my way stupid round the nightclubs and the bars and the
bathhouses and everywhere else.

There were gays on Fire Island for twenty, thirty years before, but
it felt very much as though it had only just become chic four or five
years earlier. I got the impression that Halston was just building his
fantastic place, and Warhol had just built his amazing place and there
was a sense that it was all happening. Everybody was somehow somebody. Suddenly people would turn up on your deck and it would be,
that bloke Cousins, the figure skating guy and Nureyev was around,
and there was all this sort of stuff.

All of these beautiful grey shingle beach houses with these huge
decks in amongst all this greenery ... The routine of the day was to
get up late and then you probably had staff who prepared everything
for you, so we got up around lunchtime and then you did drugs and
doing drugs was a big part of being there. You sunbathed all afternoon and in the evening they all had these silver foil things they stuck
under their chins. Suntans were very important. Nobody went in the
water, nobody swam. I always thought that was very odd.

Teatime you went to the club, back near where the little boats came
in, and you then went to the dance. After the dance you slowly
crawled back, still drugged out of your heads, back to your houses,

had dinner and then after dinner you all went back to the bar, danced some more and then rather than going home you went to this area of scrubland where everybody was fucking everybody, and so you fucked a few people and then you went home to bed.

I couldn't believe the scene in New York either. I'd only been there for a very few nights and I met somebody in a bar and they said they were going to go on to the Mineshaft. Now I'd heard of the Mineshaft when I was in London – it had a reputation. I thought, well it's now or never, so I asked if I could go with him. We walked up and it was very dramatic, because it was in the middle of nowhere in the old meat market section, and we arrived and we went up and they had a big guy sitting on a stool outside the door who sort of checked you out.

The person I'd gone with disappeared on inside and the guy stopped me and he said that he wouldn't let me in. I asked him why not, and he said, 'I don't like what you're wearing.' I said, 'How about if I wasn't wearing it?' He made me strip, stark bollock naked at the top of the stairs in the middle of this pitch dark place lit by a few red light bulbs. And then once I'd done that he let me go in and I stood there and I had never seen anything like it: fist fucking, racks, and the stench of piss and poppers and everything else and the heat and the men and the light was all red and I remember thinking standing there, adrenaline thundering round me and thinking, 'This is evil, this is wrong.' I remember being very frightened; it seemed so extreme. But later I was thinking about it a lot, and wanking when thinking about it, and the next thing I knew I was back there and within weeks it felt like home.

New York at that time ... you professed to liberation by your promiscuity: that was how you said 'We are different, this is a different lifestyle from the straight one, we're not pretending it's the same, we'll behave as we wish to.' And I took full part in it.

I never, ever once got clap, I didn't even get crabs, and how I didn't I cannot imagine, because back in London I seemed to spend my life in the clap clinic.

Eventually what happened was that I realized that I had to have some sort of work, and I started working for a tiny film promotions company in New York. I started life as a nobody. Peter Yates had made a film called *Breaking Away*, which the studio, Fox, didn't know what it was when it was delivered to them. So they handed it to our specialist outfit to try to market it. There was a little screening for the staff of this company to talk about it, and I jumped up and down and said I thought it was fabulous, and my boss turned round and said, 'Well if you think it's so fucking good, do something with it.'

I didn't actually have a clue what I was doing, but we opened it up in a cinema in New York and were lucky: the *New York Times* went and loved it and suddenly it became a hit [and was later nominated for an Academy Award for Best Film].

Peter Yates mentioned to Ray Stark, the head of Columbia Pictures, that there was this English boy who'd done this, and Stark came to New York and took me out to dinner, asked me about what I was going to do. I said, 'Why don't you invite me to Hollywood and let me find out.' Stark made me the script boy really, you know the filing clerk in the script department. I moved up, and then I came back to England when they wanted somebody to work their London office. So I did that, and I was backwards and forwards for eight years.

In 1982, when I'd been working for Columbia for a couple of years, I came back through New York and I phoned up Bob. I knew he was pleased that I suddenly had this good job and was doing well and was no longer just the little boy who ... I was staying in a nice hotel. I took him to dinner; I'd never taken him to dinner before.

I took him to the restaurant where he had taken me the very first night we'd met, and that night he said, 'Do you want to come and stay with me?' and I remember thinking he'd lost a lot of weight. I said to him, 'Yeah, OK.' We'd often slept in the same bed before and nothing had ever happened, but that night we had sex and we had quite extreme sex and I remember feeling odd about it. I remember feeling I wished I hadn't done it really; in a funny kind of way it betrayed the friendship that we'd had.

Then I went back to London and for whatever reason I didn't get in touch immediately, and about two or three months later, perhaps slightly later than that, I had a telex from his business partner saying that Bob had died and that in fact he'd been ill for some time and had never really recovered from a trip he'd made to Japan or China or somewhere and that he'd had these terrible stomach problems.

I remember a chill went through me because I knew, I was just starting to hear, about this illness that was happening in New York.

A younger man enters the room carrying supermarket bags. This is Gary, who helps with some of the chores: making lunch, driving him to the hospital. There is also a district nurse who calls round every morning to help him get up and wash. Soon they'll bring a hoist for the bath and put a frame around the toilet. He'll get a pair of tongs to help him pick things up from the floor.

I have no real way of proving this but I believe very strongly that I got HIV from Bob on that one night. I certainly don't harbour any kind of resentment or anything. I spent my night with Bob in January or February 1982 – the dates are very difficult. And then after Easter I had this strange illness, and I was just terribly tired and I felt I just couldn't cope at all. I went to a guy who was the STD consultant from St Mary's and I remember going to see him privately in Harley Street one afternoon. He examined me and he suddenly said, 'You've got a fever and you've been having night sweats, haven't you, and you've got an enlarged spleen.' He then suddenly said, 'I want you to come into St Mary's this afternoon.'

I was horrified but I knew exactly what he was thinking. I must have started to have read enough about this illness to know what the symptoms were. I refused to go to St Mary's. He did blood tests on me nevertheless, but of course they didn't have an HIV test then. I was terrified, absolutely shit scared. Later he told me that the test had come back with an abnormal T-cell count [the standard marker of the body's immune system] and I imagined I was going to die there and then.

My partner was concerned that I was being so neurotic about all of this and sent me off to a homeopath. The homeopath there and then said, 'You do not have this AIDS thing, you are fine.' That was of course all I wanted to hear and I remember leaving his surgery and thinking this is fantastic, I'm OK. And I never went back to see the doctor again.

I just got on with my life for the next few years. I was very anxious: I was all too aware that I'd lived in New York in the most dangerous time, and California too. It was all becoming mad – everything you touched seemed to be about AIDS. I lived the next years in a strange state of denial and terror. I started to get more and more paranoid, more and more convinced that I had HIV and unable to bear to look at any ... if the newspaper page had the word AIDS on it I turned over, I couldn't bear to see anything or know anything about AIDS.

But I did start to be safe. We've never had a monogamous relationship, but my promiscuity declined after I met my partner. But both of us did a lot of travelling for work and it was always understood that it was OK to meet people and sleep with people when we were away. Basically what happened for me was that I became terrified of any fucking at all, I just found it a turn off. In America I already knew of or knew a lot of people who were ill and I avoided seeing them. This paranoia continued and I started to know of people in London who were ill and in about 1987–8 I knew somebody quite well who got ill and died.

I suppose it would have been '89, spring of '89, when I got what I thought was flu which I couldn't get rid of, and then I started to get very breathless. I seemed to get worse and the breathlessness got worse, and my brother-in-law is a doctor and my sister insisted that he came and looked at me. He immediately said, 'You've got pneumonia and you've got to have this treated.' Eventually I was so unwell that one evening my sister called an ambulance and I went to the hospital. St George's.

They didn't admit me to the AIDS ward, they admitted me with suspected psittacosis [a contagious infection common in parrots, sometimes passed on to humans; in 1984 there were 410 reported cases in adults and children]. I had a parrot who was sick, so it made sense. My partner was away in America, but my family were obviously in contact with him and he was furious because nobody was doing an HIV test. He eventually phoned up the sister on the ward from California.

I insisted that I didn't actually want the test until he was back in London. So I remember one afternoon, they'd put me in a little side room with him and we sat there waiting for the doctor to come and tell us the result. We knew really what the result was going to be. It was just like something out of these awful TV doctor series: the door opened and the registrar came in flanked by a couple of his colleagues and he said, actually he was terribly nice, I like this man, and he said, 'Rupert, you do have HIV and in all probability you have AIDS.'

My feelings then were a total surprise to me, the most fantastic relief I've ever felt in my life. He then didn't stay very long, the doctor. My partner and I, we felt duty bound at that moment to cry, so we did manage to cry for about two minutes and then I realized I didn't want to cry at all, I was just so relieved, I was so … I just … there was no more pretending. I'd had eight years of whatever it was, of fear and pretence and kidding myself, and suddenly now here I was, and I had to deal with it and I remember going in for the next few days into this ridiculous state of elation.

They changed my medication and I was feeling much better, and I can remember everybody coming to visit me, my friends and family, and me sitting there, it must have been a very strange sight for them, being sort of euphoric, totally un-upset about it all. I didn't cry again about AIDS for several months. Very quickly, within a week to ten days, I was well enough to go home.

I was obviously a bit feeble but within months it was almost as if nothing had happened and I was playing squash and running and taking the dog for a walk and working, a mixture of television scripts and freelance articles.

Then my partner was also tested, and he also was found to have AIDS and a terribly low T-cell count, twenty or so [a healthy average count is considered to be above 500]. But he was mostly OK too, so I remember for a time saying to people, 'AIDS is nothing like you imagine it, it's fine.'

I didn't get ill and I didn't get tired and I didn't have night sweats, and I think I almost felt that people who were getting ill with AIDS were rather feeble. I was taking AZT [the most commonly prescribed anti-viral drug], but I was taking a very low dose and that was it and then after about a year of taking it, I was reading a lot about it and I decided to stop altogether. Then I was on no medication at all. There was just nothing wrong with me and then suddenly one day, about two years ago, I looked in the mirror and there was a tiny pink patch on the end of my nose.

I tried to convince myself it wasn't really there. Over the weeks it got a bit darker and eventually I was down seeing the doctor at the hospital and he asked me, 'What do you think that is on the end of your nose?' He said he thought it might be Kaposi's sarcoma. I walked out of the doctor's surgery and I bumped into this nurse who worked at the hospital who had the tact of a sledgehammer, and she suddenly said to me, 'Ah Rupert,' she said, 'what's that on the end of your nose?'

So I said, 'Well he's just said he thinks it might be KS.' 'Oh God,' she said, 'now we'll start seeing *much* more of you.'

I was sent off to the Marsden and sure enough it was KS. Other bits of KS started appearing and for a year it was fine, it was just skin stuff, I had topical bits of treatment. It was a bit embarrassing occasionally when it was on your face but I decided that KS wasn't really hard to deal with either.

When I was in hospital with PCP [Pneumocystic carinii pneumonia] I decided that I was going to be completely open with everybody and so I would tell work-related people and we weren't going to hide it from any of our friends. We have never, ever had a negative reaction to telling anybody. Everybody has always reacted by being very sad for us or sympathetic or whatever, but nobody has ever felt they can't deal with us any more or shocked or disgusted, well they might be shocked but never disgusted.

My mother made the decision to talk to her friends about it and now it's paid off enormous dividends because they have obviously over the years learnt quite a lot about AIDS themselves and they really are able to offer her a huge amount of support now that I'm much less well. My mother lives down in deepest Kent, lives in a fairly conventional middle-class world down there.

I've known so many people where their families haven't dared tell anybody.

Then I suppose a year or so ago, I played a game of squash, I hadn't played for a bit and I remember afterwards I had never been so stiff in my life. I knew it wasn't just like normal stiffness from being unfit; I was stiff for days and days and then I started to feel always a little bit out of breath. Then in the spring they thought that I was getting pneumonia again and treated me for that, then last April [1993] they did a bronchoscopy and they found that I had KS through my lungs.

I was told by my consultant I should recognize how serious things had got, and without saying so in so many words he implied that I should make sure I had a good summer; I knew that he didn't think I would be around by November. Initially the chemotherapy worked really well, but by October it was clear it was working less well. Whenever we walked anywhere I kept saying 'You've got to slow down.' I found myself in the afternoons just wanting to not do much. I'd go to the supermarket and carry the bags and realize that I was pretty out of puff. I also had some terrible pains in my gut and in November I went into hospital with CMV [cytomegalovirus, a virus belonging to the herpes group].

By the time I came out a month later, things had changed very dramatically. In the hospital I was no longer well enough to get from my bed in the hospital to the loo; I just sat on the loo almost in tears, trying to get my breath again. I came home and I suddenly found that all I could do was sit on the sofa. At night I was determined to get to the bedroom upstairs but it was a real fight. I began to wonder what the hell was going to happen.

I remember saying to one of the nurses, 'My fear now is dying of suffocation.' I could just see my breathing getting worse and worse, and it was happening so fast, so quick day by day. Then I'd heard about this new drug which they were using at the Kobler Centre in a very narrow trial. My consultant at St George's said there was some way in which they could make an application for the drug on compassionate grounds. It was very expensive. I don't know why but I had this obsession that this was the drug that I needed. I am now using it once a fortnight as a form of chemotherapy. It has very many of the same effects of normal chemotherapy, a feeling of nausea and unwellness for several days, but it has helped me a great deal. But I'm very breathless still, and if I got up now and went into the kitchen, I'd be out of puff. I have very bad KS; while the lung thing was happening the KS just suddenly blew up in my groin and my leg here and there. The whole of this thigh is just solid KS.

I take thirty tablets a day. I resent all of them. They discovered I had MAI as well [mycobacterium avium-intracellulare, an aerobic bacteria, another AIDS indicator condition], and so I take three lots of antibiotics every day. I take anti-sickness tablets. I take Acyclovir [an antiviral herpes treatment]. I take eight tablets of dihydrocodeine a day. What other ones? I'm probably missing out some; I just seem to take tablets all the time and I have a box here which is just filled with my tablets, and I've got a bag behind there which is just packed. I go to the hospital probably seven or eight times a week, five times for radiotherapy and two or three times for other things. I suspect I'll be dead by the summer.

I've talked a lot about dying with family and with friends. I go through different periods of feeling wonderfully enlightened and calm and then the next day hopeless and neurotic and depressed, but depression isn't the dominant feature. Shortly after I got ill, to my horror I could actually feel this illness attacking my body. But I felt that's all – I didn't feel it was killing me as a person.

I'm racked sometimes with guilt about it because I feel I'm inflicting huge amounts of pain on my family and close friends through this. I'm going home to my mum this weekend with my brother and I know she will be terribly brave with me about my not being well and finding it hard to move around her house and things, but I know that it's agony for her.

However politically correct I try to be, it's impossible not to feel that this was self-inflicted. People get furious with me when I say this. I was talking to a couple of people from the Terrence Higgins Trust the other day who were livid, saying 'How can you say that? That's what we're fighting against, to try and stop people feeling that this is our fault.' When I say self-inflicted, I'm not making a judgement, it's just that there is no denying that it was my lifestyle that led to this event.

In September 1991 he wrote an article for the Guardian *that provoked howls of outrage. He did not write specifically about his own life or illness, but about the 'inbuilt fatalism to being gay'. He reasoned that, unable to reproduce, gay men were self-destructive, 'living for today because we have no tomorrow'. It was a passionate piece, roaming the London clone scene, surveying the damage. At first, he says, gay men changed their lifestyles, lived in fear. But now fear was giving way to acceptance and gay men were again returning to the clubs, 'no longer in search of liberation but increasingly in what, terrifyingly, we are coming to see as our fate'. There were pickets at the* Guardian *offices; Derek Jarman held up the article in fury. Haselden was putting the cause back years, the letters said. 'How dare he speak for the rest of us!'*

I was very concerned about a number of young friends that I had who were finding great thrills in not having safe sex, night after night in the clubs. And I felt that gay liberation had, as I said, got stuck in the liberation phase. Unlike feminism and race issues which had moved on beyond that, in the face of AIDS we had retreated to the ghetto and to the support structures that it supplied. We seem to not have any clue of a future and nobody seems to be discussing the future, everybody's so busy coping with this awful present of illness every-where. I felt we continued to only offer one lifestyle up for inspection, which was the lifestyle of the ghetto, boys in blue jeans and T-shirts running off to the clubs and the discos, and that we were failing to reveal the range of lifestyles that gays live.

Not until the doctors and the carpenters and everybody else would stand up as doctors and carpenters and say, 'Here we are and this is me,' would we ever truly become liberated. I think that in the face of

AIDS we were embarrassed to do that. AIDS has been a very retarding force for gay liberation.

There is another side to that: I have the highest respect for the way the gay community has responded to AIDS. The fact that it has the profile that it has and that it has the understanding and the acceptance and the government money is a real testament to what gays have managed to do.

I was taken aback by the force of the anger. They called me 'self-loathing', which is nonsense; I'm proud to be gay. I got the most bizarre calls. I got one call: 'Is that Rupert? This is the Lesbian and Gay Switchboard. We're just phoning you up *vis-à-vis* your article. We had a meeting and discussed the fact that you could only possibly have written an article like that if you were seriously depressed and we were phoning to offer you support.'

I said: 'I'm furious that you're doing this, I'm not depressed, it's what I believe.'

I'm quite optimistic in some ways: but we have to move on, move on if we can. Personally I'm pleased I've lived as long as I have. It's been a fullish life, and I'm not too sad that I know it's almost over. On my medical chart there's a sticker for every year with AIDS and I've got five. When we first used to go to [the AIDS unit at] St George's we used to virtually have the run of the place. Now it's crowded. It's difficult to get the appointment you want.

At Rupert's funeral on 16 May 1994, every mourner, and there must have been at least 200, placed a long-stemmed yellow rose in a huge waterless glass vase. The funeral, in St Paul's Church in Clapham Old Town, was suffused with Monteverdi and incense. The service was taken by Malcolm Johnson, who knew Rupert well and had discussed this day with him at great length. Shortly before he died, Rupert had told him that he felt like a man all set to go on holiday, bags packed, but still waiting for the taxi. His mother spoke about her boy, about his charm and kindness and love. A friend sang the same song Frankie Valli sang after the death of Valentino. A man read Siegfried Sassoon. And his partner spoke, about their 13-year relationship and about an archway they had designed together for their garden. Shortly before he died, peering from a window, Rupert saw him lay a hollowed stone in the archway: the stone contained some of his possessions. These included a Biro to complete his long-promised autobiography, some holistic treatment to counteract the effects of chemotherapy, a condom, a box of matches from the Stonewall bar in New York, a coin commemorating the wedding of Charles and Diana and a tin soldier from his childhood. And then we all left, back for tea and more tears at his house, to the room where only a few weeks before Rupert had sat up and talked of a vanishing world.

CHAPTER 2: Subway

The blood-dimmed tide is loosed, and everywhere
The ceremony of innocence is drowned;
The best lack all conviction, while the worst
Are full of passionate intensity.
W. B. Yeats, 'The Second Coming', 1921

Don't Sleep with Americans

The club in Leicester Square was called Subway, an American name, an American concept, a quid on the door and then down to the basement, as to hell, hot no matter the month, packed even early, loud as you could bear. A disco: a great DJ, fast records, mostly imports, a lot about freedom. For this was indeed liberation, a gay bar far from home: clones, leathers, black boys, some poppers, the Village and Bay Area scene. There was a real treat at the side, a back room, a fuckroom they called it, quite rare in London, an experience you could never forget.

Perhaps a thousand men knew about it, and a few hundred went. Mostly it was the same people every night. If you didn't fancy the Heath or Clapham Common and you wanted something harder than the Burlington or Brownies and you liked the Flamingo on Berwick Street before they shut it down, then you'd come here. If you were Tim Clark and you worked as a waiter at Joe Allen, the hip media/theatre restaurant in Covent Garden, then you'd come here. 'Just a room with nothing in it,' he says. 'An ordinary sized doorway led into this black hole. One area had some sauna-style trestle seats along the walls, but that was it.'

On the trestle seats, there were semi-naked men.

If, like me, you didn't wear contact lenses and you didn't wear your glasses for reasons of vanity, it was just a nightmare, a great nightmare orgy. If you wanted somebody in particular, you just had to wait outside until you saw them go in and make sure that you followed close behind and keep them in your eyesight. It was all hands. Sometimes, if your eyes adjusted to the gloom, you could make out whether this person was under fifteen. Sometimes you would recognize halfway through the act: this person you were doing it with was somebody you actually knew.

If you were Holly Johnson, in a band soon to be called Frankie Goes To Hollywood, you came here on a weekend down from Liverpool. Taken to Subway by a friend who worked at the bar, he observed 'a room off the dancefloor that did not seem to be the toilet'. 'What's in there?' he asked his friend. 'I wouldn't go in there if I were you.' He went of course, and remembers 'flashes ... visions ... blue jeans round ankles and white vests or T-shirts scattered about or rolled up over the heads of uniformly crop-headed, moustached men'.

Peter Scott occasionally visited too, relief from his work as a college lecturer, a break from his shifts on Gay Switchboard. By the early 1980s, Scott had been a Switchboard volunteer for several years. Based in a tiny office in King's Cross, this was a service for the gay and lesbian community, one that had no counterpart in the heterosexual world. Part Samaritans, part nightclub information line, part radical grass-roots organization, it was the only national service of its kind, financed mostly by bucket rattling. It was staffed by a rota of a hundred volunteers, and fielded about a hundred thousand calls a year: one call would be a coming-out crisis; the next a general depression call; the third from someone who was bored and wanted a chat; the fourth might be someone wanting the location of the gay pubs in Southampton; the fifth about an accommodation service; the sixth a legal emergency, perhaps a child custody matter.

Switchboard was a trusted service dealing with a very young community, a community that had only developed its sense of identity and assertiveness since the 1960s. There were gay and lesbian befriending groups and coming-out groups throughout the country, and some localized help-lines, but the London Gay Switchboard was by far the biggest, the most politicized, the most efficient. If there was an anti-homophobia campaign to be launched, or a venue to be saved, or a medical crisis to deal with, then Switchboard would be the only place you could call with any confidence.

A lot of people called about sexually transmitted diseases (STDs). For a sexually active gay man in the late-1970s these were no more than an occupational hazard.

'There was everything,' Tim Clark says,

especially if you went for back-room sex or multiple partners cruising on the Heath. Syphilis, gonorrhoea, herpes, crabs – just the regular risk you ran, and you inevitably caught them with frequency. You would have regular appointments at the clinics and the treatments usually cleared things up fast. Going from injections to tablets was the big event of gay liberation as far as I was concerned. No more excruciating bum-numbing injections.

Peter Scott had a big STD file too: he reckons he's had over two thousand partners. He's had syphilis twice, and gonorrhoea more times than he likes to remember. He read a lot of medical literature and by 1980 it was clear to him that there were a range of STDs that had the possibility of getting out of hand. There was still no vaccine for hepatitis B. There was talk of strains of gonorrhoea that were becoming harder and harder to treat. There was talk of a 'gay bowel syndrome'. The understanding of what might constitute safe sex was already emerging; a few men were even using condoms.

'Who needs his lover's pick-up germs?' asked Andrew Lumsden, the editor of *Gay News* in the early 1980s.

I hear much more enthusiasm for monogamy and full-time chastity these days than for a long time past, and with one ear I'm delighted. The coming out of the randiest, cruisiest gay men has seemed at times to put an intolerable pressure on those who for whatever reasons don't want to lead a sexual life with strangers ... we've come perilously close at times to it being 'ungay' not to screw around.

Abstention would be fine for a while, the writer believed, but then he'd 'get restless, and become a romantic for anonymous sex. I maunder on about the extraordinary gentleness shown one another in this country by men making it on heath or in fuckrooms with other men.'

The word from the STD clinics was: 'If you have an STD, don't have sex,' but for many men this was unthinkable; besides, some of them had an incubation period during which the disease could be passed on unknowingly. There was discussion about what 'no sex' actually meant: was kissing OK? Was anything OK if it didn't involve penetration? As a rule, liberated gay men didn't like to be told how to live their sex lives; restrictions were seen as an infringement of their hard-won civil rights; it was no longer illegal to have sex between consenting adults over 21, and just let the new moralists – doctors, health educationists, whoever – tell them otherwise.

The relationship gay men had with STD clinics was extremely variable. Some were excellent, and men would self-refer to places like the Middlesex, St Mary's and St Thomas's, clinics that were often staffed by gay doctors. There were sympathetic centres in Manchester, Liverpool and Edinburgh too, but many sited in areas with a smaller concentration of gay men were moralizing and disapproving. Many doctors had a problem with their patients' attitude, a problem they shared with most of the general public: why, they wanted to know, did homosexual men inflict such diseases on themselves with such regularity? How could promiscuity be a birthright? And hey, they didn't even do it the *normal* way. If the doctors were homophobic, through disbelief and incomprehension as much as fear, then how would others comprehend? And how would anyone show concern in a time of crisis?

When Peter Scott first read about AIDS, it still had a variety of gay-related names. As part of his job, he heard about it earlier than most, in the reports from America in mid-1981; men on both coasts dying of rare cancers and pneumonias, all of them gay. His first thought was:

> Uh-oh, it's coming along, a bit like I expected with this super-strain of gonorrhoea that wouldn't respond to treatment. After a year it became clear that this was something that would also affect this country. This was a seriously dangerous train, some way down the tracks. And of course the tragic thing is that we didn't realize how far down the tracks it already was.

Most people didn't know of anyone who had an AIDS-related illness for quite a while. For British gays in 1981, the syndrome remained something that happened to other people, something that might never happen here, an American problem. *Gay News*, the only national gay newspaper, had a circulation of about 23,000 and sold itself on a mixture of hard news, gossip and high hedonism. In November 1981 it reported disapprovingly of the tone taken by a *New York Times* article on the 'gay cancer' which stated there was no apparent danger to non-homosexuals from contagion, and that of the 41 cases so far, none occurred outside the homosexual community or in women. 'The moral was clear,' *Gay News* reported. 'If gay men insist on having lots of sex with a variety of partners, they will have to suffer the revenge of cancer.'

The *Gay News* article, written by two Canadian doctors, suggested the disease was being used as another stick with which to beat gays for their lifestyle. The message was: Worry, but not too much. 'Undoubtedly,' it concluded, 'the factors which lead a small number of gay men to develop Kaposi's sarcoma will eventually be isolated – with or without gay-financed research. In the meantime we must endure the publicity which sensationalizes another "gay disease".'

For a while, one theory dominated. AID (as it was first known, the 'syndrome' came later) may be have been caused by amyl nitrite or isobutyl nitrite 'poppers', a recreational drug hugely popular in the gay world. Originally used as a medicinal relaxant, poppers dilated blood vessels and provided an instant rush that removed inhibitions and heightened orgasm. Widely regarded as harmless and non-addictive, poppers were on legal sale in shops and clubs, cost a few pounds per bottle and went by the name of Hardware, Quicksilver and Ram (in the United States, where their sale was prohibited, they were marketed as 'room odorizers'). Occasionally users would complain of heart palpitations or headaches, but nothing more. In this new cancer crisis, poppers rivalled promiscuity as the immediate cause, an attractive and plausible key to immunosuppression.

'The alleged connection between [poppers] and Kaposi's is analogous to the relationship between tobacco smoke and lung cancer,' an article in *Gay News* declared in July 1982, 'except that the statistical evidence on tobacco and lung cancer comes from a lot more victims and is far more conclusive.' The article then weighed up the existing evidence. A report in the *Lancet* summarized an American study of 20 men with Kaposi's sarcoma, which found that poppers were 'the only drug that 100 per cent of patients reported ever having used, although one patient reported using it only once in his life in 1977'. Further correspondence in the *Lancet* reported that two French Kaposi's patients had never used the chemical. *Gay News* noted that poppers had been around for decades without reports of serious side effects and that they were also used by heterosexual men and women. Why had there been no cases reported in Britain, it asked, where poppers were the gay drug of choice? Perhaps there was a reason: the links to cancer were thought to be with amyl nitrite, not the isobutyl nitrite more popular in the UK.

The article had a large impact on the community, not least because of its concluding paragraph. This reported that Alex Comfort, the British writer on sex, believed that 'uniquely homosexual acts, or those more often practised by gay men than by other groups, might be relevant. Until the questions [about sexual practices] are asked, no one can say he is wrong.'

'The question was, why was it just gay men?' says Linda Semple, who worked on *Gay News* and Gay Switchboard. 'At the paper we had so many theories coming in, and some really crackpot ones.' Some people thought it was caused by a strain of amoebic dysentery. Others were convinced it was airborne and 'going to get us all, like TB'. One letter ran to 17 pages in green ink. It came with a map and if you looked very carefully you could see that all the major outbreaks of AIDS in the world coincided with where the United States had naval bases.

'All hell started to break loose,' Semple says,

and the editor said 'This is nonsense, this is patent nonsense. We're not going to print these stories, we're going to try to find out what's going on.' That was good, but when we got more information the problem was how you imparted it. You couldn't scare people too much and you couldn't dictate. There were commercial considerations as well. We began to get information about attacks on the bathhouses in America and we were thinking, 'Well what's going to happen if we start publishing things saying don't go to Subway, because of the back room.' And we also had some letters saying, 'This is an American thing, why the hell are you devoting any space to it?'

At Gay Switchboard, AIDS caused huge political rifts. It was the classic debate, the same one that engaged activists in America: if you tell people to change their sexual lifestyle, is this impinging on their rights? Peter Scott says that some people at Switchboard believed quite early on – certainly by the end of 1983 – that AIDS was most likely to be sexually transmitted. No proof, 'but all the signs were there'. But advise people to use condoms in 1982 and 1983? You'd have as much chance as persuading them to be celibate, so no one tried.

The commonest form of early advice presented you with two options. If you were already in a relationship you could do whatever you liked, so long as you didn't screw around outside it. If you weren't in a relationship, then you should cut down on your number of partners. In 1983, when the HIV virus was isolated first in France and then in the United States (called at that time LAV and HTLV-III), the advice was that only about 10 per cent of people who had the virus would get AIDS, because many more people were infected than were unwell with any of the AIDS indicator diseases; most were perfectly healthy. Almost everyone was caught out by the long incubation period. 'There was even a sort of constructive optimism about it,' Scott says.

'A few people were going, "Grow up, get real, we must protect people, we must get people to protect themselves,"' Linda Semple says:

> But everyone else was saying, 'No, it's not up to us, it's up to them.' And for some time Switchboard's line was, 'It's safer than crossing the road.' That was the phrase we told new trainees to use. I'm paraphrasing, but it was basically 'If you're a really pernickety queen, then take care, but really sex is as safe as crossing the road.' There were a few people at Switchboard who were very unhappy with that line, and they left.

'In Edinburgh, gay men wouldn't sleep with Americans,' says Alastair Hume, who ran Key West, a gay bar, in the early 1980s. 'They thought if you don't go with Americans, then it wouldn't come over here, but they were actually just hiding from it, because they knew there was incredible traffic.'

Ships used to dock frequently at the naval port; there was the Edinburgh International Festival, 'a sexual delight', according to Hume, 'with people from all over the world, going like bunnies'; and then there were the cheap flights to sunnier climes.

As news from America spread, Hume and others began organizing leaflet distribution in his bar and benefits for research at the gay disco Fire Island. Key West, Fire Island: an ideal of gay nirvana. How different those places sounded now.

It was hard persuading some people. 'The other pubs weren't that interested,' Hume says:

> These days the gay scene keeps patting itself on the back for being so stunningly wonderful at practising safer sex – crap! Complete

and utter crap. You will always, in any community, get some people doing the right thing, but then you get the others who just have one drink too many, and don't give a shit. That was the attitude then.

In London, Tim Clark would still visit Subway, but he'd notice small changes:

I remember the posters going up about AIDS and condoms and poppers, but nobody paid much attention. The risk did not seem great at that stage, and we still didn't know of any English people who'd actually come down with it.

I remember the first one that I knew was a friend's former boyfriend. We didn't know anything about his diagnosis, when it happened or how it happened, but he just faded from the scene and was occasionally spotted just behaving appallingly, drunk and wild-eyed and staggering around. He just carried on drinking until he collapsed. Collapsed amongst his dustbins one night, and was carted off to hospital and died very shortly after that.

Anyone infected kept it hidden, and it was just a matter of great shame. You turned yourself into an untouchable. There was little solidarity at that stage. The impression you got was that it was somehow connected with promiscuity, and the people who got it defined themselves as being sluts. I just remember so many instances of people who kind of died fairly quickly and refused to admit it to anybody. One of them was part of the glamorous model crowd, an actor, at Joe Allen every night. He clearly died as much of shame as anything. He was one of those 'pneumonia' death certificates which were pretty common at that time. Doctors conspired in this, responding to the signals that we were all giving out.

At the beginning of July 1982, Terry Higgins, 37, was being examined at St Thomas's Hospital, London. It was the same appalling story: the doctors knew his immune system was wrecked, recognized the rare pneumonia and other opportunistic infections, but they couldn't say why or how; they knew, but they didn't really know.

Rupert Whittaker, Higgins's young lover, then a student at Durham University, remembers that Higgins had been ill for a while. Whittaker used to call him from the university and Higgins would complain of terrible headaches. Whittaker was on holiday in France when

THE END OF INNOCENCE

he heard that his partner had collapsed. He arrived at the hospital to find Higgins looking awful, grey and unconscious. He was in isolation.

But he made some progress and became well enough to leave. He became more of the person he was before: easy going and warm and supportive. It was these traits, together with his physical attractions, that Whittaker found so attractive. He was unemployed, a transitional period after leaving his job as a computer programmer.

Then he fell ill again with something else, another strange disease, up and down all the time. Whittaker suggested to Higgins's doctor that maybe it was this American thing, but he remembers all the doctors there as dismissive. 'I was not next of kin – I was not worth considering.' He says that one of the house staff said they planned to write up and publish the case and if he wanted to find out more he'd have to read it. The nurses were more supportive, but could offer little practical help.

On 4 July 1982 Whittaker met some friends in Hyde Park. He had called his lover earlier to ask what he should bring, but when he arrived at St Thomas's he found the curtains drawn around the bed:

> There were people in there doing something, there was a lot of muttering, and I stood at the bottom of the bed and asked the nurse, 'Is it all right to see him at some point?' I was taken in to another room and I had some ice cream or something and I said, 'Could you put this away for him later?' They took me into a waiting room and brought me a cup of tea, and about five or ten minutes later they came by and said, 'I'm afraid he's dead.'

No one knew anything. Nothing to read up. A nightmare funeral to arrange.

Five months later, in November 1982, some of Whittaker's grief had subsided, but the anger and confusion remained. *Capital Gay*, the newly formed London paper that was to play an important role in the dissemination of AIDS information, ran the headline 'US Disease Hits London', reporting that Higgins was among four Londoners to have died to date. It was Rupert Whittaker's friend and prominent activist Martyn Butler who first came up with the idea of a charity to raise money for research. The project was described as 'a massive entertainment machine', and it was to kick off with a themed party at the gay disco Heaven.

'Immune deficiency is already quite a problem in this country, and

Kaposi's sarcoma will take quite a few lives before long,' Martyn Butler predicted in *Capital Gay*. Another aim was to establish a widespread public health education programme, 'should that become necessary'. 'I'm amazed at the ignorance about it, even within the gay community,' Butler told *Gay News*; the paper described how AIDS was still thought of as 'a media import like *Hill Street Blues*'.

The Terry Higgins Trust would donate its first proceeds to the research being conducted at St Mary's Hospital, Paddington. A man called Floyd was organizing the Heaven party. 'I will be using my talents as choreographer and artiste to make people aware of what is happening with Sarcoma,' he said. It was probably quite a night.

Education is a slow process: while the Terry Higgins Trust and Gay Switchboard and the gay press advised and cajoled and passed on as much information as they could glean from the United States, they had little hope of reaching a wider public. Many 'non-scene' gay men were also unlikely to be aware of the severity of the crisis.

This changed a little in the spring of 1983, when first *Panorama* and then *Horizon* broadcast documentaries about the syndrome. The *Horizon* programme, 'Killer in the Village', had the greatest impact, not least because it examined the exponential growth of the epidemic thus far. The number of cases doubled every few months; if it continued at this rate, there'd be a million cases by 1989. It looked at all the theories – poppers, 'immune overload' from too many STDs, a communicable agent – and presented a sobering statistic from California to back up the latter: in a study of gay men with AIDS, nine out of 13 cases had known each other sexually. The programme talked to many patients and doctors, but they were all in the United States. For Britain, it only had a concluding question: 'Do we already have the hidden seeds of an epidemic here?'

'It was one of the first programmes that carried the message that gay men's lives are worth taking seriously,' Peter Scott remembers. 'There were practically no programmes that presented the happy healthy homosexual as a good ideal.'

The novelist and journalist Martin Amis reviewed it for the *Observer*. He listed the 'eerie invitation to diseases' that AIDS presented. 'Brain diseases carried by cats, types of TB carried by birds, "profound diarrhoea" carried by livestock: AIDS is a visitation that makes you believe in the Devil.' Amis liked the tone of the programme and echoed what he believed were its conclusions. We all knew that the more promiscuous we were, the greater our chances of catching an STD:

> With AIDS, though, it seems to be promiscuity itself that is the cause. After a few hundred 'tricks' or new sexual contacts, the body just doesn't want to know anymore, and nature proceeds to peel you wide open. The truth, when we find it, may turn out to be less 'moral', less totalitarian. Meanwhile, however, that is what it looks like. Judging by the faces and voices of the victims, that is what it feels like too.

The *Daily Telegraph* excelled itself: AIDS, Sean Day-Lewis stated, was 'newly fashionable', but there was a 'problem' with it: 'The problem remains that AIDS or the "Gay Plague" is not limited to active homosexuals.' More questions than answers, the reviewer noted, and no useful information about the British position. 'The film thus served chiefly as a warning which, in the absence of complete scientific explanation, can still be seen by those with a mind to do so as a supernatural gesture by a disapproving Almighty.'

Dr Jonathan Weber and Dr David Goldmeir of St Mary's Hospital, London, noticed other responses to the programme. In the first six months of 1983 they saw 'hundreds of patients with anxiety about the disease, and three had severe psychiatric illness with fear of AIDS as the dominant feature'. The doctors wrote to the *British Medical Journal*, noting that one of the three patients was fine until he saw the *Horizon* documentary, after which he developed an irrational conviction that he was carrying AIDS; another patient was a 32-year-old heterosexual man who said he had been sexually assaulted by a gay man in San Francisco. He then saw the *Horizon* programme, and developed acute anxiety that he was infected. He watched the video 30 times.

Gay Switchboard logged many calls after the programme, and they allayed fears as best they could. 'People called up saying they had flu, night sweats, weight loss and coughs that wouldn't get better,' Linda Semple says. 'The main problem was telling them where you could go to find out more. The STD clinic was the obvious choice, but that often had a lot of stigma attached to it. You could go and see your doctor, but your doctor was likely to know less than we did.'

So a conference was called for 21 May 1983, the first of its kind in Britain, to pool information from everyone in the field. The Health

Education Council paid for the hire of Conway Hall, Red Lion Square, and for the expenses of Mel Rosen, of New York's Gay Men's Health Crisis. Two hundred and fifty people heard Switchboard's Terry Webb open the meeting with a call to arms and a nod towards the general election less than three weeks away. 'We would like to see the great public concern translated into action by the authorities. We think the need for action is urgent, not just for homo-sexuals, but for heterosexuals as well. The actions taken so far in this country are the result of individual effort … it's just not enough.'

Dr Ian Weller, a young specialist in infectious diseases from Middlesex Hospital who had just surveyed the AIDS scene in New York, told the meeting: 'I don't think it will be very long before other grants come. The money you raise should go to other things. We must get our research funding from central government.'

Mel Rosen got personal. 'I hope you get very scared today because there is a locomotive coming down the track and it is leaving the United States. For someone who gets AIDS everything begins to fall apart, and if you're gay and you don't have a lover, you go home to an empty apartment.' Rosen explained how the Gay Men's Health Crisis provided 'buddies' to support a person with AIDS with practi-cal chores and emotional support; it provided legal advice too, and a financial aid and housing service. There were 1,361 confirmed cases of AIDS in the United States by May 1983; 520 were dead. The GMHC was getting about five thousand crisis calls a month.

'There was legionnaire's disease and a few people died … and the government put money into it,' said Rosen. 'Two hundred gay people had to die before the government responded [with small localized grants]. There is no funding if you are expendable, if you are a gay person.' New York was changing:

Every one of us knows someone who has died. It makes you old. We are learning to organize funerals. We are learning now that free sexual expression may be fatal and that indiscriminate sex may be fatal. When we go into a bar we ask people about their health … We are waking up and looking at our friends and saying, 'Thank God you are healthy.'

It was an alarming meeting; if you were complacent before it, you felt devastated after it. 'Within ten minutes of Rosen starting to speak everyone was united in disbelieving shock,' remembered Tony

37

Whitehead, a teacher just starting an MSc in education and a member of Gay Switchboard. 'I don't mind telling you I was very very scared.'

Whitehead held an informal Switchboard meeting at his flat in Marylebone. Could it cope? Was it geared up to expand to provide the sort of practical services outlined in Rosen's speech? Or should Switchboard somehow join forces with the nascent Terry Higgins Trust?

Since its inception six months earlier, the trust had organized several fundraising events, and was talking of setting up its own telephone service and printing information leaflets. But those involved, though passionate about their cause, had little experience of managing or structuring an organization of the sort the British crisis now demanded. Whitehead called Martyn Butler, Rupert Whittaker and others and arranged a public meeting for 19 August 1983 upstairs at the London Apprentice, a popular gay City of London pub; this was the second birth of the trust, fired by Switchboard experience and attended by a dozen professional gay men with some experience of the situation in the United States. The name was lengthened: Terrence sounded more formal, more serious. Within four months it was a registered company, with charitable status coming a month later.

The first trust leaflet, a scrappy folded photocopied sheet of A4, was almost a verbatim copy of those available in clubs in New York and provided the first health education information in Britain. 'Watch out for these symptoms,' it warned. 'Swollen glands, pink to purple flat or raised blotch or bump, weight loss, fever, night sweat, cough, diarrhoea.' What should you do if you had these? 'Go to a doctor who is up to date on gay health; tell your doctor you are gay; if you're not sure he knows about AIDS – ask him; if he is not familiar with AIDS, or not sympathetic – get another doctor.'

Advice on lifestyle changes was considered reasonably daring for the time, but today seems hopelessly inadequate. There was no concept of an incubation time, no suggestion that anal sex might be a high-risk activity, no mention of condoms. 'Have as much sex as you want,' it read, 'but with fewer people and with HEALTHY PEOPLE.' It stated that current opinion 'points to something like a virus that MAY BE transmitted sexually. It makes sense that the fewer different people you come in sexual contact with, the less chance this possibly contagious bug has to travel around. If you don't know if your partner is healthy – ask him directly to be honest with you about his health.' It concludes with a large message: HELP YOURSELF! The subtext of the times was: Because Nobody Else Will.

Meetings at Tony Whitehead's flat continued for the best part of the year. Robin Bell of the Gay Medical Association attended regularly, as did Julian Meldrum, an influential figure on the gay scene. Whitehead displayed commitment and charisma and soon became chair; his ability to present a respectable, measured and eloquent front to the non-gay media was one of the organization's strongest assets:

> There were about ten of us, all white middle-class gay males, I'm afraid to admit. There was a real sense of digging in, of being besieged. We were getting no help from the government, and there was a very real concern that they wouldn't deal with AIDS through education, but just by proscription, by controlling those people who were thought to be infected. It is hard to stress how deeply entrenched anti-gay prejudice was, and still is. There was all this prejudice, and a feeling that no one outside the community cared about our well-being at all. It was a war situation, but it was a war only recognized by those that were actually being shot at.

Even internally, politics battled again against plain speaking. 'Our information tried to be the most prudent we could be. The information on the first leaflets – reduce the number of sexual partners – was something I supported, but I remember being accused at gay student meetings and elsewhere of trying to further some secret agenda of putting gay men back in the closet.' A year or so later, when it became apparent that condom use might reduce the risk of infection, there were further conflicts, but for other reasons. 'The medical people in the trust believed that if we promoted condoms it would be giving the green light to intercourse, and condoms would break and we would be spreading infection,' Whitehead says. 'We won through in the end, but it became a resigning issue.'

Similar debates continued to occupy Gay Switchboard, and the recollections still haunt. 'The thing that keeps me awake at night is the worry that we weren't butch enough about the safer sex message early enough,' Linda Semple says:

> I've heard a lot of people say they worry that people died because we weren't quick enough off the mark. Whether that was because of internal bickering or whether it was because we just didn't know

enough, I don't know. In my better moments I think well, we always did say there is this information, it's up to you.

Now it's the complete opposite. A 21-year-old will call up Switchboard and say, 'I'm having sex.' And although you're not supposed to tell people how to lead their lives, someone on Switchboard will say to him, 'Right, use a condom or you die.'

By March 1983, six cases of AIDS had been reported in Britain. By 31 July 1983 there were 14. The Communicable Disease Surveillance Centre in Colindale, north London, only began recording cases in 1982, so there were probably several other cases before this date. Of the 14, all the patients were white men. There were six cases of Kaposi's sarcoma, five cases of Pneumocystis carinii pneumonia and three cases of other opportunistic infections, including cytomegalo-virus and toxoplasmosis. There had been five deaths.

The patients ranged in age from 20 to 45. All but two were gay men; one was also a drug user. The other two cases were an indication of what was to happen to the course of AIDS in Britain next. One was a haemophiliac. This man had received Factor VIII, the blood clotting concentrate, from the United States. Noting this first case, the Public Health Laboratory Service wrote in the *British Medical Journal*: 'Although the risk from blood products imported into Britain seems at present very small, further supplies of Factor VIII for this country will be manufactured only from plasma collected in accordance with the US Food and Drugs Administration regulations designed to exclude from plasma donations [all] donors from high risk groups.' In fact, by the time this reassurance appeared, it was already too late: blood products were already widely infected.

The other patient was a heterosexual, a Lancashire man who said he was neither gay, nor an intravenous drug user, nor a haemophiliac; that is, he fitted into none of the standard groups that were consid-ered to be at risk (these were the groups that had so far mapped out the epidemic in the United States, where 70 per cent of 1,800 cases were gay men, the rest mostly heroin addicts, haemophiliacs or Haitians). Britain now faced a number of questions for the first time: could the agent causing AIDS break out into the 'general' population? Were women at risk? Babies? Could it be controlled? These were enormous questions, and they would change all aspects of the debate in this country.

Some of the answers came quickly. By 31 September 1983 there had been 24 cases, ten more than two months earlier. This number included another haemophiliac, and a woman, a 33-year-old from Liverpool, neither a drug user nor a transfusion recipient, who died of both Kaposi's and Pneumocystis pneumonia four weeks after being admitted to hospital.

In time, the government would wake up to this problem. But it will become clear that the response was too slow to save hundreds, possibly thousands of lives. Money for a general health education programme, for the provision of specialist health care, for scientific and clinical research, would not be made available for three years.

Hysteria, The Early Years

'I told her, this *Mail On Sunday* journalist, that the story was so good, it had so much, she didn't need to make any of it up. Did she listen?'
Professor Tony Pinching

It was a great newspaper story, of course: sex kills you. It was even better than herpes, that last great sex 'n' health riot a couple of years back. You could pack in any amount of prejudice, moralizing and hand-wringing in a double-page spread, and because so little was known, even by government scientists (as the *Daily Mirror* observed), accuracy was a bonus, a lucky by-product. Much of what appeared before the spring of 1983 contained at least some useful information; the usual biases prevailed, but doctors were quoted at length even in the tabloids (the calming ones were of rather more use than the ones who remained 'terrified'). The tabloids then realized they'd been missing out on something great: a chance to legitimize their homophobia.

For the broadsheets it was initially a science story, culled from the medical journals. 'Mystery disease kills gays' reported the *Guardian* in December 1981; 'Cancer one of the "gay syndrome" illnesses' said *The Times* a day later. The *Sunday Times* ran the fullest report so far in September 1982:

A deadly new illness that has killed more people than legionnaire's disease and toxic shock syndrome put together is now the subject of intensive investigation ... The research has been complicated by the fact that the number of heterosexuals among the patients has now increased to about 20 per cent ... most of the heterosexuals are heroin addicts who could well have been exposed to blood by needle sharing.

In May 1983 the *Daily Telegraph* ran the news that '"Gay Plague" may lead to blood ban on homosexuals', and included an article from its 'medical consultant', a retired doctor: 'Indiscriminate promiscuous homosexuality is taking its toll through AIDS and GRIDS (gay related immune deficiency disorders). California and New York, the happy stamping grounds of homosexuals in America, are the original homes of these "wages of sin".'

The same year *The Times* and the *Guardian* both ran full-page specials. *The Times* reported all the theories and the chances of a cure; it also chastised the Communicable Disease Surveillance Centre for its inability to provide any AIDS totals outside Britain and the United States and the doctors interviewed in the story for failing to come up with 'a crack up-to-date command of the subject'. The piece was headlined 'AIDS is here'. Five months later, in November, the *Guardian* wasn't so sure: 'If AIDS is here,' it reported, 'it will surface next year', and this despite the 24 British cases to date. The article was backed up by a tough editorial:

> Our own Government's response to what may prove a major medical and social problem has so far been slow and insufficient ... Mr Norman Fowler [the Social Services Secretary] may soon have to explain convincingly why he has maintained his decision to depend largely on American Factor VIII blood for Britain's haemophiliacs, instead of continuing to buy from countries where AIDS is not prevalent, or seeking to become self-sufficient.

It concluded with the hope that the homosexual population 'should now be regarded as potential casualties, and not victims of prejudice'.

No such quarter from the tabloids. The popular press took a while to warm up; it was the classic thing: homosexuals – and drug users – didn't matter much to their readers unless they were famous, or until they threatened them. So in January 1983, as Britain faced the 'Killer Love Bug Danger' (*Sunday People*), the point was made that although it affected mostly homosexuals now, AIDS could also hit people involved in 'normal' relationships. This soon became Find the Victim. In the mid-1980s journalists would don white coats and crash the Middlesex or St Stephen's, but initially the beat was San Francisco or New York, devastated reporters sending back shell-shocked prose.

In July 1983, the *Sunday People* disclosed 'What the gay plague did to handsome Kenny'. This was an 'AIDS exclusive', revealing the 'disturbing truth' about Kenny Ramsaur, a 28-year-old New Yorker. There were two large photographs, before and after. Before, dark and dashing, his 'bright eyes show no hint of the agony to come'. After, following promiscuous sex between males, he was 'doomed' and looked 'as if he's been badly beaten up'. But 'no mugger did this to handsome Kenny'. It also reported that 'the Department of Health says that although the AIDS statistics for Britain are of concern, they are not so bad as to merit special funds to find a cure'.

Four months later, the *Sun* ran its own 'special on the disease doctors can't cure', blaming Skytrain, Freddie Laker's cheap flights, for the spread of the syndrome in Britain. The *Sun* also splashed on the two pictures of Kenny Ramsaur, again noting how 'his brooding good looks were transformed and his face blew up like a deformed football'. He died a few days after appearing on television, 'but had helped to save countless others'. Precisely how was not made clear, but there was a moral to the tale: 'Any homosexual who indulges in violent sex play, the complete sex act, and exchanges partners with regularity, is asking for it.'

The pictures of Kenny Ramsaur surfaced again more than a year later, in December 1984, when the *News of the World* ran an investigation on 'the deadly invader'. The main story was 'My doomed son's gay plague agony', a 'horrifying tale of complacency and carelessness' in which a 26-year-old man was only diagnosed with AIDS the day before he died. And this despite his 'suppurating sores', etc. But there were no pictures, so they dragged out poor Kenny, who was looking handsome as ever. That was before, of course; after, his good looks had turned into 'a grotesque swollen parody'. This always happened, the newspaper said: 'As the killer virus spreads, their faces become contorted ... until they become skeletons.'

'Fleet St does not like homosexuality,' said Derek Jameson, the editor of the *Daily Star*, on a BBC *Open Space* programme. 'They think it is abnormal, unnatural and evil because it is wrong.'

Reports of the hysteria that had affected San Francisco – dustmen reluctant to collect garbage in gay areas, bus drivers wearing gloves when handling tickets – began to appear in Britain at the end of 1983. 'Scared firemen ban the kiss of life in AIDS alert'; 'AIDS: now ambulance men ban kiss of life'; 'Policeman flees AIDS victim'. The subtext was: if people in authority are frightened of these people, imagine

43

how scared you the reader should be. A refusenik doctor would be even better, and in November 1983 they found one. Professor Keith Simpson, 76, a pathologist and specialist in forensic medicine at Guy's Hospital, London, thought it unwise to perform an autopsy on a 22-year-old gay drug addict who had died from a drug-related pneumonia (a coroner recorded a verdict of accidental death). 'I decided not to expose either myself or the mortuary staff to the risk of getting AIDS,' he said. 'How would you like to be labelled a homosexual or a drug addict if you caught the disease?' he asked, defining his own brand of social death. Professor Simpson's belief that nothing would be gained from an autopsy, since the cause of death was known, was frowned upon by Colin Berry, secretary of the Association of Clinical Pathologists. 'AIDS is far from being a well-studied disease. Autopsies might well reveal something about it.' The *Daily Express* ran an 'Expert refuses "AIDS Death" probe' story; the *Mirror* plumped for 'Top doctor shuns "sex death" victim'; the *Waltham Forest Guardian*, the paper serving the south-east London area where the man died, ran with 'Body blacked in AIDS scare', and called Professor Simpson 'Britain's most famous pathologist'. The professor was involved with the Haig, Christie and Lucan murder cases.

Priorities wavered in the hunt for treatment. 'Torture of Innocents' claimed the *Sunday Mirror* as it exposed 'Chimps in "sex plague" tests'. In other weeks, animal rights campaigners were crackpots and violent fanatics, but on 4 December 1983 they were the chosen ones. 'Healthy chimpanzees are being injected with the mystery killer disease AIDS in a new bid to find a cure for humans,' the paper said, explaining that it mainly affected homosexuals. 'Animal lovers are horrified. They have started massive campaigns to stop the research which could lead to a horrible and lingering death for the animals. They are appalled at the grim fate of the animals so popular in zoos and portrayed in such a lovable way on the famous PG Tips TV commercials.'

'It was like dealing with a foreign story: it happened to other people, in other countries. It happened in this country, but to a very foreign group of people,' says Roy Greenslade, assistant editor (features) of the *Sun* from 1981 to 1986:

The consensus that informed the debate, such as it was, was that all homosexuals are perverts. Flowing from that, AIDS appeared to be just desserts for being involved in deviant sexual behaviour. It was quickly realized that it came about due to anal sex, and heterosexual executives on the *Sun* thus fed in the fact that it was a Gay Plague. AIDS tended to suggest that it might stop all that kind of behaviour, and might lead to fewer gays being around. This might shut them away again, and if you shut them away then they wouldn't be influencing other people to 'go gay'.

At a dinner party for *Sun* top brass in early 1983, Rupert Murdoch, the paper's proprietor, mentioned that the AIDS epidemic in the United States was 'incredibly worrying'. According to Greenslade, Kelvin Mackenzie, the paper's editor, took the hint and had a look at it:

Kelvin took it as an opportunity for a good lark, like most things. There were lots of anti-gay jokes bandied about on the paper, which shut up to a great extent when Les Daly arrived (an openly gay features executive who was later to die of AIDS). Kelvin liked Les a lot, and he wasn't his only gay friend. His relationship with gays was not in any way difficult. But there were other people on the paper, in the newsroom, who regarded all homosexual activity as the devil's work.

These people were clearly in tune with their readership. 'AIDS is like everything else,' a reader wrote. 'When you mess up with nature, you have it coming to you mate. Homosexuality isn't natural. And if it isn't natural it goes against the laws of nature. It's just another plague. A homo plague.'

Les Daly would protest occasionally about one or two of the *Sun*'s wilder AIDS stories. 'Kelvin would always be rather paternalistic,' Greenslade remembers,

saying 'Well you're quite right Les, a bloody disgrace, I'm going to deal with it.' I think Kelvin hoped it would pass, and Les was realistic enough to realize what sort of paper he was working for.

And the tone slowly changed. In 1985–86, when it transpired that heterosexuals could get it, the attitude changed to 'heterosexuals couldn't get it if they only slept with one decent woman'.

Private Eye capitalized on the hysteria. On the eve of the June 1983 election, the magazine spoofed the AIDS panic and the *Daily Mail*'s breathless support for the Conservatives. 'Shock finding by doctors – AIDS THREAT TO LABOUR VOTERS'. According to its report, 'Labour voters are 90 per cent more likely to contract the horrifying cancer-virus AIDS than Tory voters.' A doctor offered advice on how best to stay healthy: 'Vote Conservative.' In another issue 'The Gays' cartoon, drawn by Michael Heath, featured one character asking another: 'I suppose you know what GAY stands for – Got AIDS Yet?'

What could you do if you took offence? Julian Meldrum, a member of the Terrence Higgins Trust and secretary of the Hall Carpenter Archives, which monitored gay media coverage, wrote to the Press Council with a detailed critique of about 60 articles published in 1983. In January 1994 he addressed a European conference on AIDS held in Amsterdam, at which he outlined a proposed code of conduct he had drawn up for the National Union of Journalists. 'We must not confuse bad news with bad reporting,' he said, but what upset him about the reporting was that so much of it had been 'untruthful, dishonest, inaccurate, incomplete, unfair to people with AIDS and to those seen as being at highest risk of contracting it'. He acknowledged that it was unlikely that his code of conduct would be rigorously enforced, believing 'the union would lose a lot of members if it were', but he read them out anyway. One, the problem should not be exaggerated; two, cut the gay plague stuff, as AIDS is not confined to any one section of the community; three, cut the plague metaphors – it is not an airborne virus, it cannot be caught casually; and four, respect the rights to privacy and dignity of people with AIDS: no hounding, no naming. He ended with a plea to use the media for beneficial ends.

Unwittingly, early hysteria may have played a part in the control of the British epidemic. In 1984, Julian Meldrum and doctors at the department of genito-urinary medicine at the Middlesex Hospital, London, conducted a brief experiment to gauge the effect of mass media coverage of AIDS on the incidence of gonorrhoea.

The sample was small and included just those men, homosexual, bisexual and heterosexual, who attended the Middlesex clinic between January 1982 and September 1983. But the results were startling. During 1982 and the first quarter of 1983, when media coverage was only sporadic, rates of gonorrhoea remained fairly constant, both among gay/bisexual and straight men. But between April and September 1983, when the researchers counted a total of 258 news items compared to 42 in the previous 15 months, rates of gonorrhoea fell markedly. In fact they only fell among gay or bisexual men, from an average of 230 cases per quarter to about 150; among heterosexuals the rate increased. The suggestion was clear: because gonorrhoea has a short incubation period of only a few days, it was possible to surmise that gay men were changing their sexual behaviour; either cutting down on partners or altering their type of sexual activity. Much of this could be attributed to the influence of gay organizations, particularly Switchboard, the Terrence Higgins Trust and the gay press. But who could say that even the most shameless expressions of tabloid homophobia didn't have at least some beneficial results?

CHAPTER 3: False Negative

At the beginning of 1981, Dr Tony Pinching was working in his lab at Hammersmith Hospital, London, when he got a call from a friend in the United States. Though he originally set out to be a neurologist, Pinching, 33, was now working almost exclusively with diseases that affected the immune system, specifically with patients who were immuno-suppressed, through treatment for transplants or auto-immune disorders. His friend in America was working in a similar field and had heard at a meeting some interesting news of specialists who were seeing rare diseases that had no apparent cause and pointed to a total immune system breakdown. They were baffled: why were these guys getting so sick?

Pinching hoped this might turn out to be a useful mystery. The biology of immunosuppression had reached a sort of plateau: so much was unknown about the immune system, about cell formation and function, about the correct use of steroids and other treatments; they needed either some more advanced techniques or some new ideas. He thought: 'This new disease, whatever it was, might tell us something.'

A few months later, after the first clinical reports of active homosexuals falling sick in California and New York were published, Pinching received two more memorable phone calls. A houseman at St John's Hospital, London, asked if Pinching could run any tests on a patient he had with a skin disease, probably a cancer infection. The second was from Willie Harris, the senior genito-urinary physician at St Mary's. Harris had heard that Pinching might soon be joining St Mary's as a consultant in clinical immunology and told him about a group of patients at St Mary's Praed Street Clinic. These were sexually active gay men, regular users of recreational drugs, no strangers to sexually transmitted disease – in fact just the sort of people who they knew were becoming unwell in America. The thinking was: if this disease is going to happen over here, we'd better get in quick and investigate what's going on. If it wasn't going to happen, then the reasons why not might also be interesting.

So Pinching joined the St Mary's virologists and microbiologists on the study, which soon included more than a hundred men answering intimate questions and submitting to endless blood tests. Funding of the study, the first in Britain, came initially from existing resources and later from the Wellcome Trust and the National Kidney Research Fund. The Medical Research Council (MRC), the government-funded body, also considered supporting the project, but eventually turned it down. The official reason was that the study was too wide-ranging, but there was another explanation too: 'They thought it would be purely an American thing,' one of the St Mary's researchers remembers. 'They said, "We haven't got anybody ill, it's not important. If we do get people, we'll fix it later."'

The initial results of the study were inconclusive, but gave sufficient cause for concern: the men studied showed none of the AIDS marker illnesses, but there were plenty of immune cell abnormalities and evidence of decreased T-helper cells (the standard marker of the body's ability to fight disease). In their report, the researchers concluded that the weakened immune systems they had detected might represent 'a latent phase of AIDS'. They didn't have to wait long to be proved right.

Within weeks, Pinching had seen his first AIDS patients. Pneumocystis, then Kaposi's, then encephalopathy, a progressive brain disorder. Most fitted the pattern: many partners, some travel to the States, some previous STDs. Many died within weeks of admittance.

Within St Mary's, most of Pinching's fellow doctors found it hard to come to terms with this syndrome; it was still an American thing, still a freakshow. So he decided to bring a patient along in person to one of the hospital's case presentations, a regular forum for rare disorders. Often this kind of thing was just done with slides, but Pinching discussed it with one of his patients, and explained that it might help demystify matters:

I just wanted them to know that this wasn't a Martian, this was an ordinary bloke, only he happened to be a gay man, so what. So he came in, and I can still hear the drawing in of breath, the hush that descended. Here was the moment of reality for that audience; this wasn't just a strange disease that we read about in the journals with a strange sort of people who do bizarre things. This was an ordinary bloke, you could have met him anywhere, and he was terribly straightforward.

Across town, at the Middlesex Hospital, Professor Michael Adler, a genito-urinary specialist, was also seeing his first patients. 'I can remember his face,' he says of the very first, 'I can remember every sort of skin lesion he had.' And he can remember the prejudice shown towards his patients:

It was very difficult to get them hospitalized, it was very difficult to get patients treated as normal human beings. People were frightened, they thought it was contagious, the patients had to be put in side wards, you couldn't get the domestic staff to go in, you couldn't get the porters to go in. We treated people extremely badly. It was like medicine six hundred years ago.

Dr Ian Weller worked in the same department. Weller was still relatively new to infectious disease, but in February 1983 he had attended the first post-graduate course on AIDS in New York, where he had visited the Memorial Sloan Kettering Hospital and the Veteran's Hospital and had seen the growing toll first hand. One of the first things he read on his return to London in March 1983 was a brief note in the *Lancet*. The headline read: 'Acquired Immunodeficiency Syndrome: No UK Epidemic'. It explained how serious AIDS had become in the United States, but quoted the Communicable Disease Surveillance Centre saying that in its work to date it 'has not so far detected an important problem in England and Wales'.

The following week Weller met Carl and Ray, his first AIDS patients in the clinic. In the hospital he recalls

enormous problems with staff at all levels. Every step of the way was a battle. The fears then were not necessarily unfounded, as we didn't know what we were dealing with. There were doctors and surgeons deciding not to do a certain procedure because it was deemed to be 'inappropriate'. This was largely influenced by an anxiety or fear. This fear would go right across to the domestic staff. One night I was sitting in a patient's room, and this hand came round the door with food on it, and just dumped it. I laughed with the patient, who said 'It happens all the time.' Within five minutes a bunch of flowers flew across the room – whoosh! That time I didn't even see the hand.

Whenever that happened we just got a hit squad together to deal with the specific problems when they occurred, just to explain to people. At one hospital there was even a move to have a committee of three wise men who would meet to decide whether a given operation was appropriate or not. As if the physician looking after the patient couldn't tell.

In July 1983 Weller, Adler and others applied to the MRC to fund a cohort study of men at their clinic; they were seeing about 115 homosexual men each day. Again the MRC turned it down. They reapplied and a year later were awarded £160,000, about £110,000 less than their original request. It was an intensive study, examining many aspects of natural history and immune abnormalities, and it attempted to establish an antibody test for markers which might identify patients at risk. As in all these early projects, the patients were open about their lifestyles and eager to help. 'Like us,' Weller says, 'they were optimistic at that time that the people who were dying were going to be the minority. They thought, "It's not going to happen to me." There was a wonderful optimism. Slowly, as the natural history studies published their results, we saw the doubling time of the cases, and you suddenly realize what sort of epidemic you have.'

It wasn't long before these doctors began seeing women with AIDS. The first Tony Pinching looked after was a heterosexual English housewife who had one partner – her husband:

It turned out he'd been having a few others, mainly in Africa, on the side. And she told us lots of things about herself and it was quite clear that she'd just had conventional, heterosexual intercourse and she'd never injected drugs, and everything was unremarkable. That told us that there was going to be a heterosexual epidemic. I didn't need any more convincing, though it took a lot of people a bit longer to convince our health officials, and possibly quite rightly so. But as a clinician you're in a privileged situation of hearing very early exactly what was going on.

In October 1983, the Medical Research Council called the first meeting of its Working Party on AIDS. To date it had received four applications for AIDS-related research and its staff had realized two things: first, the procedure for allocating grants was slow and cumbersome, involving approval by several boards and peer groups. Many applications would have to wait four months before receiving a response. This was a necessary process to ensure that any research it backed was both necessary and cost-effective, but it might also prove a handicap in a health crisis when a fast-track response was needed. Even more significant, perhaps, was the fact that because AIDS was so new, few people at the MRC knew what was good research and what wasn't; in fact, very few people knew what was going on at all. Those who did were the very people applying for grants.

The Working Party, consisting initially of 12 members and several observers from the MRC and Department of Health and Social Security, was convened to smooth out these problems. All the familiar faces attended: Dr Pinching, Professor Adler and Dr Harris, as well as Dr Robin Weiss of the Institute of Cancer Research and Dr Richard Tedder of the Middlesex. Of the others, almost all would also do critical work in the coming years. The meetings were chaired by Dr David Tyrrell, the director of the MRC Common Cold Unit.

On 10 October 1983 they met for the first time at the MRC's Regent's Park headquarters to guide policy and compare notes. In summary, this is roughly what those doctors knew at that time:

1   AIDS is a profound impairment of the immune system, first recognized in the United States five years ago, first reported in the journals three years ago. About 3,200 cases have occurred in the US; 30 cases have been confirmed in the UK, of whom half have died. Hardly any patients lived for more than two years after diagnosis.

2   The two most common early manifestations of the disease are the tumour Kaposi's sarcoma and Pneumocystis carinii pneumonia. Because of the general impairment in immunity, other infections are common. There are a number of early marker diseases that are either AIDS in a mild form, or a precursor to it. This AIDS-Related Complex (ARC) may be characterized by persistent generalized lymphadenopathy (PGL – an enlargement of the lymph glands), diarrhoea, fever and weight loss.

3   The immune defect appears to be the result of reduction in the T-cell population (a type of white blood cell also known as T-helper lymphocytes or T4 lymphocytes), and an increase in T-suppressor cells.

4   In the US, gay men account for about 70 per cent of all cases. Other groups at risk are haemophiliacs who receive Factor VIII concentrate, intravenous drug users and recipients of blood transfusions. The pattern of transfer is thus similar to the hepatitis B virus, which can be transmitted sexually and through blood.

Women can contract AIDS and it is thought likely that babies may be infected *in utero*.

5 The cause of AIDS is not known, but it is thought most likely that it is a virus, possibly a mutant strain of a recognized condition: those being studied include Epstein-Barr virus, cytomegalovirus and two retroviruses called human T-cell leukaemia virus (HTLV) and lymphadenopathy-associated virus (LAV). AIDS has a long incubation period, anything from a few months to four years, during which the patient is unaware he or she is carrying but may pass it on.

6 There is no effective treatment. All that can be done is to treat specific diseases, but as these are often very advanced upon presentation and often accompanied by many complications, effectiveness is severely limited. Drugs such as interferon and Interleukin II can be used on an ad hoc basis to boost the immune system, but any minor beneficial effects are strictly short-term.

7 The disease may have originated in central Africa. A mild form of Kaposi's sarcoma has been endemic there among young men for many years. While these cases have mostly been benign, a more virulent strain, similar to that found in the West, has recently been diagnosed.

The first MRC meeting noted that AIDS posed fundamental, new and unexpected questions of basic science. Those present had never been so helpless in the face of a new condition: the playing field was so wide, the rules as yet unexplained. Were the cases they had seen so far the tip of an iceberg? Had they recognized the problem early enough? Would the American epidemic give them the breathing space they needed? No one could say for sure, but as they returned to the wards that afternoon and in the following weeks, their hopes that their experience would be confined to a handful of cases seemed increasingly remote.

Two months later, the doctors gathered again. There was no good news. Dr Pinching reported back from two other meetings he had attended in recent weeks, at the New York Academy of Sciences and the Royal Society of Medicine in London. These meetings, precursors to the big annual international AIDS conferences, were by now regular occurrences, marked by much excitement and initially little professional jealousy. Pinching found no major new findings at these particular gatherings and noted that although there was much scientific activity some of it was not well thought out.

Professor Adler had been to the World Health Organization meeting in Denmark in October 1983, where it was reported that there were 268 European cases. Dr Palmer, of the Public Health Laboratory Service (the parent of the Communicable Disease Surveillance Centre), had visited the Centers for Disease Control in Atlanta, where he learnt that the wife of a haemophiliac had recently developed AIDS, confirming that heterosexual transmission was not only possible, but likely.

It was up to Tony Pinching to write up the minutes. He knew these were terrible times, but professionally it was also the most exciting period he had known. He split his time between the lab and the filling wards, where he attempted to allay the fears of those around him. AIDS tended to attract those clinicians who didn't feel threatened either by the infection risk or by young people dying. Pinching had previously looked after patients with suspected Lassa fever and had worked in renal units which were only just recovering from the Edinburgh hepatitis outbreak, in which many patients and staff became sick and died after the contamination of dialysis units.

That episode had tightened up guidelines on the handling and cleaning up of blood. He tried to remember them as best he could when he dropped at St Mary's a bottle of blood from a contact of a patient who had AIDS in the States. He scrubbed the floor and his hands and it was only later, while he was driving back along the Westway to Hammersmith, that he saw a deep cut across his finger. He remembers thinking: 'Mmm ... I wonder what *was* in that blood.'

As yet there was no way of knowing, but the announcement in April 1984 that the viral cause of AIDS had been isolated would change everything. The precise sequence of events would later become the subject of litigation, because it soon emerged that the HTLV-III retrovirus that American oncologist Robert Gallo isolated in his labs at the National Cancer Institutes, Maryland (a retrovirus that was shown to destroy T-cells and was present in 88 per cent of the AIDS patients he tested), was but a variant of LAV, the virus that was isolated months earlier by Luc Montagnier at the Institut Pasteur in Paris. To the bulk of the medical world the value of the discovery was never in doubt (even though some questioned US Health Secretary Margaret Heckler's optimism that a vaccine was now perhaps only two years away). Gallo swiftly developed a test for antibodies to HTLV-III (the human T-cell leukaemia virus type III, which changed its name to HIV, the Human Immunodeficiency Virus in 1986).

In Britain, clinics such as James Pringle House, the genito-urinary department of the Middlesex, soon found it hard to handle the number of tests being conducted on patients. A meeting of AIDS colleagues held at the hospital in February 1985 recorded that 'the demand for antibody-HTLV-III testing has been such that Virology have not been able to cope with current staffing. Routine testing is to be reduced to a minimum'. Blood donor centres filled up too, not so much because people wanted to give blood, but because since all donations were being tested it was the easiest and least embarrassing way of finding out whether you were HTLV-III positive. Subsequent meetings at the Middlesex noted other problems: the considerable number of 'false positives' and 'false negatives', the latter consisting of individuals tested too soon after infection, at a time when the virus was undetectable by the first primitive screening methods; these people might unknowingly infect others. And then there was counselling, or the lack of it: how did you tell a patient that there was a chance they might soon die?

'We were obviously very naïve,' says Ian Weller:

We performed a large number of anti-HTLV-III tests without written consent. Blood was taken from patients with AIDS, patients with lymphadenopathy, patients with multiple sexual partners, and controls. What we told the patients at that stage was that 'We don't know what this test means. It may well mean that you've been infected with the virus and you've recovered. You've got antibodies, and you may be immune.' That shows how little we knew.

Originally doctors thought the situation might be similar to that of hepatitis B, in which only a small proportion of people infected actually get sclerosis of the liver. In early 1984, the common belief was that out of one hundred people infected, perhaps only one would develop AIDS. Five years later, that figure would be revised to about 90 per cent.

In September 1984 the results of the first significant British study of the prevalence of HTLV-III was published in the *Lancet*. Nineteen doctors from seven different clinics and labs had helped conduct the survey, carried out with a prototype of the test which became commercially available only a year later. Two thousand people were stud-

55

ied, the vast majority in London, but some also in Manchester. In one sense the results were reassuring: only those groups previously identified as being at risk (gay men, haemophiliacs, drug users) were found to have high levels of antibodies to HTLV-III; out of a thousand random tests on blood donors outside these groups, none was HTLV-III seropositive. But in another sense the results were extremely worrying: 30 out of 31 patients with AIDS tested positive, which was to be expected, but 89 per cent of those with persistent generalized lymphadenopathy, the pre-AIDS marker, also tested positive, which was considered high. Of gay men tested who believed they were well and had no symptoms of illness, 17 per cent were found to have the virus. Less than 2 per cent of drug users tested were positive, but the figure for haemophiliacs was 34 per cent; the tests on haemophiliacs were conducted on sera stored since 1982. The doctors stressed that 'it would be unwise to presume that AIDS will necessarily develop in seropositive subjects', but their optimism was short-lived.

'What happened then,' says Ian Weller, 'was that we started to see that the people who had antibodies started to get sick. Then the virus detection techniques improved, so more and more people were found to be virus positive, and the whole atmosphere around the patients changed once we knew what it really meant.'

Shortly after the test became available, Tony Pinching took the test too, still curious about that cut on his hand. His test was negative.

What could you tell people who had tested positive? With no cure and no effective treatment, and with newspapers daily muddling the number of virus carriers with the number of AIDS cases, how could you convince anyone that their life wasn't as good as over? Some patients convinced themselves that optimism was all there was; this wasn't self-deception, it was what their doctors believed too. There were advantages in early diagnosis: warning signs could be heeded, new drugs tried.

In mid-1985 Charles Farthing, a research registrar at St Stephen's Hospital, London, wrote a draft advice paper for people who were HTLV-III positive. It was a type of written counselling, perhaps the first of its kind in Britain. It explained what being antibody positive meant in terms of health expectancy and again struck optimistic chords: 'Hopefully the majority of HTLV-III antibody positive individuals will never become unwell, let alone develop AIDS ... Take care of yourself. Think positively. Do not transmit this infection to others. Soon, perhaps very soon, there may be a successful treatment for this new disease.'

Meanwhile, there could only be practical advice and lifestyle changes: report any opportunistic infection early; get plenty of rest; exercise, but don't overdo it; balance your diet; limit the alcohol and cut out the cigarettes; don't share a toothbrush or razor blade; don't carry an organ donor card; and don't have any live vaccines for things like yellow fever or polio.

People were advised not to be frightened of asking questions about new drug trials, and to be aware of the potential side effects. The Terrence Higgins Trust and the Body Positive self-help group were promoted as good sources of support, but the word was not to tell many friends or your employer of your positive result: they might turn 'nasty'. And telling your GP might affect applications for life and medical insurance.

And then there was sex. Dr Farthing provided the most thorough guide yet to what was known and what was considered unsafe. Exactly which sexual activities transmitted the virus were unknown, but surveys of gay men provided some good indications of relative risk. 'Men who are only passive in anal intercourse are much more likely than others to be HTLV-III antibody positive,' Farthing advised. Active anal intercourse and oral sex were considered to be less of a risk, though there were many HTLV-III positive individuals who swore that they had never had passive anal sex. 'A condom, whilst probably a reasonable protection if it remains intact, can break easily with anal intercourse, and if it does there is no protection at all. It is surely important therefore to restrict active anal sex only to those partners whom you know for certain to be also HTLV-III positive.' Clearly this presented other risks, such as impairing immunity through contracting another STD.

The only way to be absolutely certain of not transmitting infection was to have 'entirely non mucous membrane contact or "dry" sex'. Kissing was deemed to be very low risk, although 'live virus has been isolated from semen and saliva and therefore considerable saliva exchange or any semen exchange could theoretically transmit the virus'. The choice was yours, the guidelines said, while noting that 'restricting anal sex only to an already regular partner or to partners whom you know to be positive, cutting down on the total number of partners or having only "safer" or entirely safe dry sex with antibody negative individuals is what most antibody positive individuals decide'.

57

This advice had a very limited circulation, reaching only those already infected. The Terrence Higgins Trust was also beginning to provide similar information. But education for the general public was far less detailed and far more coy. In January 1985 the Health Education Council, a government-financed organization, issued a pocket-sized pamphlet (numbered STD 21) that set out the basics. There was no mention of anal intercourse or details about kissing or safe sex; understandably, since for most people such events did not exist or were considered repulsive and sinful. Politically, it was unimaginable to discuss homosexual sex in anything approaching an intricate or frank manner. This rendered the leaflet's information of very little specific value to gay men, the group most at risk: specifically it stated that 'it's not yet known whether the way you have sex affects your risk of getting AIDS', a far less assertive comment than that already present in medical literature.

The leaflet was available primarily in STD clinics and GPs' surgeries, its purpose clearly to settle nerves and ease the fear; you can't get it from shaking hands or sharing glasses. Before setting out the symptoms, the leaflet stated 'Now hang on ... as you begin to read this list of symptoms you might start thinking "Yes, I've got that ... and that ... and that ... Oh no, I've got it." Well, perhaps, but most probably not.' The original draft of the leaflet ended with the comment that 'There is a lot of research being done in the USA.' This was later amended to include the words 'and other countries', suggesting that the UK was playing its part too. There was another, more significant change. The second draft of the leaflet, prepared in June 1984, contained the observation: 'In a very small number of cases AIDS has been passed on from the mother to the newborn child.' It was deleted from the version printed six months later, despite widespread knowledge of mother-to-baby transmission at the time. This was not an oversight but a conscious decision not to unduly alarm pregnant mothers.

The timidity of the pamphlet provided a significant pointer to what the Department of Health and government ministers considered to be politically acceptable when dealing with such intimate matters. The tone of the leaflet and much of its contents resurfaced in the first nationwide government AIDS education campaign more than a year later.

In December 1984 there were 96 reported cases of AIDS in the UK,

421 in Europe, predominantly in France and West Germany, and 6,993 in the United States. The British number was still small but growing rapidly. By the end of February 1985 it had risen to 132. The headlines were still hysterical – we were to have a hundred thousand cases of AIDS by 1990, we were to have one million people infected. It was the unique cases that now aroused most tabloid interest: the AIDS grandmother, the AIDS pilot or the AIDS nurse. In February 1985 the newspapers got wind of a terrible accident, first reported in the *Lancet*. While caring for a woman who had lived in central southern Africa and was later diagnosed with AIDS in a Hampshire hospital, a young female nurse received a 'needlestick' injury to her finger when she was resheathing a hypodermic needle on a syringe containing blood freshly drawn from an artery. Thirteen days later she developed a severe flu-like illness with sore throat and headache. Then a rash. Then severe pains in her joints. Then generalized lymphadenopathy. The woman's first HTLV-III test was negative. Three weeks later another test showed she was positive, the first recorded case in the West of a hospital worker contracting the virus from a patient.

This was the ideal tabloid story, the perfect tragedy: young nurse, a member of a caring profession, inevitably pretty, gets infected not by sleeping around or indulging in other detested activities, but simply by doing her job. There should be hell to pay, because this was an innocent victim. The next big story, about the blood supply, also carried the heavy subtext of innocence and guilt. By March 1985 there had only been three reported cases of AIDS among Britain's five thousand haemophiliacs, a cause of some relief and not a little complacency. What no one knew then was that approximately 1,200 haemophiliacs had already been infected with the virus. Many of them had been carrying it for four years.

CHAPTER 4: The Fridge That Day

As a boy, Simon Taylor couldn't do much. A normal haemophiliac among some five thousand in Britain, but an abnormal life. He was one of about two thousand who suffered severely, a bleeding episode every ten days or so, every other day off school, no sport, no travelling, or travelling only to specialist hospitals where they'd hook him up to machines and change his fluid.

This was an excruciatingly painful life, these bursting vessels, these bleeding joints. His older brother didn't have it, which initially made it worse. Some boys at school imagined a Sam Peckinpah movie; one scrape and they'd be swimming in it. In fact you would just disappear for a bit, cry off for a plasma transfusion when things got very bad, when the swelling or bruising started or a pseudotumour or arthritis threatened. All this turmoil, and then you die young, 40 if you're lucky.

It's genetic, a lack of clotting Factor VIII, or in some cases Factor IX, (haemophilia A, far more common, means you lack Factor VIII; haemophilia B, also known as Christmas Disease, means little or no Factor IX). When Simon Taylor was born in the mid-1950s there was very little treatment. Plasma transfusions were time consuming and difficult and expensive, and not very rich in clotting factor; if you were lucky you'd just about stop the bleeding. There was a slight improvement with the arrival of cryoprecipitate in the late 1960s, a more concentrated form of plasma pooled from a number of donations, but it was essentially the same process for the patient – the hospital, the hook-up.

In 1973, everything changed. They'd worked out a way to fractionate the clotting factors from the pooled plasma of thousands of donors and then freeze-dry the concentrate, so you could take it home in packages, in Safeway bags. Because you only needed such small quantities, you could pump it in yourself. This was great science and it transformed lives. You could travel, have a normal education, hold down a job. You could treat a bleeding episode more quickly, so there would be fewer after effects and less pain. You could even use it preventatively. Simon Taylor, 16 at the time, could see himself going to university, America even. 'It was like someone had suddenly changed their mind. "Here, you can have a decent life after all."'

There were a few problems. It was expensive, a few thousand a year per person, but the NHS looked after that. And it was in short supply. Until the mid-1970s practically all of England's blood plasma was supplied by the National Blood Transfusion Service, but demand now far exceeded supply; everyone wanted to treat themselves and they used far more. The good news was the Americans had plenty to spare. Besides, what they couldn't make in Oxford now they would be able to make in a few years. David Owen, the health minister, said so in 1977: self-sufficiency in all blood products, just as in Scotland. It was mostly a matter of money, of investment in new plant.

Then quite a few people began to fall ill. Since Factor VIII had become so much more concentrated, its manufacture changed dramatically: for every batch of concentrate, plasma from upwards of 3,500 donors would be needed. This was pooled in a huge bloody vat; if one donation was infected, they all were.

And then, Simon Taylor says, 'People started asking, "Where does all this plasma *come* from?" And we discovered that of course in the United States they didn't have the same wonderful system where blood was just donated.' Plasma was acquired on a paid-for basis, only a few dollars a time, but if you had no money, selling a litre or two was an easy ride. Plasma companies would sell it on for a profit, and they weren't always discriminating about how or where they got their supplies. This was commerce: you'd cut the corners if you could, wouldn't screen donors and wouldn't heat treat your product to rid it of infection. It was blood, but it could have been diesel. And who was to tell them that intravenous drug users couldn't donate; it was a service, the companies argued, and they were helping the needy at both ends.

'We didn't know what the risks were,' Taylor says, 'we just thought this isn't a terribly good idea. But it wasn't like we were going to stop taking the concentrates. If severe haemophilia went untreated, it could be fatal,' and there was little likelihood of picking up any infection that could be as bad as that.

The worst you could get was hepatitis. In fact, almost all haemophiliacs using concentrates, both NHS and commercial supplies, developed antibodies to some form of hepatitis, if not them all: hepatitis B, hepatitis non-A or non-B. But most shrugged it off, became vaccinated, or fell ill and then recovered; only two British haemophiliacs died from hepatitis between 1974 and 1980.

In 1980, 60 per cent of all Factor VIII used in Britain was imported. Most of this came from the United States, or rather from companies licensed in the United States; there was no guarantee that all the donors actually came from the US and in fact some evidence to suggest that plasma had been gathered in Mexico and central Africa.

When the first American haemophiliacs were reported to have acquired AIDS in 1982, Britain's haemophilia centres (of which there were about a hundred) and the Haemophilia Society showed concern but not alarm. A year later, with haemophiliacs representing one per cent of all American AIDS cases (17 cases out of twenty thousand with haemophilia A), the situation was not much changed. No haemophiliacs had contracted Kaposi's sarcoma and it was thought that they might have an entirely different disorder from that seen in homosexuals. Rather than an infection by a viral agent, it was widely believed that they contracted AIDS as a result of repeated antigenic challenge to their immune system; this view wasn't that far from the 'immune overload' theory with gays. And then there was the other familiar logic: American companies and the NHS were beginning to heat treat most of their product and recipients in Britain should benefit from the time lag of the American experience. In November 1983, in a written response to a question from Edwina Currie, the health minister Kenneth Clarke felt confident enough to say that 'there is no conclusive evidence that AIDS is transmitted by blood products'. The early science of AIDS, much of it breathless guesswork, has always been short of conclusive evidence; you ran with what you believed. For the politician this would frequently be a useful tool, but Mr Clarke would soon regret his reassurance.

By the beginning of the next month, the National Blood Transfusion Service and the Department of Health and Social Security had drawn up new donor guidelines and printed a new leaflet detailing high-risk groups. By the end of December 1983 two haemophiliacs had been diagnosed with AIDS. In the same month the *British Medical Journal* ran a leading article which noted that when AIDS was first linked with haemophilia, some British centres curtailed surgery and home treatment, but most had then reverted to their routine service. 'Throughout the world the opinion of the majority is that the risk of haemorrhage and its complications far outweighs the risk of developing AIDS or chronic liver disease.' It was still thought wise to treat severely affected children with cryoprecipitate to lessen the risk further. 'The most important precaution of all,' the article concluded, 'is to maintain a high level of surveillance of the haemophilic population'.

The article was written by Dr Peter Jones, the director of the Newcastle Haemophilia Reference Centre. He did maintain a high level of surveillance and the emerging picture was devastating. Based at the Royal Victoria Infirmary, Newcastle upon Tyne, Dr Jones's centre served a population of 3.1 million. His staff saw 143 patients on a regular basis, not just haemophiliacs, but their families, and on a social as well as a clinical level. As so much treatment now took place at home, Jones got to know his patients as friends, often from birth. He'd be invited to their weddings.

Although he was clearly anxious about their health status, little could be done to determine whether they might be infected until the test became widely available in mid-1985. Jones's staff then spent a few weeks testing everyone, analysing stored samples that had been kept frozen for years and samples provided in the last few months. Ninety-nine patients with severe haemophilia A were tested for antibodies to HTLV-III and 76 were found to be positive. All except one had received commercial Factor VIII concentrates. Eighteen patients with haemophilia B were also tested (recipients of NHS-produced Factor IX) and all were found to be anti-HTLV negative. Three patients had already died from AIDS and a further 30 had AIDS-related complex or lymphadenopathy. All 68 health care staff were negative.

There was one more disturbing feature: three out of 36 sexual partners of HTLV-III positive patients were also seropositive. This had profound importance for haemophiliac families and wider implications for heterosexual transmission of the virus in the general population.

The results were presented in the *BMJ* in September 1985. The authors of the report – Dr Jones, his staff and several immunologists and microbiologists from other hospitals and laboratories in Newcastle and London – concluded with a plea: 'To cope we think it imperative that the medical, nursing, social work and laboratory support provided to every centre treating people in any group at risk, including haemophilia centres, should be assessed as a matter of urgency. Extra support is also needed by the voluntary societies concerned with the care of patients with AIDS in the community.'

Two weeks after these results appeared, Barney Hayhoe, minister for health, announced that AIDS 'is a very serious disease'. He recognized that 'it is vital to do all we can to control the further spread of the disease and to help those who have already been exposed to the virus'. He talked of taking a long-term view, of co-ordinating the response, of a programme of public education as a 'lynch-pin' of the strategy. All this was in hand and would come soon, he said, but for now he was happy to announce that his department would be allocating new funds. These would include grants to help haemophiliacs: £20,000 for the Haemophilia Society to advise its members (this was in addition to the £15,000 the society had received a few months ago, reward for what Mr Hayhoe said was 'invaluable work'). And there was more: £90,000 was earmarked for counselling at haemophiliac reference centres, working out at about £900 for each centre or £45 for each individual. At the end of his announcement, Mr Hayhoe declared that his government 'fully understands public concern about AIDS'.

'I guess the most traumatic ones were the young married couples and the children.' Dr Peter Jones remembers breaking the news; he had to do it a lot. There wasn't any counselling, no advice about life insurance, just the blunt stuff: terribly sorry, you're positive.

> Of course you have remorse. You feel very, very upset in terms of individuals – everybody has their favourites. You see a child who five years ago you knew was going to live a normal lengthy life and a high quality life, and he's suddenly infected and dying.
>   You feel anguish for a nurse who's taught somebody how to inject themselves, or has injected them herself, and then she realizes she must have been injecting the virus at the same time. And it must be horrible to be a mother who's done that to her son.

Peter Jones told himself that medicine has always been like that, and that if he didn't maintain some pragmatism, some objectivity, then he'd be useless to people. Haemophilia gets you used to horrible things, to foul disorders, to premature death.

'My wife later admitted that she was frightened, and that was true of all the partners. They were frightened that we were in the midst of a new pandemic that we didn't understand properly.' At first Jones was disarming. 'I told her I'd puddled around in blood for years and was probably immune.' Occasionally, though, some of the anxiety would get through to him. His first patient diagnosed with AIDS shared his care with another centre, and rather than call the ambulance to take him for some treatment one day Jones drove him himself. 'I knew that the ambulance staff would get dressed up in biological warfare suits and frighten the shit out of everybody. Later that day I put my youngest son, who was three and the apple of my eye, into the same car seat as the man with AIDS had been in two hours earlier and I felt this little tremor of fear: was I doing the right thing?'

To allay the fears of his patients and others who didn't have access to the latest scientific updates, Dr Jones wrote a booklet, 'AIDS and the Blood: A Practical Guide'. Published in 1985, it answered basic questions in a simple way, things like 'Should I modify my haemophilia treatment?' and 'Can AIDS be spread by ordinary social contact?' One page posed the question 'Am I alone in feeling dirty and depressed about my transfusions?' Not at all, but you shouldn't believe some of the misinformation flying around: it's true that some concentrate was donated by drug addicts and homosexuals, but 'some patients began to worry that the [drug] addiction itself could be spread by blood. This cannot, of course, happen. Neither can homosexuality be spread by blood.'

Another portion tried to answer the question of what an adult should tell their children. Depending on their age, you should tell them a) 'AIDS is like hepatitis and we have coped with that', b) 'Like hepatitis, doctors are working on a vaccine to protect people', c) 'Treatment is already being made safer by heating it, and I expect there will be other ways to make it better soon', and d) 'It isn't catching to other people like a cold'.

These were common concerns and it was regular advice. This was before AIDS care became almost routine at the Royal Victoria Infirmary, a time when the local crematorium kept the body of a haemophiliac back until last, to the end of the day, lest the AIDS virus infect other dead bodies; in one case they burnt an empty coffin and incinerated the body away from the regular furnace. But they got used to it after a while.

By the beginning of 1994, about half of Dr Jones's infected patients would be dead:

I've had anger directed at me by one family only. They don't like me and keep away from me for that reason, and I understand that. What I find incredible is not that, but the fact that everybody else still comes. The mothers of some of the children who died still come. We still get Christmas cards, they still come to weekends we hold for our patients. It's a family thing. Haemophilia always has been a family thing.

In the first months of 1985, Dr Jones constructed his own theory as to how his patients and other British haemophiliacs had become infected. Five years earlier he had found that plasma for the manufacture of Factor VIII and Factor IX had not only been bought from paid donors in the United States, but also from donors in central Africa. It was an indirect purchase, because when demand outstripped supply in the US, international plasma brokers were called upon to meet the shortfall. These brokers, working principally from offices in Zurich and Montreal, would draw on numerous supply sources: many situated precisely in those areas in central Africa where Kaposi's sarcoma was now endemic – Kinshasa, the capital of Zaire, as well as Ghana, the Congo, Ivory Coast and Senegal.

Dr Jones wrote a lengthy letter to the *BMJ* in March. 'Given the long incubation period for AIDS,' he wrote, 'these facts suggest that the disease was introduced into the United States not by sexual transmission, but via plasma obtained in endemic areas. The exposure of a population with no natural resistance to the virus and with a proclivity for promiscuity resulted in spread.'

He noted that if plasma from these endemic areas was still being used, then the current system of screening would be inappropriate. Heat treatment may make safe Factors VIII and IX, but other blood products, particularly intravenous gamma globulin derived from multiple donations, should still be considered as potentially infectious. He called on the companies and government agencies concerned to come clean and state the country of origin of all their plasma on every pack.

The letter caused some concern and drew strong criticism. Writing to the *BMJ*, Dr Donald Acheson, the Chief Medical Officer for England, assured him that on the basis of confidential information in his possession, he was confident that none of the plasma covered by UK licences came from areas where AIDS was known to be endemic. Robert Reilly, of the American Blood Resources Association, went on the offensive. He claimed Dr Jones's opinions were factually and scientifically incorrect, stating that all US blood products manufacturers must be licensed by the Food and Drug Administration, 'and it can be easily verified that they do not rely on plasma from Africa'. He questioned why, if AIDS was introduced into the US by foreign plasma and not from sexual contact, the disease was not visible only in the recipients of plasma. In a final flourish, Mr Reilly stated that Dr Jones 'discredits his otherwise fine reputation and discredits the commercial industry, which strives to meet a diversity of national blood product requirements with the highest quality of products'.

Dr Jones would have none of it. In another letter he noted that

all that the major companies engaged in the collection and fractionation of plasma have to do in order not to be bound by FDA rules is to set up subsidiaries outwith the United States. Examples known to regulatory bodies in Britain and other countries include the longstanding contract between a multinational company and a plasmapheresis centre in Lesotho in Africa and the facilities run by at least two companies in Mexico.

Mr Reilly's contention that AIDS did not enter the US through blood products because of the low incidence of related disease was dismissed on the grounds that albumin has always been heat treated, and that this process inadvertently also killed off HTLV-III.

And so it went for a while, back and forth. These days, Dr Jones maintains his beliefs, with slight modifications:

I knew and I know that there is no international law which prohibits the use of plasma from developing countries. There should be. I also knew that the whole thrust of what was known as AIDS was that this was a gay plague initially and that somehow this had got into America. There was very little evidence of the plague being anywhere else in the world at that time, particularly in the developing world, except Africa. And I knew that plasma had been collected in Africa for use by the people who manufacture blood products. So it was natural to think that this might be one of the ways in which this particular infection had got into the blood supply and I still think that.

I think that we will one day be able to prove, through the make-up of HIV, that the African connection is true. Now obviously it came in other ways too. Probably by air travel and the ways you know about already. But I know that plasma was collected in Africa, both in South Africa and Central Africa, and was used for the making of blood products at the time when HIV first came to light.

67

The logic, he says, is simple enough: the companies dealing in plasma regard it as a resource which they can buy cheap and sell expensive just like any other. Dr Jones says he has talked to people who have collected plasma in Africa. Of course the industry denies this – why should they admit it? 'The key point is that neither industry nor the health authorities answered the main conclusion that I made and that was that if you're going to use plasma it should be labelled properly and we should know where it's coming from. We still don't.'

As a doctor prescribing blood products licensed in this country he is dependent on the licensing authority which takes evidence in secret; doctors have to rely on the authority's word and on what the manufacturers tell them:

A rep from a blood product company can walk into my room now and tell me that he has an accredited herd of donors in a particular part of the United States and that he does A, B, C and D to each of these donors and the plasma comes from nowhere else, and I don't believe him.

There's written evidence of the blood collection in Lesotho. I've also met the doctor who worked in Zaire, which of course was the epicentre of HIV, perhaps is the epicentre of HIV. Now, if plasma was coming out of there, then obviously it was infected. And no amount of rebuttal can take away the fact that somebody who is qualified and who's actually been there and done it, has told me. Again, it all comes down to commerce.

In Koblenz, western Germany, at the end of 1993, a small blood-supply company called UB Plasma was found to have been failing to screen its product adequately: health officials tracing unexplained cases of HIV discovered that while the firm had processed about 7,000 units of blood since 1992, they had only purchased 2,500 testing kits. For Dr Jones this sort of practice came as little surprise; the economics of the international trade in blood products is only revealed every time there's a crisis, he says.

'I've seen documentation of lying by major blood companies. I've seen evidence that plasma was imported into this country outside the authorities, outside licensing. Which is why I don't have very much, well I don't have total faith. I have a lot of faith, but not total faith in licensing procedures.'

What can be done? One solution would be to treat blood products like jam: label them, with country of origin, precise contents. The fact that this should have happened decades ago, but hasn't, is blamed on the expediency and self-interest of Western governments.

Dr Jones's is still a minority voice; but his confidence is persuasive. Soon, he says, blood typing will show that the virus in people with haemophilia can only have come from Africa or the Middle East. 'We can type HIV around the world. And the link is there.'

Most haemophiliacs in Newcastle probably became infected between 1979 and 1981, before anyone recognized AIDS. Simon Taylor, who was not one of Dr Jones's patients but was treated in London, thinks he also seroconverted at this time. He remembers an illness, probably in late 1980: erratic temperature and a loss of appetite, nobody knowing what was up. This lasted a couple of months off and on and then suddenly he had an incredibly severe reaction, a fever of 104, was seriously ill for a day and was then fine. The classic conversion process, though at the time he hadn't a clue.

In 1984 he read an article saying that in America it was assumed that almost everyone with haemophilia who had used these blood products expected to become infected. 'So in my heart I think I knew really. Virtually everybody with haemophilia A had been treated at some point with imported products. People had been quite lackadaisical: there were various companies producing different commercial products, and then there was UK-produced product, and to some extent when you went in for your supply you got whatever was in the fridge that day.'

In 1985, when his doctor found out his test result from stored samples, Taylor was in the process of buying a house. At his request, the result was kept from him for a few weeks so that he could fill in a life insurance policy with a clear conscience. Later his doctor said, 'Well, as you've probably guessed, yes you are positive.' 'No great shock then, but I've been told that some people were just tested and then told by letter: "Dear Sir, You've got AIDS. Yours faithfully".'

By the end of 1985 there were reports of 721 people infected by bad blood in Britain, the vast majority haemophiliacs, but some also as a result of a transfusion or tissue replacement during an operation. By the end of 1986 this figure was 1062; at this time there were 2,625 reports of HTLV-III infection by all modes of transmission. A paper in the *BMJ* in July 1986 from virologists in London and Manchester showed that non-commercial British blood products were far from free of contamination. Out of 166 patients tested who had only used British concentrates, 18 were found to be positive to anti-HTLV-III (11 per cent). Unlike most recipients of imported concentrate, all but one of those infected by British products seroconverted only after 1983. This allowed some damning speculation: that they had been infected after AIDS was recognized, at a time when those already infected by other means were able to contaminate supplies which were then not adequately screened or treated. In fact, routine screenings of all blood donations were not introduced until October 1985.

At the beginning of 1987, the Haemophilia Society estimated that 1,200 people with haemophilia had been infected. The society's newsletter called it 'the single biggest disaster in the history of the National Health Service. Never before have so many been affected so terribly by treatment which was intended to help them lead a normal life'.

There was also a strong belief that the companies producing the blood concentrates could have done much more to protect their supplies far earlier than they did. 'They could have screened for hepatitis,' says Simon Taylor, now an official of the Haemophilia Society. 'Most of the donations infected with hepatitis were later also found to be infected with HTLV-III. Also, heat treatment products had been developed but hadn't been implemented, and these had been shown again to be effective against hepatitis. So we could have used hepatitis as a sort of surrogate marker for HIV. If they'd done that, we probably wouldn't have had anything like the problems we did, and do. However, it's always easy to be wise after the event.'

As with gay men, haemophiliacs faced widespread discrimination whether they were infected or not. When treatment had been poor in the 1960s and early 1970s, many haemophiliacs had covered up, hiding it from employers if they could. People 'came out' more when the concentrates made even severe cases manageable, but in the mid-1980s many ran back to the closet. 'Haemophilia itself became a marker for having AIDS,' says Simon Taylor. 'All of a sudden people in factories would say "Hang on, it says here in the paper that everybody with haemophilia's got AIDS. Bill, you've got haemophilia haven't you?"'

There was no support mechanism outside the family or haemophilia centres – unlike with the gay epidemic, there was no 'haemophiliac community'. And it wasn't concentrated in London: whereas three Thames regions carried the burden of about three-fifths of all HTLV-

III infections, haemophiliac cases were spread evenly around the UK. Cue panic in hamlets.

In September 1985, over two hundred parents gathered in a hall in Chandler's Ford, Hampshire, to be told that a nine-year-old haemophiliac at the local school had tested HTLV-III positive; the boy was not 'outed', but alongside his parents revealed his status openly. The boy attended Scantabout County Primary School, from which about one quarter of pupils had been kept at home by anxious parents. The headmaster stressed that the boy did not have AIDS, talked about an incubation period and outlined the small infection risks. Tony Pinching drove down to address the meeting, ran through the medical stuff and advised that the boy had enough to face without this sort of stigmatism. He played not just the expert, but the dad too: and yes, on reflection, he would allow his own kids to attend a school with an HTLV-III positive child. One parent who was keeping his child at home wanted cast-iron proof that if his kid collided with the boy in the playground, he would not get infected. Pinching wasn't in the business of issuing guarantees, but he weighed up the risks. 'I asked how many roads the boy crossed on the way to school, and whether he used rear seat-straps if coming by car. I said the risk of the child being killed or seriously injured in these situations was orders of magnitude more than the scenario he had painted.' The point went home.

For a while, the boy got real star billing: Hampshire County Council sent along two staff to keep him under observation throughout the school day. According to *The Times*, they would leap into action the moment he cut himself or began bleeding, though what this action would be was not specified. All but a handful of parents eventually returned their children to school and the boy made several new friends. In retrospect, the incident was a model of crisis management. At the time, of course, it was yet another unique AIDS drama, a broad terror of the unknown. Within days there were reports of eight similar alarms at schools throughout the country: parents wanted to know whether you could catch it from chewing pencil tops, from running barefoot, from sharing wind instruments.

A Little Advice

In September 1985 when the media descended on Chandler's Ford, the commotion was understandable: no one had told these people anything. Unless you were gay, or a haemophiliac, and if you lived out-side London or Edinburgh, the virus was unlikely to have touched your world. Your information came from the newspapers and television and, although there was much balanced reporting, the emotions AIDS induced in most people were probably those of fear and horror. Aside from a waiting-room booklet produced by the Health Education Council, government departments of health or education had produced no information for the general reader. Three years on from the first reported cases, with estimated numbers of infections ranging from ten thousand to a hundred thousand, there had been little debate in the Commons, little investment in research, no health education campaign. And financial compensation for infected haemophiliacs? Out of the question.

But there had been a number of promises. In November 1984 junior health minister John Patten reaffirmed what Dr David Owen had first announced under a Labour government in 1977 – that it was the intention of the Health Department to ensure self-sufficiency in blood products in the immediate future. Three months later, in February 1985, Kenneth Clarke, Secretary of State for Social Services, conceded in the Commons that the programme of heat treatment had meant that such a timetable had to be re-examined. Nine years later, self-sufficiency was still some way off.

Limited legislation reassured some, but horrified others. The Public Health (Infectious Diseases) Regulations 1985 made the disease subject to some of the provisions of the Public Health (Control of Disease) Act 1984. Announcing the new measures in a written parliamentary reply in February 1985, Kenneth Clarke stated that people with AIDS, or those suspected of being infected, could be forced to undergo medical examination and be detained in hospital. There had been some disquiet from backbenchers about his previous statement that AIDS would not be made a notifiable disease lest it discourage people from coming forward for tests, and this new measure was to provide a safety net to be used as a last resort. It was a move intended to protect the 'general public against the spread of the disease', Mr Clarke announced, a legal constraint against patients 'in a dangerously infectious state ... We are satisfied that we need to take powers now to be in a position to protect the public in the event of such a risk arising'. This was hardly the compassionate action that people who had recently tested positive or their carers were looking for. Clarke went on: the new measures also required local authorities to take 'all reasonably practical steps' to prevent people coming into contact with the dead body of a person who died of an AIDS-related illness. It was only a matter of months before the new regulations were employed.

In mid-September 1985 Manchester city magistrates ordered that a 29-year-old man should be detained against his will at Monsall Isolation Hospital. The city's medical officer had informed the court that the man was 'bleeding copiously and trying to discharge himself'. The man's solicitor claimed that 'the order should not have been made, as it led to his virtual imprisonment ... the trust between doctor and patient was affected by the element of compulsion'. Ten days after the initial court order, the Terrence Higgins Trust appealed to Manchester High Court and won: a judge heard new evidence that the man's condition had improved, and said he was now free to go. It was then reported that he had changed his mind and would now stay put for further treatment. According to Les Latner of the Terrence Higgins Trust, 'Now he knows he can leave, he is quite happy to stay. Once people had explained to him that he was in no condition to leave, he agreed that hospital was the best place for him.' Mr Latner expressed disquiet that doctors couldn't have persuaded him to stay in the first place, 'instead of rushing off to the courts. His parents didn't even know he had AIDS until they read the court report'. He said that the news of his enforced detention would almost certainly deter other people from seeking hospital treatment or presenting for a test.

Comprehensive testing of all blood donations was introduced a month later, when it was estimated that two million samples would be examined in the next 12 months. Potential donors were presented with an updated leaflet outlining the procedure: before any blood would be accepted it would first be tested, not only for the HTLV-III virus, but also for hepatitis, syphilis and signs of anaemia. You were not advised to give blood if you fell into three categories: practising homosexual and bisexual men (with no account being taken of the incubation period); injecting drug users; and the sexual contacts of these two groups.

Testing was now also to be made widely available at STD clinics and other centres. Commercial screening kits had been available in the United States five months earlier, but their introduction in Britain had been delayed owing to the high number of false readings.

The two approved kits were made by Wellcome Diagnostics, an off-shoot of the British pharmaceuticals giant, and Organon Teknika Ltd, a Dutch company. Both employed variations on the enzyme-linked immunosorbent assay (ELISA), a complex colour-change control test involving up to eight stages and taking three hours. Any positive results would then be confirmed by the established Western blotting technique, whereby the constituent proteins of the virus are separated and identified by their relative molecular mass.

The delay in finding a suitable kit would be seen in some quarters as a callous reluctance by the government to grant licences until the test from Wellcome was ready (the test was developed at the Middlesex Hospital and the Institute of Cancer Research); but these allegations surfaced only rarely, and were dismissed by health officials who cited an independent report in the *Lancet* which mentioned the unreliability of earlier commercial screening kits.

The evaluation of the kits was conducted by the Public Health Laboratory Service (PHLS) in north London, the network responsible for the monitoring of infectious diseases. The 52 laboratories that made up the service were credited with a key role in reducing the incidence of typhoid and tuberculosis since the Second World War, and were more recently employed to control the spread of legionnaire's disease and salmonella. It was the cause of some embarrassment, therefore, when two notable microbiologists revealed in September 1985 that they had been employed to advise on the effects of the break up of the PHLS. The DHSS was examining the possibility of transferring central responsibility for the service to local authorities; it was claimed this would save much of the £37 million annual running costs. The leak provoked outrage, not least among doctors in the AIDS field who petitioned the Health Department to change its mind. This caused such embarrassment for the government that two weeks later Norman Fowler, Social Services Secretary, conceded in a television interview that it was never intended as a cost-cutting measure. Further, he said that his department had decided not to abolish the present system after all.

On 1 October 1985 Dr Donald Acheson wrote to all doctors in England informing them of the introduction of the HTLV-III antibody test and its attendant protocol. The key point was that people who believed themselves at risk *should not donate blood* just in order to be tested. This had indeed been happening for the past few months, causing considerable alarm, because even a reliable test cannot detect the earliest stages of infection. Besides, there was counselling to consider. Dr Acheson wrote that this would be provided by health

74

authorities; employees were being given specific training at that very moment at St Mary's, Paddington.

Dr Acheson's letter arrived with a slim blue booklet giving further details of the test and how best to advise patients. It covered issues of confidentiality and anti-discriminatory advice to be given to employers. It was a cool-headed report, a clear attempt to dampen panic. In contrast to some of the hysterical predictions from other sources (including a representative of the Royal College of Nursing who predicted a million British infections by the end of the decade), the booklet viewed it as unlikely that most GPs would be called upon to deliver bad news. It stated: 'Positive results are expected to be very rare.'

Slowly things were moving. Largely through the influence of Dr Acheson, ministers began to take heed of what was happening. By the end of October 1985 there were 241 reported cases of AIDS in Britain (three-quarters in London); the most common estimate of the number of people infected was twenty thousand. In a rough comparison, the total of British AIDS cases ranked third in Europe, about 340 cases behind France, 60 behind West Germany; Britain had about 45 more cases than Italy, 70 more than Spain.

On 2 December 1985 Norman Fowler announced that AIDS was indeed being taken seriously by his government. In a written parliamentary answer to Roger Sims (MP for Chislehurst), Mr Fowler said that he had allocated £6.3 million to combat the spread of AIDS and to help those already infected. The package worked out like this:

£2.5 million for a national information campaign to begin in March and run throughout the year. Most of this would be directed at the public in general. The necessary preliminary research was already underway.

£2.5 million for the three Thames Regional Health Authorities who would continue to carry the heaviest burden (north-east, north-west and south-east); the money would go towards treatment and counselling.

£750,000 for the recently rescued Public Health Laboratory Service, to continue its testing work.

£270,000 for the six principal English haemophiliac reference centres in England.

£100,000 for training health professionals in counselling work;
this would continue at St Mary's in London and expand to
Birmingham and Newcastle.

Two months earlier, the Terrence Higgins Trust had received a
grant of £25,000; this brought its total government grant, for the
three years it had been running, to £35,000.

These millions were regarded by some in parliament, and many
outside commentators, as a little excessive. It took Mr Fowler just
nine months to realize how inadequate they would be.

The motivation for these grants came from a few individuals in the
DHSS, none more forceful than the Chief Medical Officer. In June
1985 Dr Donald Acheson, an experienced epidemiologist, prepared a
confidential paper for Norman Fowler. Entitled 'HTLV-III infection,
the AIDS epidemic and the control of its spread in the UK', it made
sobering reading. It estimated that people were becoming infected at
the rate of 50–100 individuals per week, and warned that 'this degree
of infectivity may persist indefinitely'.

Dr Acheson revealed that about 20 per cent of gay men attending
one London sexually transmitted disease clinic were known to be
seropositive. The proportion among gays attending STD clinics outside London was believed to be 5 per cent.

He noted: 'The key issue which will determine the eventual scale of
the epidemic in the absence of effective preventive action is the facility with which transmission of infection tales place as a result of heterosexual intercourse.' This was language government ministers could
understand: the question, still, was whether the general public, the
straight nation, was at risk.

Dr Acheson had a little evidence: a small number of female partners
of bisexual males and of haemophiliacs had become infected, which
indeed suggested that male-to-female transmission, presumably by
semen, was possible. As for female-to-male transmission, there was
conflicting data. In New York City, in spite of a large number of
AIDS cases in female prostitutes (some of whom would also be using
drugs), only 28 out of 3,354 cases had been reported in males who
said they did not take part in anal intercourse, use drugs intravenous-
ly, or form part of a high-risk group (haemophiliacs, Haitians). Then

again, the epidemic of HTLV-III infection in sub-Saharan Africa appeared to affect men and women equally. While it was not certain to what extent transmission had been due to tribal scarification and dirty needles in this region, Dr Acheson wrote,

> heterosexual intercourse cannot be excluded as a possible means of transmission. Although the American data suggests that homosexual intercourse is the most important means of sexual spread of HTLV-III infection in our present state of knowledge, it would be wrong for policy to be based on the assumption that heterosexual intercourse will not in the long run assume a significant role. This point should be taken into account in formulating a preventive strategy.

What form this strategy should take was presented to Mr Fowler in the broadest terms. Each of the high-risk groups should receive specifically targeted education. For homosexuals such a programme 'will require their co-operation'. One 'favourable point' was that because the epidemic was currently concentrated in London, there was 'still an opportunity to curtail its spread to the provinces'. The possibility of offering immunization against hepatitis B as part of a general package of health education was raised. As for intravenous drug users, every effort should be made to get the message across in clinics and elsewhere that AIDS was a serious potential threat. Generally, Dr Acheson advised that education should be directed to the general population and to pupils in secondary schools as part of their sex education.

He concluded his report with a warning; if alarm bells hadn't rung in the secretary of state's office before, they were certainly ringing now. The personal and social implications for an infected person were 'calamitous'; no vaccine for at least five years, little effective treatment, indefinite infectivity, mother-to-baby transmission, discrimination, ostracization ... and then you probably die.

Within nine months the government would have some general adverts in the newspapers; within 18 they'd have images of tombstones on the television. An education campaign targeted at drug users would appear in over two years. Specific government campaigns aimed at gay men would not appear until 1989, almost four years after Dr Acheson's report.

Apart from Dr Acheson, the most important source of advice came from a group of doctors who had been meeting in private in Health Department rooms at the Elephant & Castle. The Expert Advisory Group on AIDS (EAGA) first met on 29 January 1985 and had 22 members. Most were doctors, including several specialists who had dealt clinically and scientifically with the epidemic since the beginning: Pinching, Adler, Tedder, Weiss. Other physicians came from blood transfusion or related services in Birmingham, Manchester and Edinburgh. There were also many representatives from the department, including the chairman Dr Abrams and Dr Acheson.

This was the most influential body to advise government ministers throughout the first decade of the epidemic. Some members would leave and others be appointed, but there would hardly be a week without an EAGA sub-committee chewing over policy or debating new services and treatments.

One important sub-committee met regularly to consider the health education campaign. Hospital doctors were augmented by specialists in community medicine and gay men with relevant experience, including Tony Whitehead of the Terrence Higgins Trust and Dr Heath of the Gay Medical Association. Other committees met to consider infection control for drug users and haemophiliacs and their families, but the emphasis of this one was on gay men. By the time of a meeting in July 1985, the estimated proportion of gay men attending STD clinics who were infected had increased to 30 per cent. The minutes of the meeting noted that 'although AIDS was a general public health issue, health education policy in this respect should be concerned primarily with those people who were most at risk'. One of the doctors stated that 'nothing could be accomplished without the commitment of the homosexual community'. Tony Whitehead now regards this comment as extraordinary, given the levels of self-education conducted within the British gay world for the last two years, which he described as 'essentially a crucial survivalist policy formulated by a community that believed it was being left to slowly die'.

At the meeting, various strategies were presented. It was agreed that, in asking people to modify their sexual lifestyle, health education faced an enormous challenge: it was one thing alerting people to the dangers, quite another persuading them to change the habits they'd had for years. Several approaches were highlighted: Professor Anthony Coxon, a behavioural scientist, observed that 'illustrated lectures on the subject had been given in Cardiff's homosexual club'. The preferred method of the Terrence Higgins Trust was a gay club 'road-show', employing traditional cultural entertainments such as drag acts. The Chief Medical Officer suggested that a campaign to encourage the use of condoms should be initiated, the first time this had been mentioned in such a meeting. He suggested that such a campaign would have to be 'both sensitive and sophisticated'.

Other EAGA meetings discussed at length the implications of testing and the provision of adequate counselling. It was agreed that the person or service instigating the screening test 'must take responsibility for the consequences'. Widespread counselling provision and training were likely to cause strain on existing resources, but their importance could not be overstated.

It was a wise conclusion: no preventive education would help those who tested positive. These meetings were already too late for many thousands who took the test in the months that followed its introduction in October 1985. Six months later, at a meeting at the Institute of Medical Laboratory Sciences in London, Dr Don Jeffries of St Mary's said that there had been several cases of people committing suicide or attempting suicide on receiving a positive antibody result. 'We still don't know exactly what the results of the tests mean,' he said. Dr Pinching was at the same meeting. He said it would be foolish to assume that everyone who is positive will necessarily develop full-blown AIDS. 'Not everyone who gets chickenpox goes on to develop shingles.'

Caroline and Tim

I didn't go for a test, it was just done without my knowing. I went to the doctor feeling very run down and he took blood and thought it was glandular fever. My glands were up and I said they'd been up for quite a while. But then slowly things started coming back to me and I remembered the man I had slept with in Australia in 1983. His boyfriend had gone down with a kind of rash and no one really knew what it was. I knew that the man I slept with was very active sexually and was bisexual. That's where I got the virus.

I went back for the results of the glandular fever tests and they were all negative, but the doctor there, a locum, was very keen and said that he'd requested a test for the AIDS virus. I said he had no right to do that and that I wanted the test stopped. He said it was too late, so I said in that case I didn't want to know the results. But two weeks later my own doctor turned up one night at my house. I knew the minute I opened the door. He said, 'I've been told you don't want to know the results, but you're too intelligent not to know that it was positive.'

Caroline Guinness, late thirties, with a soft South African accent, lives in north-west London. She's been HIV positive since 1986. She has an 11-year-old daughter, Lee, from her second marriage. Her first marriage was to Tim Clark, a gay journalist who has written about HIV and AIDS since the mid-1980s.

TIM CLARK: I was there when she got her diagnosis, when the doctor came round. I kind of answered all her questions as best I could whenever things got ... she would get hysterical a few times. Not surprisingly. It wasn't just her she was worried about, it was Lee as well. Initially all kinds of things sent her into a cold sweat, like 'Oh my God, what if Lee's used my toothbrush when I haven't been looking!'

Obviously it was a complete shock to me. Of all the people I'd known who had been diagnosed ... I was appalled. Not least the fact that we'd both had sex with the same guy who infected her, at different times.

She needed people to talk to, but she was paranoid about confidentiality. She didn't want anybody to know at that stage, especially her straight friends because she knew that they would treat her in the way that us gay people had treated the first suspects in our community – these strange alien creatures who would then become pariahs. They'd become objects of wonder and awe, rather than just normal people who'd got an infection. She was quite right: the newspapers would have been round like a shot.

CAROLINE GUINNESS: There was nothing available on positive women at all – no research, no groups you could turn to. Most of the support I got was from my gay friends, although very few people knew about my status. Just before Christmas 1986 a good friend of mine died, the actor Douglas Lambert. Tim and I had helped look after him because he didn't want to waste away in hospital. It was very draining and it affected me badly: I could see myself going terribly like that, just losing everything so quickly.

Just before Christmas I got a call from someone I knew at the Terrence Higgins Trust saying she was organizing a fundraising event with music and could I help organize it. I'd had a fair bit of experience. I'd left South Africa when I had just turned eighteen, mostly for political reasons. Tim was one of the first people I met and we lived together in this big hippie house in Portobello Road. It was the first time that I realized I could say whatever I wanted without getting arrested for it.

I started off working for Bill Curbishley, who was managing The Who and others, first as a receptionist, but I was soon involved in everything. I then worked for another manager, who had no money, and did Motorhead, Hawkwind and a lot of American bands – not really music I liked, but I learnt a hell of a lot, organizing all the tours. And then I started working with Russell Mulcahy, when pop video was just beginning. We got £2,000 pounds from a record company to do two videos for OMD and we thought that was a fortune. Within a year we were getting budgets of £150,000 to do Elton John. Then I crossed over to film, working with film music, and that's when I got diagnosed. There was no way I could continue or cope with it, so I stopped. My source of income dried up and I didn't know what was going to happen. I was actually terrified. Lee was at nursery school and I couldn't tell anyone for fear of what might happen to her.

But I got this call, asking me to do this concert, which was supposed to raise money and awareness, and that's when things started to change. Tony Whitehead was running the trust then still from a tiny office. It became very apparent very quickly that the trust knew nothing about music at all, and they said things like, 'Oh, let's have it somewhere like Wembley ...' This was in December '86 and they said the concert had to be on 1st April, which was then International AIDS Day.

I couldn't do it on my own, so I asked a girlfriend who worked in the music business to help. She knew about my diagnosis, but nobody else working on the concert did apart from Tony and his boyfriend. The Marquee in Wardour Street gave us little offices and it was absolutely shambolic. We started contacting everybody, managers, agents, musicians, and none of them wanted to know. The managers and agents said they couldn't help because it was about AIDS and they didn't want their artists to be seen as gay. I used to hear really stupid things: I remember going to LWT and speaking to some producer who said, 'I recently met someone with AIDS and I thought "What do I do? I might end up sitting next to them." And I thought,

"Well, you're sitting next to someone right now!' There was such ignorance. It certainly didn't encourage me to be open about my status.

But I badgered a lot of journalists to give us some publicity, and then George Michael stepped in, which I actually thought was pretty brave of him, because there were all these rumours about him being gay. He was brilliant and he started badgering other people. Some other people had come in straight away – Holly Johnson, Boy George, Jimmy Somerville, the obvious ones, the gay people. But we were very aware that we needed a cross-section if we were to reach a cross-section of society. Aswad came in early as well. But all the real biggies were initially reluctant. Queen absolutely flatly refused, wouldn't even return calls. John Entwistle of The Who was the MC, a good choice because he was so unflappable and there were a lot of prima donnas to look after. The promoter wouldn't even commit himself until the very end, until the big artists were in.

We had some brilliant volunteers who organized a lot of smaller events in bars and clubs, but we had some pretty hopeless ones too. One man working on the club events liked young boys very much – he called them his bunnies. The place was full of Michael's bunnies. It got to the point where the Marquee got really upset because they'd walked into the boardroom and found two of his bunnies bonking on the table. Complete madness. I remember George Cant, Tony Whitehead's boyfriend, coming in after that saying, 'Uh-oh, trouble in the warren!'

Two weeks before the event, it just turned, because we suddenly got a deal for worldwide television coverage, and then suddenly all these other names came in. It turned out to be a brilliant night. I think it raised £250,000; a lot of money went on administration costs. People were spreading the safer sex message and I think it changed a few things. [The show, called The Party, was held at Wembley Arena. Lots of free condoms, safe-sex messages on T-shirts and reworking of old songs. A Capital Radio DJ wanted everyone to fight 'this *incredible* disease called AIDS'. Elton John sang 'Will You Still Love Me Tomorrow'. Several fledgling organizations received vital cash.]

Elton said he'd do it with days to go. Then Herbie Hancock and Meatloaf appeared from somewhere. And a lot of the people who said they'd be unavailable because they'd be out of the country or in the studio were in fact hanging around backstage.

TIM CLARK: In 1985–6 I went to that hospital on Hammersmith roundabout. They have a GUM [genito-urinary medicine] clinic there. I had rung up Gay Switchboard to find out which places I could anonymously walk into without an appointment. I wanted to do it on the spur of the moment, whenever I actually screwed up my courage to do it.

I went in there and was just paralysed with embarrassment. I'd been to clap clinics before, but not for quite some time, and now with all this haze of guilt and fear hanging over the place it was right back to the good old days of the late 1960s: shuffling in as a guilty school-boy. There were a few other people with their heads buried in maga-zines. They did the blood test. I think there was a little bit of coun-selling first – very earnest and well meaning. Then I had to come back for the result two weeks later.

I was scared shitless, but at the same time I was convincing myself that I'd be all right. I went in for the result and the doctor sat me down and peered closely at the form. He said: 'Er well, I'm really sorry, but it seems to be positive and I haven't a clue what I'm sup-posed to do now because it's my first day on the clinic. Just sit here while I go out and find out what it is I'm supposed to do now. You're the first one I've done.'

So he left me there and it felt like I was in an elevator where the cord has suddenly snapped. My jaw hit the floor and I went very cold and started shaking and sweating and my mind was spinning. 'Fuck! What now?'

About five minutes later he came back and said, 'I'm very sorry, I've misread your diagnosis. It's negative.'

I didn't know whether to hit him or kiss him. I wanted to grab him by the throat and shout 'Don't ever do that to anybody again!'

At the same time I was so grateful to be suddenly free. He then insisted on sending me in for further counselling about my sexual behaviour. Clearly if I had come for a test I was at risk. It was fairly primitive counselling but I wasn't listening to a word at that stage. So we went through the motions. I just kind of nodded and said, 'Yes, yes, yes, of course, thanks for the condoms.' I couldn't wait to get out of there.

The strange thing that happened after that, at least in those days, was this strange euphoria of this reprieve. You think, 'Well, you can probably lapse a bit now and again and it'll be all right.' Because the test was negative on the basis of your appalling past sexual behaviour, you get this appalling false sense of security that you've just taken well-judged risks. What bollocks, but you can convince yourself of almost anything if you try hard enough.

I do know of some people who claim that after having a negative test they vowed never to put themselves at risk ever again and maybe they've stuck to it. They claim to have done. Personally I found it impossible. I also know lots of people who have finally admitted they have slipped. Even people who are high up in the gay community say privately, 'Well, yes, of course I've not been safe myself on a few occasions.'

So inevitably some while later I felt compelled to go for another one.

CAROLINE GUINNESS: At this time I was still trying to find out more about how it affected women, to see how many other women were infected. I'd heard of this doctor at the Royal Free who specialized in women and children. Of course I was very interested and so I went for this meeting with him over lunch at the Royal Society of Medicine. His name was Tom Courtney and he was pretty convincing, a real smoothie but rather weird ... instinctively you knew there was something wrong about him. On the other hand he was very knowledgeable and said that he was doing this research into dextran sulphate, which was the thing at the time.

I remember going to see him in late 1987 at the Royal Free – a regular office with his name on it. There was nothing at the time to suggest he was a fraud. He asked whether I would help set up this organization called WOMB – Welfare of Mothers and Babies. Together with a few people who helped on the concert, I said we would.

At that time I got a call back from an organization called Positively Women, a group I had heard of through the Terrence Higgins Trust. It was from Sheila Gilchrist, who set it up. Sheila was pregnant, and they had no organization, just this belief that something should be done. They'd just lost the room where they held their support groups and the next one was going to have to be in a pizza restaurant. Sheila and Kate Thomson, a full-time student, had done some groundwork, but there was no funding, nothing.

This WOMB charity stuff was bubbling away and it became increasingly obvious that Tom Courtney was an appalling fraud. As soon as he knew that I had met this group, he was after Positively Women in a big way. He was claiming outrageous things, like he was treating 666 women – just the number should have told us! He was claiming that all the patients at the Royal Free were his, but then we met Margaret Johnson [the consultant in HIV at the Royal Free] and found that he was claiming all her patients. When we rumbled him we got on to everyone – lawyers, the Charity Commission – and no one would listen. Meanwhile the guy was getting in a lot of funding. At this point he was becoming abusive and aggressive. When the Royal Free eventually investigated him they kicked him out, but he still wasn't struck off. He set up in Harley Street, which is where he finally got done for rape [in November 1992 he was found guilty of two rapes and two indecent assaults and received a seven-year prison sentence]. He hated Sheila and I because we created such a ruckus about him. We tried to set up Positively Women on a firm footing, but very privately, to keep it away from him. Sheila and I went to see Margaret Jay who had just started at the National AIDS Trust. She had heard of Tom Courtney, so she was aware why we were trying to set up with such subterfuge, without this monster coming crashing in. She told us to give her a budget, which we did on the back of a cigarette box then and there, and she okayed the grant immediately. We got £10,000, which meant we could start properly.

We got offices in Gray's Inn Road from the Terrence Higgins Trust and started doing posters and leaflets. I was basically on my own for the first three or four months: Sheila was having her baby. Everything was new: there was still nothing available for women, certainly nothing from the government despite their recent campaigns saying AIDS can affect everybody.

We started doing a lot of publicity, though I didn't tell the press I was positive. But our group was run exclusively for positive women by positive women, so how the media didn't pick up on the fact that its director was positive I find absolutely extraordinary. It became very obvious that because I didn't fit the description of what they thought someone with HIV should look like, then there was no way that I could have been.

Once people knew about us, people started coming thick and fast from all over the country. Most of them were saying, 'Thank God there's something at last.' The support group became a weekly thing. There was one-to-one counselling and a lot of campaigning. A lot of statutory organizations were beginning to get AIDS money from the government and were developing their policies on HIV and AIDS, and we had to make sure we weren't forgotten. I've never worked so hard in my life. Sir Donald Acheson, the Chief Medical Officer, was tremendously supportive and became a personal friend of Sheila's. I was asked to help write a speech for him that he gave at a conference in Paris.

Princess Diana was a great help too. She opened our new premises in Islington and I remember her strict instructions that her aides should wait outside, she just wanted to talk to the women. She stayed for ages, not just chatting about HIV, but anything. One of the women asked her how *she* coped. She met Lee, who was completely tongue-tied. She made Lee laugh. Then I met her again two years later, at a thing for the International Council of Women, and she came up to me and said, 'How are you doing? How's Lee?' She remembered exactly what Lee was interested in. I thought, 'Wow, you're a lot more with it than anyone gives you credit for.'

There's an enormous difference between Diana and Princess Margaret, who also appears at various AIDS things. Princess Margaret really does appear to be in it for the social side. She comes out with the most appalling statements that really upset people. The Royal Academy of Art held a pop art exhibition and gave some money to Positively Women. So Princess Margaret came to this special evening. Sheila was there, with her daughter who presented the flowers. And there were also some Ugandan women there. And Princess Margaret actually said, in very loud tones, 'Well it's not surprising there's so much AIDS in Africa, considering …' She didn't actually say 'considering they fuck like bunnies', but words to that effect.

She then said: 'All positive women should be sterilized.' Sheila replied, 'You know the little girl who presented the flowers to you? Well her mother has AIDS.' And Margaret said, 'Well, it's no excuse, she should have been sterilized.' Sheila said, 'And *I'm* the mother.' I thought it was going to come to blows. But Margaret's very unaware. She surprised me because her best friend, Lady Glenconner, lost a son to AIDS.

The last time I met her she was fairly out of it. Again it was another art thing, some money being raised for the Haemophilia Society. She said to me, 'Are you married?' I said, 'No, I'm divorced.' She said, 'Oh. *I'm* divorced you know!'

TIM CLARK: I had my second test about two years later. For that one I went privately to Harley Street. It was advertised in the back of *Time Out*: 'HIV tests, 48 hours' and so on, sixty quid, seventy quid.

86

That again was negative but they again wanted to offer me more counselling but I just said, 'No, I know exactly what I'm doing and you can't tell me anything I don't know, because I've been researching things myself.' Quite arrogant, but they kind of accepted that.

I lied of course and said I just slipped up once.

By this time I was in a longish-term relationship. He was very neurotic about becoming infected, because he's never been promiscuous, he's always been a one-man guy. As far as he was concerned all of his previous relationships had been monogamous. He was very neurotic about me infecting him, so it was nice to be able to present him with this certificate.

Sometime later I went to Harley Street again. This time I was positive. That was in 1989. I just wanted to get out of there and think about it.

Suddenly I felt I had to put my foot on the accelerator and do something or I couldn't face it at all. I went to Paris to get away from it all. By that stage I knew a lot of people who had died or were unwell, a stream of illnesses one by one, and it was just all getting rather wearing.

Caroline wanted me to start doing things her way, which was taking it easier, getting support and financial help, and kind of ease up on the workload and I didn't want to do it that way. We did have quite a few arguments about that. She said, 'All these deadlines and adrenaline and journalism stuff is going to do you in,' but I would say, 'No, I'm sure it's the adrenaline that keeps me going.'

She accepts it now but there was a time when I'm sure she thought I was in denial, that denial syndrome that is supposed to afflict everyone.

And I suppose she was partially right. I just wanted to blot it out and put it to the back of my mind. I didn't want it to be a burden on anything I did, apart possibly from sex.

So I went off to Paris and there was nothing there for positive people at all, despite the fact that the numbers were enormous. I had been involved in Act-Up in London [the AIDS activism group] and there was a nascent Act-Up group in Paris, but they didn't have a group like the Terrence Higgins Trust. After a while I fell ill and got misdiagnosed by a doctor who said I had cancer of the stomach. He said a big lump had shown up on my X-ray. In London they examined me and it turned out it was a lump of fat.

CAROLINE GUINNESS: All the spontaneity about Positively Women has gone now. It's been crippled by political correctness. Now the funders dictate how you run the organization, but before we were working much better when it was running instinctively. We expanded from one to three offices and we got a lot more organized. More and more women began dropping in and a real pattern started emerging. We started off with mainly drug users or ex-drug users, but then came more and more women who had contracted the virus sexually. The transmission was all one way: from straight or bisexual men to women, never the other way round. We started doing our own research, compiling our own list of symptoms, tying to get it to be recognized. I went over to America to see what was there, but they didn't know much there either. In New York it was mostly connected with poverty, with women drug users or prostitutes.

We were seeing a lot of women from other parts of the world, a lot of African women. Initially we were told, 'Oh, you'll never get any black women joining, you're all white and middle class,' but that didn't tally in any way with what was actually happening. One of the original women involved was from Uganda and did a lot of work amongst Ugandans over here. We found that because some of the women were from the north of the country and some from the south, they liked having a buffer between them. They didn't want anyone in their community to know they were positive and then they'd come to meetings and meet other people in their community who'd also been hiding it.

Then the PC thing came in, about 1988–9, people saying we should have a drug-users group, and an African group, but I felt that there weren't that many of us with the virus, that we could afford to split up.

When money began coming in from local authorities, which meant that we had to have a management committee, that's when the war started. I think the PC lobby did untold damage. Because we'd been given this money by an authority, they wanted to come in and see how the money was being spent, which is OK in practice, but causes problems because we were an organization only for positive women, which is why women felt so relaxed there, and we didn't like people from outside sitting in. We also began to be seen as a good research facility.

Then the lesbian thing started, which was very distressing. We started getting our first frauds turning up at the support group. We

had a lot of very young mixed up lesbians, wanting some sort of protection, claiming to be positive, and we found out they weren't. That's
devastating when people are opening up their hearts and then finding
out there are frauds there. There was this hidden message from some
lesbians: 'We want to be involved. We want this virus!' Then there
were funding restrictions: 'What work are you doing for lesbians?'
They said, 'Oh, you have to do leaflets, you have to do safer sex for
lesbians,' and it was hard enough trying to get through to heterosexuals who were more at risk. Then it got to the point where a lot of the
people in charge of the funds were lesbians. It was all turning into
something it wasn't and I resigned in 1991. Sheila, Kate and I were
absolutely fed up, and then it soon became an organization that wasn't
run by positive women. By the time I left we had probably about four
hundred women who had been in contact with us and about 99 per
cent of them were heterosexuals with real problems. I continued to
give lots of talks around the country about the organization's work and
clearly I still support most of the service they offer, if not the way it's
run.

A few of us then started the International Community of Women,
again for positive women. This offered no support services, it was just
a group for women from all over the world who wanted to exchange
information.

Last year I was asked if I would go on to the board of directors at
the Terrence Higgins Trust. Through the years the trust had helped
me a lot. I hoped to help develop welfare support for women, stuff
like that. I was pretty unimpressed with their literature, but I don't
have the energy to throw myself into it as I used to. I am slightly
tokenistic as the sole woman on the board. There's a lot that's wrong
with the trust, but I'm happy to be involved in all the good stuff it
does. When I first joined the board I said I'd like to meet all the staff,
so I spent a day going round asking everyone what they did. It was
pointed out to me that this was the first time a director had ever done
that. I can see myself bringing in a few changes like that.

There are a lot of ghouls around. There was one person I knew
who had an absolute obsession with positive people. He was constantly
turning up socially and then he tried to seduce every positive woman
he could. There's another side to AIDS that attracts people with
problems and I haven't quite figured out why. I have acupuncture at
the London Lighthouse and I do see a lot of it there. We call them
the spot the victim brigade. They're always being given tours.

I've had the virus for ten years now and I'm doing pretty well. I think alternative medicine such as acupuncture has actively helped me. I think there are some doctors, too many doctors are still thinking of AIDS purely in terms of traditional treatments. For example, I'd been to Turkey on holiday and I came back feeling very depleted, very tired. I started losing weight. I went to see my doctor, had a few tests and my T-cell count had dropped to 150. Officially this meant I had AIDS – the new definition is anyone with a T-cell count below two hundred. So my doctor said, 'Well, we have to start talking about this,' and I knew she was going to start talking about prophylaxis and stuff like that.

Instead I just went to an acupuncturist, went on some herbal medicine and when I went back to my doctor four weeks later it had jumped up to 260. My doctor said, 'Ooh, it must have been the holiday.' I said, 'No, if you remember it was after the holiday that my count dropped.' I told her about the acupuncture and treatment and she said, 'Well we mustn't get too excited.' I thought, well, I went from an AIDS diagnosis to out of an AIDS diagnosis within four weeks. If she had put me on AZT and I had jumped up by 110 it would be hailed as a miracle. They think it's good if AZT produces an increase of twenty.

We do not really speak honestly in this country about treatments, or sex. It makes me very suspicious of all these studies and surveys. Many people I know dabble in recreational drugs. They have a lifestyle about which they're not telling their doctors. I've got a girl-friend who just went on a three-month binge on ecstasy, and at the end of it her T-cell count had gone up by five hundred. Now of course I'm not saying that ecstasy is good for T-cells, but I said to her, 'Did you tell the doctor?' 'Of course not.' They're doing all this intricate research, with these endless tests, and people aren't telling them the truth.

It was the same when they were doing research into male/female and female/male transmission – so many people lied, all these men saying they got it from one-night stands. I went for a time to the heterosexual support group at the Lighthouse. There was a guy there who had gone on television and said he'd got it from a one-night stand in Torremolinos. In the support group, though, he was very honest. He'd really been having an affair with a drug-using woman, he probably tried it a couple of times, he'd had anal sex, he'd had herpes.

I thought, why the hell did he go on television and do the little innocent victim number? Probably because he was paid.

Tim Clark returned from France to work on the Fifth International Conference for people with HIV and AIDS. One of his several duties on the men's magazine Arena *is writing the AIDS Update column. In June 1994 he was in good shape, and for six months he had been in a relationship with a man who was antibody negative.*

Caroline remarried in New Zealand on Christmas Day 1993. She was hoping they could find a long-term project they could work on together. In June 1994 she was feeling 'better than ever'.

I only told Lee I was positive a few months ago. She reacted very well. For years she knew all about HIV and AIDS. I've always tried to teach her about fairness, so she was already a real campaigner on any civil rights issue. Her favourite event of the year is Gay Pride. She said, 'Why don't the press put anything in? There were fifty thousand people there.' Her father, who lives in Los Angeles, pays her school fees. It's a progressive school and I felt very confident in being able to tell her teacher and headmaster and I told them before I told Lee so that she'd have the support there, and there was a counsellor at the school who was primed up for it as well. She was a bit overprotective for the first week or so. 'Are you all right Mum?' every five minutes. I told her she could help in little ways, like tidying up the house. She went off that idea very quickly.

Sheila died recently and Lee insisted on coming to her funeral. I tried to warn her what to expect. She was OK when Sheila's coffin was out, because that was the place to cry. But as soon as she saw another friend of mine who was really unwell, she'd gone blind and no weight, that really upset Lee. It was a lot closer to home. Since then she's gone back to this 'Are you all right, Mum?' thing every five minutes.

But some things don't really change. A few weeks ago Lee came home in floods of tears, saying one of the kids had told other kids and she was being treated badly. The teachers sorted it out, but now I'm uneasy about going to the school, because I constantly feel I'm being gawped at, mostly by the kids. You know, this strange alien with this dreaded disease.

CHAPTER 5: Shooting Gallery

At the City Hospital, Edinburgh, in January 1985, nothing much happened that hadn't happened before. The usual collection of folk gathered in outpatients with minor ailments, mostly the poor and elderly. Stuck away in the southern reaches of the city, in Morningside, the hospital was not one of the most prosperous and attracted little attention to itself. Doctors who worked with infectious diseases were regarded by most of their colleagues in other specialties as either reckless or insane: for there was a history here, a terrible memory that had haunted the Edinburgh hospitals for years.

In the early 1970s a sudden and fatal outbreak of hepatitis hit not only patients but hospital staff too; at the Royal Infirmary it struck a registrar, a nurse and one of the women who worked in the labs – a receptionist who had no direct contact with patients. Some of the spread was attributed to contaminated dialysis machines, but some remained inexplicable. Months after the lab worker got jaundice and died they worked it out: part of her job was to open the blood bags and take the tubes out; the bags had staples, and careless contamination was easy.

Hospital staff couldn't forget how their colleagues died. A regional hepatitis unit was established at the City and staff adopted stringent new care procedures. The outbreak has not been repeated; the vast majority of the cases they saw in the late 1970s and early 1980s were confined to injecting drug users.

When Dr Donald Acheson delivered his confidential report to Norman Fowler in June 1985, he noted that there was only one reported British case of HTLV-III transmission amongst intravenous drug users (IDUs). The risk was there, he noted, and it was a serious one, not least because it presented an obvious link, through the sexual contacts of drug users, into the wider heterosexual community. But there might still be time to limit it.

Dr Ray Brettle, a consultant at the City Hospital 400 miles away, could have dashed those hopes four months earlier. Brettle, an Englishman who had trained in Scotland, had spent much of 1982 and 1983 in North Carolina, where he had seen his first few cases of

AIDS. Before he returned to Edinburgh he received a request to bring back everything he could on the syndrome; no one had really seen any cases, but it seemed like an unnerving condition. Brettle came back with some slides and spent a fair amount of time giving little presentations to those who were interested. 'The blood transfusion people were very worried,' he remembers, 'but most other people thought I was mad and a lot of my talks met with indifference.' Time passed; the city had a small share of gay cases, diagnosed at STD clinics or at other hospitals near the centre of town. The Scottish AIDS Monitor, formed in 1983, did much to issue preventive advice and helpline support. But there was no such service for drug users, not least because it appeared there was no need. The drug users who frequented the City presented with the same ailments they always had, although it did seem there were more of them: more hepatitis B, more heart disease, more abscesses on the arms, all the obvious results of injecting drug use. Staff saw more cases of heroin overdoses, too. But still: it did seem that HTLV-III had passed them by.

Then in February 1985 Brettle received a phone call from a haematologist to say that the Lothian region was setting up an informal AIDS group; would he come along? Some testing kits had been obtained from the United States and been used on stored sera from local haemophiliacs. This was really just a precautionary thing, as Scotland had been self-sufficient in blood products for several years. But the results were startling: several samples were positive. Amid much confusion at the blood transfusion service, clinicians ran the tests again, this time with control groups of gay men and injecting drug users. Then it hit: the drug users came up positive. They thought, 'Ah, silly, we've mixed them up ...' So they ran it again and all the drug users came up positive again.

The first rumblings that Edinburgh might have an epidemic on its hands appeared in a letter to the *Lancet* in mid-August. George Bath of the Lothian Health Board and four doctors from the bacteriology department of the University of Edinburgh Medical School screened 106 serum samples collected from drug users in 1985. This consisted of 62 men (average age 27) and 44 women (average age 24). Sera from 24 men and 16 women were confirmed as HTLV-III positive, a total of 38 per cent. Rough comparisons were made with other parts of Europe: in West Germany the rate was considered to be 6 per cent; in Italy between 20.3 and 22.5 per cent; in Switzerland between 32 and 42 per cent; and in Austria and Spain between 44 and 48 per cent. In

93

England the rate varied from 1.5 per cent measured from frozen samples in 1983 to 6.4 per cent in 1985. The letter noted that the 38 per cent in Edinburgh included several female prostitutes.

One week later, the situation looked even worse. The trade magazine *General Practitioner* announced that Dr Roy Robertson, a young Edinburgh GP, had tested the intravenous drug users whom he treated regularly at his West Granton Medical Group. He found that over half were HTLV-III positive. In Dundee, 20 of 35 IDUs were found to have antibodies. According to virologist Dr George Urquhart, four had already developed swollen glands.

In February 1986 Doctors Robertson and Brettle and five others published a report of their ongoing researches in the *British Medical Journal*. They had tested stored blood samples from 164 drug users and found 83 (51 per cent) to be positive. The doctors noted, however, that because of the age of some of these samples, which were originally taken to monitor hepatitis, the true rate of infection might actually be as high as 85 per cent. The figure most commonly quoted at the time was that the city had about two thousand positive drug users, the majority sexually active.

In their report, the doctors noted that it was likely that the epidemic had struck Edinburgh because of three concurrent events: the increasing popularity of heroin; the methods by which heroin was injected; and the frequency of sharing equipment owing to the difficulty in obtaining sterile needles and syringes.

'It was a peculiarly local thing,' Ray Brettle says. 'That was the tragedy.' After the general psychedelics drug culture of the 1970s, somebody began to target young people with heroin. There was a lot of cheap heroin that flooded on to the UK market and the stuff was always landing on the east coast, and Edinburgh was an ideal distribution point: great links with London and other major cities. Suddenly also there was a great shortage of cannabis. At parties there would often be one guy who knew what he was doing, and he would draw it up for others.

Some drug users can remember a new American face appearing on the scene in the early 1980s, a man with a lot of supply and a skilled technique. No such man has ever been isolated. But there are some other theories: Ray Brettle thinks the virus entered Edinburgh via Spain. Certainly it was true that a lot of the more adventurous users would go over to Italy and Spain to bring back heroin; cutting it locally would more than pay for their trip. When one of these people came back from Spain in December 1982, he checked in at the City Hospital with jaundice. By January 1983 he had hepatitis B and, because his blood had been frozen, retrospective tests could be done which showed that he was also infected with HTLV-III. He stayed in Edinburgh for about the first six months of 1983, telling Brettle subsequently that during this period he shot up with lots of people in various areas. 'He told me names of people who were now patients. This guy was not the only one, but I'm sure he was one of the key people. He came back to Edinburgh a few years later, and he was referred to me, and he's now dead.'

The history of drug use is littered with stories of one or two people dropping into a group. In Washington DC in the 1940s an outbreak of malaria was later traced to shared drug equipment. Widespread HTLV-III infection in Spain and Italy started among drug users in 1981 and then spread rapidly, some two years before the Edinburgh explosion. One theory blames the United States Air Force: in Aviano, Pordenone, near the Italian Dolomites, there is a US military base, and the story runs that prostitutes who came on to the base would shoot up with drug-using soldiers who were already antibody positive. Around the base there was a lot of seropositivity and in other areas there was none, or the incidence was very low. The story also runs backwards: that prostitutes infected the airmen. Either way, unsurprisingly, there is no record of how many top guns, if any, were positive.

When the virus reached Edinburgh, the method used to inject drugs was one particularly likely to pass it on. The drug was washed out of the syringe into the bloodstream by repeatedly drawing back the plunger and injecting the user's own blood: a system known as 'booting' or 'flushing', and almost certain to transmit a virus if that needle was shared. Further, it was common usage to rinse equipment between shots in a communal bowl of water, water that would swiftly turn crimson with blood.

Heroin use probably peaked in 1983. And it was in 1983 that Brettle observed a strange practice at his hospital:

Whenever we took blood from someone on the wards we had special boxes to throw the needles away, because we'd learnt our lesson about hep B. But then we had to design a system whereby you could lock it, because patients' friends would come in and all the needles and syringes would disappear. At that time I couldn't understand why they were nicking these things, because we'd never

95

seen it before. We should have responded by saying, 'Here, have lots of needles and syringes for free – clean ones,' but we went along with it all and locked them up. And of course all the needles they took were infected, because the people we saw were all in with hep B, and goodness knows what else. So these needles would then be used for their friends to shoot up again – not a bad way to guarantee the spread of disease.

The Lothian and Borders Police had been tough on drugs for years. By the early 1980s not only would drugs be seized and users and suppliers arrested, but any drug paraphernalia would also be confiscated. Occasionally the possession of needles or syringes, even without drug possession, would be sufficient for charges to be brought. Chemists and other surgical suppliers would also be prosecuted if it was believed that equipment sold would be used by drug addicts. 'It was a ludicrous idea,' Brettle observes. 'It was like saying you were going to rid people of alcoholism by taking away their drinking glasses.' What happened instead, of course, was that drug users shared their gear around. One story has it that on one estate in Muirhouse one needle was passed around for three months.

At the end of 1983 there were 11 officers in the drug squad; at the beginning of 1984 this had increased to 21. Dealers got wise. It was common practice for users picked up for possession on the street to be cajoled by police into naming their dealers in return for more lenient prosecution. Dealers would soon learn to insist that, once an addict had come to them for heroin, that person would not leave the dealer's flat until they had shot up; you couldn't be done if you weren't carrying anything, no matter how stoned. And thus were shooting galleries created: addict after addict using one dealer's kitchen, one dealer's works.

In March 1987, some months after the scale of the epidemic had been acknowledged, the House of Commons Social Services Committee heard evidence from Mr W. G. M. Sutherland, Chief Constable of the Lothian and Borders Police, and from Detective Chief Inspector Douglas Kerr, head of the Lothian Drugs Branch. The policemen were proud of their efforts in the battle against drug abuse. 'We have been hard,' said Mr Sutherland. 'We have put a lot of effort into this problem, and it is fair to say we will continue to do that.' But he did not believe that his force had been tougher on drug users than other forces and he had worked in five of them. Neither man would take responsibility for what had happened with the spread of infection; they were just following the law, the guidance from the Lord Advocate.

When asked whether his force's policy had been modified as a result of the epidemic, Mr Sutherland said that in many cases clean needles would not be confiscated if there was no trace of heroin, 'but there will be times when we will take possession of the needles, and I think that must be understood by all'. He acknowledged that 'the AIDS problem is a much more serious one than the drug abuse problem' and yet if they could stop drug use they would be making a great contribution to solving the AIDS problem. 'Certainly in the Edinburgh situation that would have been the case – if we had clamped down on it earlier, we might not be in the situation we are in today.'

At the end of September 1986 a groundbreaking official report was published by the Scottish Committee on HIV (AIDS) Infection and Drug Misuse. This document, referred to as the McClelland Report after its chairman, the head of the Scottish Blood Transfusion Service, recommended that it might be necessary to issue syringes and needles on a one-for-one exchange basis to drug users in order to control the epidemic. There were other suggestions too – safer sex advice, family planning, an increase in funding to monitor spread and care for those infected – but it was the needle exchange that got them flustered in Westminster. The Scottish Secretary, Malcolm Rifkind, opposed the recommendation on the grounds that anything that encouraged drug abuse would be likely to accelerate rather than reduce the spread of AIDS. John MacKay, Scottish Office minister with responsibility for health, thought the idea outrageous: 'AIDS is a totally self-inflicted illness,' he told the Commons, 'and it is so much more morally reprehensible when it is inflicted on children.' SDP health spokesman Charles Kennedy noted that Mr MacKay's comments showed 'a callous disregard for human misery and political ineptitude for a major issue of public concern'. This, he said, was 'a rare combination'. But there was no clear party divide: two months before the McClelland Report a motion appeared on a Commons order paper also suggesting the adoption of needle exchange, and signed by a former Conservative health minister, Sir Gerard Vaughan, and the long-serving backbencher Sir Bernard Braine.

Roy Robertson and Ray Brettle supported it, of course; in fact they'd been doing it themselves on the side for a while. A letter signed by Robertson in the *Lancet* observed that in London and Glasgow the incidence of HIV infection among drug users was relatively small (less than 5 per cent), and that the problems of needle sharing in Edinburgh were so particular and so acute that users would ask regularly, 'If the virus is really being spread by needle and syringe sharing, why don't doctors make them available to us?' or more damningly they would say, 'If doctors really wanted to help us, they would give us clean needles and syringes.' The *Lancet* also ran a letter from Amsterdam, singing the praises of its own needle exchange programme that had been running smoothly since 1984.

A sub-committee of the government's Expert Advisory Group on AIDS also met to consider the problem. These meetings were attended not only by the usual doctors and DHSS people, but also by representatives of the Terrence Higgins Trust, the Standing Conference on Drug Abuse (SCODA) and the Institute for the Study of Drug Dependence (ISDD), organizations which had already collaborated to produce some plain-speaking advice leaflets for users. The consensus favoured needle exchanges, but noted that reaching those users who needed them most was fraught with difficulty. There were other recommendations too, principally that the DHSS should conduct a drug-related public health campaign. Here was another political bombshell: the main tack of previous campaigns was 'Stop. Drugs Kill You' (or, once the ad people had got hold of it, 'Heroin Screws You Up'); this didn't allow room for behavioural modification. The EAGA minutes note one spark: 'The use of a pop star in a campaign was discussed.' When the last general 'just say no' drugs campaign was being developed, in October 1985, the idea of using a pop star had been tested and had not been found effective. 'Drug abusers tended not to have idols among pop stars, and there was also the difficulty of finding an individual star who would have an appeal across the age range. Another angle was to place an article on AIDS and drug abuse in a magazine such as the *New Musical Express* ...' As things turned out, there was to be no specific AIDS and drugs campaign for two years, until September 1987.

In January 1987 the government announced that pilot needle exchange schemes were to be established in nine UK cities, including Edinburgh, Glasgow and Dundee. These would be based on a strict one-for-one swap and be accompanied by some form of education on 'safe drug misuse'; their success would be closely monitored before they were extended to other areas.

When the schemes were launched it was acknowledged that they might form only part of the solution. The exchanges would be established in the area where sharing and infection were considered highest (in Edinburgh this meant one morning a week in Leith), but it was unlikely that addicts from a different area would travel far just to obtain clean works. Besides, in Spain and Italy needles and syringes could be bought off supermarket shelves, yet HIV infection amongst drug users was the highest in Europe. (Admittedly this was mostly down to the fact that in these countries the incidence of injecting drug use was also the highest in Europe.)

Needle exchanges were not new to Britain. Though never sanctioned officially, informal schemes had existed for years in Liverpool, where the pattern of injecting drug use was also high, and at a centre behind Tottenham Court Road in London, which attracted mainly long-term users. But it was estimated that only about one in five addicts would use a service. Hugh Dufficy, a worker at SCODA and formerly at the Blenheim Project in West London, believes that one of the reasons the government sanctioned the official schemes was because ministers and health officials had become alarmed at the spread and influence of voluntary organizations beyond their control:

It had been clear to anyone working on the ground that the official policy of stipulating total abstention wasn't working. Politically it was attractive, especially to ministers who had personal experience of drug use in their family, and it showed voters that they were trying to deal with the problem. But the way you knew it wasn't working was because every year the figures would go up and up.

Ray Brettle, attending the Paris International Conference on AIDS in the summer of 1986, had listened to several presentations suggesting that the more heroin a user injected, the more their T4 cell count reduced. A logical deduction, perhaps, but one that the supply of clean needles might do little to improve. Oral methadone, a heroin substitute, had been prescribed for many years before AIDS appeared, most often as part of a short-term detoxification programme, but it now took on a greater significance. Brettle started to prescribe it at the City Hospital and the word soon spread. It caused chaos, because suddenly his Edinburgh clinic was swamped as never before.

Prior to this, he had seen a lot of users coming in for their tests, many of them dealers. After receiving positive results many of them left with doom in their hearts: 'Well I'm positive, so I may as well carry on using.' They made appointments to come in again a few weeks later, but most never showed. All this changed when word got round that Brettle had become Mr Methadone and the line stretched right down the hall. Having had the tacit support of his colleagues before, Brettle now became the object of scorn. 'You could understand it,' he says. 'You'd be dealing with Mrs Smith from Morningside, and some guy would stumble down the corridor bawling, "I want my scrip [prescription]! Where's this bloody doctor?"'

Throughout 1987, about a hundred addicts would come to the City regularly. Not all had cut out heroin use; some used their methadone to supplement their habit; others sold it. But once they came, health and sex education could be administered with their chit. The staff found that you could only teach them about HIV once you'd first heard about their other problems, principally financial.

Some users were still unduly careless: needles would be left in corridors and on seats. To limit confrontation, users were seen in segregated specialist clinics on certain days. Not that this helped official relations very much. 'The health board hated what I was doing,' Brettle says. 'They may say they were happy now, but at the time they did everything they could to stop me prescribing.' He went through a year's supply of pink prescribing pads in three months and was hauled up before Scotland's Chief Medical Officer. The complaint was partly moral, partly on grounds of cost, which came back directly to the hospital, about £3 per day per prescription:

They didn't want all this cost and all these hospital resources going to what they saw as a bunch of wasters. My impression was there was an incredible moral outrage, though they knew they couldn't say that. Drug users had traditionally been the responsibility of psychiatrists, and there was some embarrassment that if you were positive in Edinburgh you got methadone from me, and if you were negative you got damn all ... a crazy situation where it seemed as though you were almost encouraging people to catch the virus so that they could get access to the drug.

In the long term, the ideal situation would be a combination of needle exchange, methadone maintenance, education and counselling, as each situation demanded. This would be expensive and resources were initially quite insufficient. The House of Commons Social Services Committee heard evidence from Roy Robertson that demand was most often met by a telephone helpline. 'For me as a GP, I think that it is quite a sad betrayal of people's expectations of their medical services that they have to go into a telephone booth and phone up a tape which might give them some advice about drug abuse or about AIDS. We should be getting face to face contact.'

What was initially a theoretical dilemma soon became a practical one. No matter how much methadone he prescribed, inevitably Brettle's wards began to fill up. At first the Lothian Health Board thought it best to spread to several hospitals the load of those people who were HIV positive and had fallen unwell, but as in London centres of excellence developed to take the lion's share. The City saw few cases of gay men – unless they also happened to be drug users – but its beds soon contained many of the drug-injecting men and women it had first treated as outpatients. Brettle liked to tell a joke about the other places: 'When they came to us the first thing some of them said was, "Oh, it's nice to see a face. All the other people wore masks." You would ask patients how they were treated, and they said, "Pretty badly, and the worst thing was the food. We only got Ryvita." "Why Ryvita?" "It was the only thing they could slide under the door."'

Brettle soon spotted a gentle irony: 'A lot of my patients hated having needles put into them. You ask them how they get it, and they say, "Someone else always had to shoot it in."'

Some money to deal with this increasing caseload came after a while, but Brettle's initial applications for research into the natural history of the epidemic and its consequences for the heterosexual population were turned down (at the beginning of 1987 there were 22 babies who had been born in Edinburgh to mothers with AIDS antibodies in their blood. At least ten partners of infected drug injectors were also positive). 'I was jumping up and down and I still couldn't get any funding,' he says. 'The Scottish Home and Health Department ran me and a colleague around for a year. Then they said: "You should have gone to the Medical Research Council because we don't have the money."' Brettle's earliest funding came from the United States, from the American Foundation for Aids Research (AmFAR) which had witnessed the devastation AIDS had had on addicts in New York; Britain's Medical Research Council produced some money a few months later.

In the mid-1980s it was feared that Glasgow would experience drug-related infection rates similar to Edinburgh's, but it was an overestimate. Drug users injected less, there was a greater supply of needles, users may have been more territorial and less mobile and the virus may simply have been introduced later than in Edinburgh or Dundee (where, by 1987, up to a third of drug injectors were believed to be HIV positive), thus ensuring greater effectiveness of needle exchange and health education programmes.

A needle exchange was established at the gatehouse of Ruchill Hospital, where it met with fierce local opposition; local women came along with their children in buggies and stood outside the door jeering people who came to use the service. Users would be ferried by bus from Easterhouse several miles away, to be told that they were giving the area a bad name and that their used needles were a threat to the young. The exchange soon shifted to Easterhouse itself.

Pharmacists who distributed equipment were dealt with less harshly than in Edinburgh; one, near Possil Park, though also the target of local opposition, supplied up to 30 users a day.

Between 1985 and 1987 the situation in Glasgow looked set to mirror that of the east coast, albeit at a slower pace. When testing began in 1985 the incidence of infection among drug injectors was about one per cent; two years later it was almost 5 per cent. Andrew Moss, a statistician from San Francisco, arrived in Glasgow to help assess the future scenario; he forecasted more doom: hundreds of infections and AIDS cases were expected in the next three years. 'It was projecting what now seemed to be ludicrously exaggerated numbers of people,' says Dr Laurence Gruer, a consultant in public health medicine who works at the HIV centre at Ruchill. A study of 1,786 drug injectors from the Greater Glasgow area examined between 1986 and 1989 showed that only 66 had been infected, or 3.7 per cent. At the International AIDS Conference in Berlin in 1993, the Glasgow experience was singled out as one of the relatively few examples worldwide where an epidemic of HIV among drug injectors may have been averted. (The incidence among gay men was also low.)

'It must have been very, very touch and go,' Gruer says, 'because if you look at the levels of hepatitis B and hepatitis C among drug injectors in Glasgow, they were tremendously high. About 70 odd per cent of drug injectors have got evidence that they'd been exposed to hepatitis B and more than 80 per cent are infected with hepatitis C.

So it's certainly not the case that blood-borne viruses had not been spreading.'

Gruer believes there is another important element which may explain why HIV has not spread as rapidly as these other viruses:

HIV just doesn't seem to be quite so infectious, quite so easily transmitted from one person to another. In particular it looks as though HIV, once it gets into your system, multiplies rapidly, so for the first few weeks or months you're very, very infectious, and then it goes into a more latent phase and you become less infectious. If someone is only sharing relatively infrequently, they may not actually transmit the virus to anyone or to just a very few people.

Back in Edinburgh, the wards were filling up. But there was a little hope, a sign of slender progress, because the overall trend of infection was down. After the devastating impact of the first test results the rates slowed down markedly. At the end of June 1987 there were 1,239 reported cases of HIV infection; by the end of September 1987 this had increased to 1,381; and by the end of June 1988 the figure was 1,504. As a comparative marker, the figures for the same periods for the North West Thames region increased from 1,800, to 2,151, to 2,410. The figures for the North East Thames region more than doubled within that year, from 525 to 1271.

Of the Edinburgh figures, about a half were due to injecting drug use, a quarter to homosexual sex, and the final quarter to contaminated blood products and other routes of transmission. By far the greatest of these other routes was heterosexual sex. Largely because of the drug-injecting epidemic, Edinburgh had more cases of HIV contracted through heterosexual sex than anywhere outside London.

This may be explained partly by patterns of prostitution. The logic is straightforward enough, though there is little hard evidence: to finance a drug addiction some women (and in fewer cases men) turned to prostitution; if infected and indulging in unprotected sex, it was thought that they could pass the virus to a client. It worked the other way, of course: an HIV positive male, infected perhaps through drug use, could transmit to a prostitute. Perhaps prostitutes shared needles. Infected prostitutes could pass on the virus to their babies. A reporter writing for the *Sunday Times Magazine* in 1986 came across a woman called Karen, a 26-year-old prostitute with an £80 a day habit. 'AIDS doesn't bother me,' she said. 'I went to the City Hospital two months ago for the test ... the doctor told me I was positive ... I asked him when I was going to die, and he said maybe two years, maybe five, maybe it would never develop. I was really upset then, I went right out and had a hit ... I'd rather die of heroin than of AIDS.' Karen conducted much of her business, at £20 a time, behind a wall behind a carpet shop in Coburg Street. Was she worried about passing on HIV to her clients? 'No, why should I? They're all just dirty old men. We call them the creep show.'

An infected drug user could pass on the virus 'vertically' to her children as well as 'horizontally' to her (or his) partner. Ray Brettle and Roy Robertson had identified at least ten partners with antibodies by the end of 1986, and the trend was clearly upwards.

For some people, and many legislators, this was the nightmare scenario, far more threatening than the infection of drug users by themselves: the route to the general population. Others denied it. Ray Brettle remembers people voicing the opinion that if you were stupid enough to sleep with a drug user then it was your own bloody fault if you became infected. 'Any excuse would be constructed to show it wasn't a real threat to them. If a partner of a drug user gets it it's not really important, but if Mrs Smith down the road gets it by sleeping with someone upstanding she met at a party then it's something else.'

It wouldn't be long before health officials, the moral right and some media commentators would accuse Brettle and Robertson and many other doctors in the AIDS field of empire building: as soon as they dealt with one problem, they said, they would create another to keep them in business. 'They say, "Oh, you just want to get more money,"' Brettle says:

In fact by talking about the potential of the spread and encouraging a public education campaign, I'm trying to limit my aggrandisement; if I said nothing, or if I said, 'Don't spend money on prevention, it's all rubbish,' then I'd be laughing: I could just sit back and watch them roll in.

People keep on telling me it's not happening, but often a woman will come in who had a boyfriend three years ago, someone I know, someone I've treated, a drug user. It's horrible when someone says to you, like a girl said to me, 'I'm not going to make thirty, am I?' She was twenty-five, and you have to say, 'No, you're not.'

Brettle worries about his own children:

Obviously for most people it's never a problem: they have sex, and they're never going to catch anything. The problem is, I keep seeing these patients ... What makes me despair is that 30 per cent of my patients, about a hundred people, went into a relationship knowing that their partner was positive. If people will do that, if people will have sex without a condom with somebody who's openly positive, then how the hell are we going to persuade two people who are probably *negative* to use a condom 'just in case'?

CHAPTER 6:
A Plague on Both Your Houses

> Three people are arguing amongst themselves as to which is the oldest pro-
> fession in the world. The first, a landscape gardener, says 'Well, the first
> people in the world were Adam and Eve, and they worked in the garden of
> Eden, and that's what I do, so I must represent the oldest profession in the
> world.' The person next to them, who organized conferences on HIV and
> AIDS, said, 'No, no, before God made Adam and Eve he brought order
> out of chaos, and that's what I do, so I must represent the oldest profession
> in the world.' 'Wait a minute,' said the politician who was standing next to
> them, 'Who created the chaos!?'
> Joke retold by Chris Smith, Britain's only openly gay MP

'I would be grateful for your early advice on a matter which gravely
concerns me.' So began a letter received by a west London GP from
one of his patients. The letter suggested that the battle against AIDS
was not being won. The writer explained that his wife regularly visited an 80-year-old woman who lived alone in a nearby flat. In the flat
above hers lived two homosexuals; another lived in the basement. The
gay men had been good neighbours and had run lots of errands, but
now, 'in view of the increasing incidence of AIDS', the writer had
great anxiety that his wife might be at risk from visiting the old
woman. The letter concluded with a plea for advice: what precautions
could his wife take to avoid contamination from this dreadful disease?

In February 1986, this letter had found its way to Donald Acheson.
The Chief Medical Officer had seen this sort of correspondence before
and it made him wonder. How would people learn?

The letter was distributed at a meeting of the Expert Advisory
Group on AIDS (EAGA). At the same meeting, the assembled
doctors and Department of Health officials were presented with a
script from the advertising agency TBWA. Perhaps this was the
answer Acheson had been looking for; perhaps this advertisement, the
first stage in an unprecedented public campaign, would make the
general public aware of how one became infected; just as important, it
would explain how one could not. 'Are You At Risk From AIDS?' the
title read.

Clearly, some progress was being made. Dr Acheson felt some relief that at last his message was getting through. This new campaign was still in its infancy, but it was already a great improvement on what had gone before.

Six months earlier, Barney Hayhoe, the health minister, had announced that a paltry £100,000 would be spent on an unspecified health education project. The trade paper *Doctor* announced that 'Brave Barney has declared war on AIDS', and the minister himself promised to 'provide reliable, responsible information for those at greatest risk and for society in general', but in fact his spending limit bought him little more than some small regional press adverts and some more leaflets from the Health Education Council.

Before being shuffled out of the Department of Health in 1985, John Patten had also been considering an AIDS advertising campaign. The under-secretary had spent several days in the summer of 1985 discussing the epidemic with doctors and community leaders in New York and Washington and was convinced that something should be done in Britain. Initially, Norman Fowler, the Secretary of State, was not hugely supportive, unsure of the scale of the problem, busy with other things. (As one official at the Department of Health saw it, Fowler liked to concentrate on one issue for months at a time and throughout most of 1985 he had little time for AIDS.)

When Fowler did first express interest in mounting a preventative campaign he found no interest among his cabinet colleagues. Indeed some were directly hostile. Margaret Thatcher believed it to be a small problem and one confined to homosexuals; best to let them sort it out themselves, she thought. Kenneth Clarke, once a health minister himself, referred to John Patten as 'the Minister for Gays'.

Patten was the first well-known political figure to shake hands with a person with AIDS and the television news made much of the event. Patten hoped it would destigmatize the condition and he was relaxed chatting to 'Bill' off camera. Bill spoke openly about his lifestyle, telling the minister that he had probably had about 200 partners in his lifetime. Patten nodded. After the encounter, on the way back to the department, he turned to an official and said, 'Did he really say two hundred? You wonder where he got the energy.'

In November 1985 there was a sea change. Norman Fowler announced that it was time to take things a little further. British AIDS cases only numbered about 250, but the rate of increase had begun to suggest that we might be witnessing a rate of growth similar to the United States, albeit with a delay of two or three years. In addition, there were signs that the crossover into the heterosexual community was now more than a distant threat. So £2.5m was to be allocated for a national information campaign. 'Prevention is the only vaccine we've got,' he said. His vaccine trials were to be in the form of two national press adverts.

These were not snappy and creative examples of the adman's art. They consisted of practically nothing but closely worded text, resembling nothing so much as a prospectus for a share offer. What is more, every word had been pored over for hours.

The early drafts were very different from the final copy that appeared in the papers. The wording went back and forth between the Department of Health and Social Security, the Expert Advisory Group and Downing Street, an endless stream of scribbled amendments, deletions and questions. At one point Acheson and his team sent for some inspiration from the United States, in the shape of the gay newspaper *New York Native*. Because copies were often seized by HM Customs, they were shipped over by diplomatic bag.

Margaret Thatcher had serious misgivings about the campaign, although she had finally been persuaded by Acheson and then Fowler that something was necessary. 'The Department tried to keep her out of it as much as possible,' one civil servant remembers. 'At one point, after she had seen a draft, we got a message from Nigel Wicks [her Principal Private Secretary], which said, "She wants to know if they have to go in the newspapers?" We asked him where else they were supposed to go. He said, "She was wondering about lavatory walls – like that old information they used to have about VD."'

Professor Anthony Coxon, director of the Social Research Unit at University College, Cardiff, sat on a newly convened DHSS Advisory Group on Health Education and AIDS. Recalling the newspaper ads, Coxon noted that 'a high proportion of our unanimous suggestions were ignored or over-ruled'.

'The whole thing was deeply frustrating', Fowler says. 'The advertisements had to go through H Committee [the weekly home affairs cabinet meeting], which allowed everyone to give of their views of the subject, without any great knowledge of what we were trying to do. And when [the advertisements] finally appeared they were not effective; most people didn't take any notice.'

Even when all copy was finally approved, there were further delays.

'I can remember one meeting in the Health Department,' says Dr
Charles Farthing of St Stephen's Hospital:

> The advertisements were all completed, and the minister came to
> the meeting for the first time to congratulate the committee and
> said it would be running in two or three months' time. I responded
> with horror. 'What do you mean, Minister, two or three months'
> time? Do you realize how many people will get infected and die in
> the interim?' The minister was horrified. Everybody was hushed,
> and it ran in two or three months' time.

What readers finally saw when they opened their papers on Sunday
16 March and the following day differed substantially from the fifth
draft submitted by TBWA only a month before. In fact there was
hardly a line that remained intact. The opening statement, 'AIDS has
attracted an enormous amount of attention from the media', was
changed to 'AIDS is a serious disease'. Then came a warning, signed
by the four Chief Medical Officers, that what followed 'may shock
but should not offend you as we are talking about an urgent medical
problem'.

The text then split into sections, each headed with a question. In
the section headed 'What Is AIDS?', the printed advertisement omitted an observation in the draft regarding the likelihood of a person
infected with the virus developing AIDS: 'On present information,
three-quarters remain fit and seem to suffer no ill effects'. But the
approved advertisement did contain a box with a strange diagram,
with various parts labelled A, B and C. A caption underneath, which
bore no connection with anything that followed, contained bastardized
scientific text: 'A: AIDS nucleoid containing the biological message to
cause damage. B: Lipid membrane (very fragile). Packages virus and
allows movement between cells. C: T-helper cell/white cell.'

The next column contained a section headed 'How Is AIDS
Spread?' The newspaper version reported two ways: sexual intercourse
with an infected person and blood-to-blood transmission most common through needle sharing. What it omitted was the intricate detail
present in the draft: 'During sexual intercourse, minute breaks may
occur in the walls of the vagina. It is through these that the infected
semen passes. As the rectum is far more delicate than the vagina, it
is more easily damaged. This means anal intercourse is the easiest way
of becoming infected.' This information was excised on the firm

instruction of Margaret Thatcher, and in a simplified version the term 'anal intercourse' became first 'back passage intercourse' and finally the approved 'rectal sex'. (Tony Whitehead of the Terrence Higgins Trust informed *Gay Times* readers that he had another workable phrase: 'Why not use words like bum fucking? There would be no ambiguity about that.')

The advertisement made one mention of the word 'sheath' reducing the risk of AIDS, but it had a foggy notion of the concept of safe sex: 'Any sex between two people who are uninfected is completely safe'. (How did you know? What about the incubation period?)

Concluding, the ad asked 'What of the Future?' The printed version observed that 'Doctors and scientists around the world are searching urgently for a vaccine or cure', which replaced: 'Governments around the world are spending vast amounts of money in their search for a vaccine or cure.'

Perhaps more lives would have been lost if it had not run at all. But the adverts were not attractive, had no visual impact and demanded a lot from readers casually flicking their way to the sports news. The Social Services Committee, which reported in May 1987, judged the advertisements 'fine examples of how important and useful information can fail to be conveyed through poor presentation'.

A few months after the campaign appeared, the *BMJ* printed the conclusions of a survey conducted at Southampton General Hospital. It was a small, random sample of public opinion (about 300 people), but it produced startling results. Respondents were questioned before and after the press campaign. Only 31 per cent had seen the adverts, but it appeared that the campaign caused confusion rather than dispelling it. Before it, 5 per cent thought there was a vaccine against AIDS; after it, 10 per cent did. Before, 10 per cent believed the infection was spread by sharing washing, eating and drinking utensils; after, this had risen to 14 per cent. Before the campaign, 48 per cent didn't know what the initials AIDS stood for; after it, 59 per cent didn't.

To counteract such adverse publicity, the Department of Health issued the results of its own, larger survey of about 1,850 people, conducted by the British Market Research Bureau, which suggested that a greater than normal percentage had seen the adverts and noted their contents. These days, however, Norman Fowler acknowledges that the advertisements 'frankly I think had next to no impact whatsoever'.

Following the campaign, the government came under continued

pressure to do more. Predominantly gay groups, particularly the Terrence Higgins Trust and Body Positive, ran powerful lobbying campaigns, increasingly stressing the 'equal opportunities' element of the virus, the message that it was infecting more and more heterosexual people who did not take part in high-risk activity. 'It wasn't a wholly cynical move,' says Tony Whitehead, chair of the THT, 'but it was clear that the button you had to press to get more money was the one labelled "everyone is at risk". That was true, of course, and it was the line that permeated the campaigns.' Having worked for years in a vacuum, the gay organizations were now providing Acheson and the DHSS with much invaluable information. 'We were tolerated because we were needed,' Whitehead says. 'As soon as they found a way of not needing us very much then old homophobic attitudes did re-establish themselves.'

The Expert Advisory Group also continued to press the government to step up the campaigns; doctors began talking of imminent 'burn-out' if the government continued to regard AIDS and its prevention as low priority. Their views were echoed increasingly by the medical journals. A *BMJ* editorial stated that Britain had a chance to act, 'but time is running out. Despite the claims by the DHSS, publicity in Britain so far has been unimaginative and of little impact'.

The College of Health went further, suggesting that £30m should be spent on public health education, and that this would be cheap compared to the NHS bill in five years if nothing was done. The College of Health had operated a telephone helpline in the wake of the newspaper campaign, receiving on average 95 calls per daytime hour in the first five days. The Labour peer Lord Young of Dartington, the college's chairman, said that the advertisements had been most welcome, but if that was the full extent of it, it would be 'too little too late'.

For Acheson and Fowler not all of this pressure was unwelcome. There had never been an 'emergency' health campaign like this. The only comparison Acheson could make was that one of his predecessors, Sir Wilson Jamieson, had talked on the radio during the Second World War about the risks of gonorrhoea and syphilis. Acheson's fear in 1986 was of a moral backlash, and even though the newspaper adverts had largely been 'made safe', he woke up on the Sunday they appeared expecting a barrage of angry phone calls. But the phone didn't ring. 'I spent the quietest weekend for many months ... You will be interested to see the signatures of the four UK Chief Medical

Officers in the top left-hand corner of the advertisement. There is no doubt as to which heads would have rolled had there been public outrage.'

Recriminations about the ineffectiveness of the first campaign continued at meetings of the Expert Advisory Group. Simpler, more explicit language was recommended, with more detailed descriptions of what were considered safe and unsafe sexual practices. One document prepared for a meeting in July recognized that 'whilst these advertisements may have to be Government funded, it may be possible to have them placed by non-Governmental bodies and to avoid any specific Government attribution'.

One dilemma was how to reach gay or bisexual men who were not part of any scene and did not regard themselves as homosexual. Gay-specific campaigns of the sort mounted by the Terrence Higgins Trust would be unlikely to reach them. The DHSS had identified eight separate target groups as being at risk: heterosexuals, undeclared homosexuals or bisexuals, high-risk homosexuals, long-term intravenous drug users, 'experimenters' with homosexuality or intravenous drugs, recipients of blood products, travellers to and from high-risk areas and sexual contacts of these travellers. This list seemed to include everyone apart from sexually inactive children and lesbians, the latter considered to be at very low risk. How could general national advertising hope to reach them all equally, unless by fear?

On 2 July 1986 Sir Donald Acheson wrote privately to members of the Expert Advisory Group. The delay in producing further campaign materials since the first newspaper advertisements was due to 'taking stock' of the market research. There now were some new half-page national press ads ready to roll, rather less cluttered than the previous ones, but still avoiding any contentious language and dealing only with the basics: no need to worry about infection from shaking hands, touching and hugging, or from swimming pools, restaurants, doorknobs or clothing. Ignoring the hundreds of infected haemophiliacs (who would soon launch a politically embarrassing claim for compensation), the adverts said: 'Most people who have the AIDS virus caught it by having sex with an infected person. Almost all the rest have caught it by injecting themselves with drugs using equipment shared with an infected person.' Acheson wrote to his advisers that the wording had been kept within the bounds of the earlier campaign 'so as to allow it to be placed quickly ... I recognise that what is said about sexual practices is not as explicit or detailed as many have advocated and believe is necessary. There will always be limits to what can be said in national advertisements'.

But even this bland language was too much for some. Lord Hailsham, the Lord High Chancellor, wrote to Margaret Thatcher and several cabinet ministers objecting to the use of the words 'having sex'. 'I am convinced there must be some limit to vulgarity!' he wrote. 'Could they not use literate "sexual intercourse". If that is thought to be too narrow, then why not "sexual relations" or "physical practices", but not "sex", or, worse, "having sex".' For Lord Hailsham, 'sex' meant either male or female. 'Nor does "having sex" mean anything at all.'

This letter was copied to Norman Fowler, who needed no reminder that the obstacles he faced were still huge. Even in 1986, AIDS was 'not being taken seriously ... people didn't know the risks, people didn't know what might happen'. He saw himself isolated in cabinet. 'I was accused of getting a bit obsessed with this subject.'

Fowler had been Social Services Secretary for over five years, and says he had known for some time that the campaign he was being urged to mount by external forces was an impossible thing to achieve within the present set up. 'There is a mechanism inside government, there's a Home Affairs Cabinet committee, but if AIDS just happens to be one issue on the agenda, in amongst three or four others, it gets pretty limited thought, and pretty limited discussion.'

Margaret Thatcher was not an ally. The Prime Minister had met Acheson and listened to his warnings, but expressed little interest in leading any sort of campaign herself. Indeed this would have flown in the face of the forceful back-to-the-family campaign at the centre of the Conservatives' moral rearmament. If the traditional family was to be reclaimed as the backbone of British life, it necessarily followed that any 'deviant' behaviour was to be condemned. This applied to anything that was seen to have been invented in the 1960s: promiscuity, homosexuality, drug-taking. For some backbenchers, and others who influenced party policy, AIDS couldn't have come at a better time. Geoffrey Dickens, MP for Littleborough and Saddleworth, suggested in a television interview that homosexuality should be made illegal again. James Anderton, the Chief Constable of Greater Manchester, claimed that God had been speaking through him when he issued his famous comment that homosexuals were 'swirling around in a cesspool of their own making'. Sir Alfred Sherman, who had retained a close relationship with Thatcher ever since they had founded the Centre for Policy Studies in the 1970s, wrote to *The Times* in a language of his own generation: AIDS was a problem of 'undesirable minorities ... mainly sodomites and drug-abusers, together with numbers of women who voluntarily associate with this sexual underworld'.

The Prime Minister was a great personal supporter of what became known as Clause 28, an amendment to the Local Government Bill introduced in 1987, which forbade councils and their schools from promoting the acceptability of homosexuality. Publicly she said next to nothing about AIDS and in her memoirs, *The Downing Street Years*, she made not one mention of the biggest health challenge of her government.

'She could only watch with pursed lips what was going on,' Edwina Currie says. 'And disapprove. She was preoccupied with other issues. She was sorting out Europe, she was moving on to the royal stage, was Margaret; she had more important things to do. And there was an element of not sullying herself. If the thing went wrong she would have sacked Norman Fowler and then dusted her hands off.'

Currie and the health minister Tony Newton joined the DHSS in September 1986, displacing Hayhoe and Ray Whitney. Currie claims that it was this reshuffle which created the environment Norman Fowler needed to make headway.

'My impression is that my predecessors were not only not interested, but actively hostile. In which case you couldn't make any progress at all. You certainly couldn't have a campaign on an issue as sensitive as that without the full support of ministers.' After September 1986, Currie says, 'you're talking about a different world'. With the economy performing well, 'there was a feeling that the nation could cope with moving on to more complex issues and taking on board something difficult. People were beginning to recognize the seriousness of the situation'.

But there remained some vocal opposition within Currie's own party, notably from the Conservative Family Campaign. This group included several influential backbenchers and peers, as well as Michael Alison, Margaret Thatcher's Parliamentary Private Secretary. The Campaign had its own solution to AIDS: the isolation of all those infected and the recriminalization of homosexuality.

In October 1986 many were persuaded by the publication of a report from US Surgeon General Everett Koop. Koop was an ultra-Conservative, just up Reagan's street. His was a doomsday scenario, and he emphasized the importance of widespread public education;

if any doubts remained in the minds of health ministers or the moral majority right in Britain, Koop's report should have hustled them away.

Another dramatic despatch arrived from the British High Commissioner in Zambia. Despite the fact that the local government was denying the existence of the problem, the High Commissioner had obtained evidence that as many as one in five of the urban population was already infected. 'With remarkable clarity of vision he predicted the dire future social and economic consequences which have subsequently come to pass in Zambia and neighbouring African countries,' Donald Acheson says. 'At the time I was asked whether I thought the figures were accurate. I said I thought they were. Then I was asked whether I thought the same thing would happen here. I said I thought it would not, but there was no doubt that heterosexuals were at risk.'

In the same month, Fowler found a new way forward. With the help of Ken Stowe, his permanent secretary, and Robert Armstrong, the Cabinet Secretary, he helped convince Margaret Thatcher that as she wasn't particularly concerned with AIDS, she should appoint a cabinet committee to look after the issue and report back. 'I think she felt probably that we were overreacting, or at least there was a prospect that we could overreact,' Fowler says. 'So she obviously wanted in charge a senior minister who could keep us on track.' Willie Whitelaw, the Deputy Prime Minister and one of Thatcher's most trusted friends, was an inspired choice as committee chairman: he would show level-headed commitment to the problem, while at the same time keeping Thatcher away from the issue. Thatcher was influenced most by Robert Armstrong, who was himself influenced by Donald Acheson. The late journalist Peter Jenkins recalled a lunch with Armstrong in October 1986 at which 'anal sex was mentioned during the avocado, buggery in Her Majesty's prisons as we ate our beef.' Armstrong said he feared 'catastrophe', and admitted that nothing had caused him greater loss of sleep in the whole of his long career as a public servant.

After months of effort, Fowler couldn't believe his good fortune: the Cabinet committee contained almost everyone of significance, excepting the Prime Minister – Home Secretary Douglas Hurd, Education Secretary Kenneth Baker, Defence Secretary George Younger, Welsh Secretary Nick Edwards, Scottish Secretary Malcolm Rifkind and John McGregor, Chief Secretary to the Treasury. Cabinet committees are normally secret things, but Fowler was so gleeful that after its first meeting he announced its formation on the steps of 10 Downing Street, where he also preached about the importance of safer sex. This was his moment, his main chance. He was doing the nation good and he was doing himself no harm either. 'At one stage Margaret Thatcher said to me that I should remember I was "more than the minister for AIDS",' Fowler wrote in his autobiography. "But it seemed to me that here was a life and death battle in which the Government could do something to determine the outcome. I did not want people in five years' time to turn round and say "if only they had done more in 1986".'

Fowler also had a secondary agenda, and with hindsight hints at a personal interest. 'I had been in the DHSS for a long time,' he says. 'The best part of five years. I had done the social security review, we'd gone round the financing of the health service for the 55th time, and now there was an opportunity of demonstrating the possible effectiveness of the health service without spending billions of pounds – and we could have effect. That was not an unimportant factor to remember.'

The Whitelaw Committee met seven times between its first meeting on 4 November 1986 and Christmas and considered all the big issues: anonymous nationwide testing, funding, condom distribution, health education. The comparative speed of the operation (compared to the lack of progress that had been made hitherto) was reflected in the conviction of Fowler's speech in the Commons on 21 November. This was the first time AIDS had been discussed at length in Parliament.

A poor turnout heard some important news. The government regarded AIDS as such a serious threat, Norman Fowler announced, that £20m would be spent in the next year on public education. There would be more newspaper adverts, some posters, a leaflet dropped through the letterbox of every home in the country and a radio, television and cinema campaign.

Thus the response to AIDS 'went ballistic'. Michael Meacher, shadow Social Services Secretary, observed that 'we have gone as a nation from hardly talking about AIDS at all to scarcely talking about anything else'.

'AIDS: The New Holocaust' ran a headline in the *Sunday Telegraph* two days after the Commons debate. For the *Mail on Sunday*, Jeff Ferry reported back from America that 'the greatest danger facing Britain is not unemployment. It is not poverty. It is not even nuclear war. The greatest danger today is the growing epidemic of the killer disease AIDS'. The United States, said Ferry, is 'a country where it is already too late'. The *Sunday Times* ran a large picture of the Average Family: two parents, two teenage children and a baby. 'They look happy and healthy. But from what we now know about the way the AIDS epidemic is developing, all are potential victims.' Reporters Peter Wilsher and Neville Hodgkinson stated that 'most strikingly, ordinary heterosexual intercourse between men and women – including husbands and wives – is now clearly established among the areas of risk. The absolute figures are still small – only a handful, seven men and nine women here – but careful contact-tracing has left no room for doubt'.

But there was doubt about how many people were already infected. Sir Donald Acheson left no one much the wiser when he announced 'our studies show that for every person who has AIDS, there are 50 carriers. We estimate there are 30,000 carriers, but only 4,000 of them are known because they have had blood tests. We can't be certain, though. It could be many more than 30,000, or it could be less'. In January 1987 the broadsheets made calculations of their own. On 9 January *The Times* believed 40,000 might be infected; on 12 January the *Independent* plumped for 60,000; and within three days *The Times* had increased its estimate to 100,000.

The government's new campaign would have two simple messages, Fowler said: 'Stick to one partner, but if you do not, use a condom' and 'Do not inject drugs; if you cannot stop, do not share equipment'. This made it sound like more of what had gone before, but the opposite was true. The newspaper and magazine advertisements resembled more a snappy hard-sell campaign, less an operator's manual. The pay-off line 'DON'T AID AIDS' was joined by 'DON'T DIE OF IGNORANCE', and the ad people came up with a concept or two: in one the word 'AIDS' was gift wrapped in festive paper, and beneath it ran the words 'How many people will get it for Christmas?' Another showed a T-shirt with 'Sex & Drugs & Rock 'n' Roll' scrawled across it; beneath was the message 'At least rock 'n' roll can't give you AIDS'. Yet another appeared in the shape of a heart: 'Your next sexual partner could be that very special person ... The one that gives you AIDS'.

The poster campaigns relied on stark typography and simple messages. There was no science here, no statistics: 'AIDS is not prejudiced. It can kill anyone. Gay or straight, male or female, anyone can get AIDS from sexual intercourse. So the more partners, the greater the risk. Protect yourself, use a condom.' One hoarding featured the word 'AIDS' in giant letters and beneath it the question, 'How big does it have to get before you take notice?' Simon Watney, a gay activist, lecturer and critic who has written widely about HIV and AIDS, remarked in March 1987, 'it is far from clear what we are expected to take notice of, beyond the poster itself ... The question which we should be asking some five years into the epidemic is, how big did it have to get before *they* took any notice?'

The government failed to provide specific material targeted at the gay community, believing that its funding of the Terrence Higgins Trust would be sufficient; the trust received just over £100,000 for all its work for 1986-7. Subsequently, however, Edwina Currie would claim that much was being done behind the scenes. 'Many people didn't see the hot material because we told our health care workers and everyone necessary to get out to gay groups, including promiscuous gay groups and get material to them that would persuade them to start changing their habits.' Challenged over the fact that much habit-changing had already occurred, Currie claimed that 'a lot of the people who were in the underground scene then, indeed as now, were reckless people, crazy people'.

The educational material produced by the Terrence Higgins Trust caused some embarrassment when ministers at the DHSS consulted it for clues as to how to prepare the text for the mass leaflet drop. 'You could tell how far the material had got [around the table] as the eyes popped,' Edwina Currie says. 'I will admit I learned things that day as I read the information; I cannot for the life of me imagine how people could get pleasure from some of the practices described'. Norman Fowler's own comprehension of sexual practices also came on in leaps and bounds; certainly he had a firmer grasp on the issues now than some months before when he is supposed to have asked a colleague at a press conference, 'Oral sex? I had no idea you could get it from talking dirty.'

At one meeting to discuss the wording of the leaflets, about 20 people had gathered around a conference table at the DHSS. Oral sex came up again. 'Oral sex? Do we know how many people *do* this sort of thing?' asked Norman Fowler. People looked away, looked at their notes, at their dusty glasses of water. The silence was broken by Donald Acheson. 'About 60 or 70 per cent,' he said, never less sure in his life; very little research had been conducted into this area. After the meeting, two of the DHSS officials turned to each other and smiled. One said, 'I wasn't sure if Norman was asking because he thought that everyone else did it but him, or whether he thought he was the only one.'

Another official remarked of one minister that he 'had real problems. He was deeply ignorant about sexual matters – he was unable to pronounce "vagina". You've no idea what a problem it is to talk to someone who doesn't believe in sex anyway'.

A similar leaflet drop had already been tried in West Germany. In Oxford, the local health authority had also sent AIDS information to every home, but the results had not been encouraging. 'We used the post office for mailing, in the same way the DHSS is planning to do,' Dr Alison Hill, a registrar in community medicine, told the trade magazine *Pulse*. 'The leaflet would arrive at homes with a bundle of other commercial leaflets – it all got chucked in the bin.'

The DHSS planned to counteract this by sending the leaflet in an envelope with the words, 'Government information about AIDS', and the fact that 'it deals with matters of health and sex that may be disturbing', a come-on if ever there was one. The wording of the leaflet went through almost as many changes as the first advertisements. Currie believes that it was John Major, Social Security Secretary, who pointed out that it would be helpful if they could all decide on the same meaning for some of the more important words. How would people define 'promiscuous'? One minister defined it as sleeping with more than one person. Currie, recalling her student days, believed it meant more than five a year. 'It was clear,' Currie concludes, 'that we had no idea what view the general public would have, and we were going to have to take a real leap in the dark.' Or as the *Lancet* put it a year later: 'Medical science knows more about the molecular structure of the HIV virus in a leucocyte than it knows about human sexual behaviour in the bedroom.' Determined that we should never learn more, in 1987 Margaret Thatcher cancelled a survey of the nation's sex habits, because, in the words of Norman Fowler, 'That was beyond the pale for her. She felt we were getting a little bit too deep into it and losing our perspective.'

In the end, not just one, but two leaflets were produced for mass distribution. The first was printed in November 1986 but then scrapped. It was very different from the one delivered in the two weeks from 12 January 1987. 'Avoiding AIDS: Government Information 1986' was a far more explicit pamphlet than the one finally approved. 'A copy of this leaflet has been sent to every household in the country,' the introduction ran. 'If you are a parent, remember that as children grow up they may experiment with drugs and sex. They may need advice sooner rather than later.' What followed would have outraged many parents. 'Anal sex,' the leaflet explained, 'when a man's penis enters his partner's anus (back passage), nearly always causes damage. This means it is easier for the virus in the semen of an infected man to get into his partner's bloodstream than in other kinds of sex.' Then, in bold capitals, 'AVOID ANAL SEX'. Next up, another capitalized message: 'DO NOT TAKE PART IN ANY SEXUAL ACTIVITY WHICH MAY DAMAGE THE PENIS, VAGINA, ANUS OR MOUTH OF YOU OR YOUR PARTNER'. Other paragraphs dealt with drug use, travelling abroad and the risks from unsterilized skin-piercing equipment.

The rewritten leaflet made no mention of the words 'penis', 'anus' or 'back passage' or any activity which might cause skin trauma. The first leaflet did not include the words 'homosexual' or 'gay', but the approved version stated that AIDS 'is not just a homosexual disease', confirming that the virus can be passed 'from man to man, man to woman and woman to man'. According to Jonathan Grimshaw, a gay HIV positive man who sat on the public education committee advising the DHSS, Sir Donald Acheson often repeated his concerns that if incorrectly handled, the whole campaign could cause a huge backlash against all gay men for 'causing and spreading' the virus (i.e. unleashing even more prejudice than existed already).

Throughout November, ministers wavered on whether to go ahead with the leaflet at all. In part the decision was made easier when it was found that a junior civil servant had already ordered the printing of 23 million envelopes without official approval; this would have been a costly mistake to explain away. There was talk too of not sending leaflets to the elderly; before this was ruled out as too impractical, there was talk of withholding the guidelines from anyone whose first name was Gladys, Albert or Daisy.

'We were a bit scared as to how the public were taking it,' Edwina Currie says. 'It was a heart-stopping operation. We were following those opinion polls with the greatest care, I can tell you. It could have been a big joke. It could have been badly handled. It wasn't badly handled.'

Just before the campaign started, even those who had been instrumental in its inception began to get cold feet. Sir Donald Acheson called up Tony Pinching: 'Are we doing the right thing?' Would such an unprecedented campaign spread more panic than enlightenment?

If Norman Fowler had similar fears, they were set aside by two overseas trips. In November 1986 he visited the World Health Organization in Geneva and met its AIDS project director, Dr Jonathan Mann. Here he learnt of the WHO's estimate of the scale of the epidemic worldwide: 100,000 AIDS cases to date; five to ten million HIV infections; up to three million deaths expected in the next five years. Six weeks later he was in San Francisco, reviewing the devastation. He toured Ward 5A at the San Francisco General, met his first AIDS patient and learnt about the effectiveness of community care, needle exchanges and public education.

He returned with greater resolve and his enthusiasm inspired others. Now it was his health minister, Tony Newton, who said, 'I'd rather have a few people offended by words which they might prefer not being used in public than a significant number of dead teenagers.' There were almost certainly already many dead teenagers in the AIDS figures released by the DHSS in February 1987: 686 AIDS cases and 4,000 deaths predicted by the end of 1989.

The government's campaign received a mixed reaction. The *Financial Times* reflected a widespread commendation in the national press, noting that Britain's campaign was being copied by Belgium and Italy: 'For once the advertising world has managed to act for the public good with a unity that has won it approval and respect.'

Religious leaders were less impressed, the Catholic Church disapproving of condom promotion, the Anglicans expressing doubts about the lack of any accompanying moral guidance. Sir Immanuel Jakobovits, the Chief Rabbi, presented Norman Fowler with a long list of misgivings. The campaign 'encourages promiscuity by advertising it', Sir Immanuel wrote. 'It introduces to many children and decent young people ideas on sex and marriage entirely unknown to them ... It tells people not what is right, but how to do wrong and get away with it – it is like sending people into a contaminated atmosphere, but providing them with gas masks and protective clothing'. The Chief Rabbi had his own message: 'Say plainly: AIDS is the consequence of marital infidelity, premarital adventures, sexual deviation and social irresponsibility – putting pleasure before duty and discipline.'

The Terrence Higgins Trust had rather different objections. Appearing before the Social Services Committee, Tony Whitehead praised the campaign for creating awareness, but in his regular column in *Capital Gay* he suggested that the trust had been exploited. He claimed the trust's helpline number and that of the London Lesbian and Gay Switchboard were printed on the leaflets without consultation or any extra funding to cope with the large increase in calls. 'The very least the Government could do would be an upfront thank you and a large cheque.'

In February 1987 the trust was receiving about a thousand calls a week to its helpline. In a memo, the organization detailed the course of action the government should take. This included the establishment of a national body to co-ordinate all statutory and voluntary services, the setting up of advice and counselling centres in every city, a 'massive' expansion of existing services and the grant of more money to the trust – 'the minimum of which to be £5 million'. Government grants to the Terrence Higgins Trust did increase; in August 1987 £300,000 was allocated for 1987–8, a threefold improvement on the previous grant but dismissed by the trust as quite inadequate for its burgeoning supply of services.

The leaflets were accompanied by the first of two portentous advertising campaigns on television. The first featured an exploding mountain, a tombstone on which was chiselled the word AIDS, and a bunch of flowers. They didn't tell you much, other than that something terrible was going to happen and that something was going to come through your letterbox. Maintaining the geological theme, the gravelly voiceover was by John Hurt. AIDS is a danger to us all, he said. Anyone can catch it through sex with an infected person. You can't always tell if someone is infected. You should protect yourself against it. You should be getting a leaflet about it soon, which you should read. Don't die of ignorance.

'I wanted advertisements that brought people up sharp,' Norman Fowler says. 'Adverts that were shocking and hard sell. We told the agency that's what we wanted, and that's what they produced.' This shock factor went a little too far: originally the tombstone adverts had a loud hooter at the beginning of them, like those found on old steam trains. The thinking was that this noise would jolt the viewer out of cosy slumber. 'That went,' Fowler says. 'It was slightly difficult to know what the hooter related to.'

The advertisements were principally the work of Sammy Harari of the agency TBWA, a young but rising star in the advertising world. When Harari had been with the agency Yellowhammer he had masterminded the 'Heroin Screws You Up' campaign, the accompanying posters from which soon became collectors' items in student bedsits. Home Office minister David Mellor and Norman Fowler had liked Harari's work, particularly the great efforts spent researching his campaigns, and were pleased to learn that he had joined TBWA in mid-1986. TBWA handled the account for blood donors and had been responsible for the poorly received first AIDS press campaign; the rumour was that the agency was about to lose the AIDS account before Harari arrived.

Harari had regular meetings with Fowler, Acheson and Romola Christopherson, the senior civil servant at the DHSS in charge of information. Together they would present their work to the cabinet committee. Most of the posters and youth press advertisements got the nod, but there were worries about the television campaign. 'There was one very senior member of the committee who said, "I do not think that the word condoms should appear on TV screens",' Harari says. Harari had a bet with Acheson that they'd win through eventually; he still has a framed £5 WH Smith gift voucher on a wall.

Harari concedes that the approved campaigns, which also included the notorious 'icebergs' image, were 'maybe a bit too Hollywood, a bit too doom and gloom', but points to a far greater miscalculation. 'We were about six months late,' he says, suggesting that in the period between the conception of the advertisements and their broadcast, the public had learnt a lot about AIDS from other media, and were thus ahead of the game:

Here was this huge latent soft putty waiting for an imprint to land on it and I think the imprint could have been harder. Six months previously they were actually spot on, but the preceding hysteria about AIDS in the press was unbelievable, things like 'Rabbi gave me AIDS', 'Rabbits gave me AIDS'. But for a campaign of that sort I think you only get one bite at it.

In retrospect, Harari regrets that the cabinet committee did not feel able to run a bolder campaign. A year later it was comparatively easy to gain approval for his more explicit behavioural and drug-related campaigns, even the one which read 'It only takes one prick to give you AIDS'. But election-year consensus politics was a nervous thing to watch. Harari was in a cabinet committee meeting shortly after James Anderton had delivered his 'cesspool' speech, and remembers everyone saying 'the guy's a complete loony, gone off his rocker' and laughing at his 'direct line from God' claims. 'But in the next two weeks the *Daily Mail* carried out an opinion poll and they found that 55 per cent of people in this country by and large agreed with his views. And then suddenly the committee had to take his views into account.'

The Tombstone and Iceberg advertisements came in for much flak, not least from the advertising industry. The director of one London firm concluded that the only certain way of stopping the spread of AIDS was to persuade everyone to give up sex. 'The problem is that selling celibacy is like trying to market empty cans. If you try hard enough, you may get a few takers. But it is never going to catch on.' The UK creative director of the international agency SSC+B Lintas said after the first broadcast, 'just about the only thing that can be said in its favour is that it is better to show this than to show nothing'.

The doctors at Southampton General Hospital who had earlier reported local confusion following the March 1986 newspaper campaign repeated their survey nine months later. They found that 44 per cent of respondents could not name one symptom of AIDS and that one person whose first language was not English had seen the Tombstone advertisement and thought that AIDS was associated with the use of pneumatic drills.

Yet the DHSS was encouraged by the results of its own research into the effectiveness of the whole campaign. Ninety-five per cent of 900 adults polled agreed with the comment that 'the Government is right to be doing advertisements like these'. The research was conducted in three waves. The proportion claiming to know a 'good amount' about AIDS increased from 42 per cent in November 1986 (before the onslaught), to 52 per cent in January 1987 (midway) and 61 per cent in February (after the Tombstone and Iceberg and leaflets). Eighty-one per cent considered AIDS of 'great concern' in February 1987, but only 46 per cent were very or a little worried that they or someone they knew might catch AIDS (a 10 per cent drop from a month before). There was still a little confusion: 14 per cent believed the virus could be transmitted by kissing, 13 per cent by using the same glass and 9 per cent from sneezing. The proportion who agreed strongly that 'people can considerably reduce the risk of catching AIDS by using condoms' increased from 70 per cent in November 1986 to 78 per cent in February 1987. Awareness at the

DHSS may have lagged somewhat behind that of the public, however. The department's 1986 Christmas cards featured a man selling mistletoe telling a passing shopper: 'I just can't seem to shift it; what with all this AIDS about'.

Another poll, conducted some months later by the Cancer Relief Macmillan Fund, found that almost one in three adults questioned regarded AIDS as their biggest health worry, behind cancer but ahead of heart disease. Among single people, half gave AIDS as their biggest concern. The fears clearly bore no relation to death rates: of 531,000 deaths in England and Wales in 1986, heart disease claimed 187,000 and cancer 140,000. At the beginning of 1987, the official toll from AIDS was still under 700. Thus fear remained the key, for good or worse. As Sammy Harari was used to pointing out in all his meetings with ministers, there was likely to remain a huge gulf between attitudinal change and behavioural change.

Harari's campaigns were certainly inspiring to some. In January 1987 the Football Association wrote to every professional footballer and club amateur with health guidelines of its own. For the burly midfield general or the tricky winger, the government's information was clearly insufficient: what they needed was 'AIDS and Injuries in Football'. The FA's medical committee, headed by Dr John O'Hara, a 79-year-old Sussex GP, concluded that it had done all it could to persuade players to stop kissing and cuddling when celebrating goals, but what with this new fatal thing going round, enough was enough, Brian. 'Now we aim to frighten players into it.' An AIDS awareness charter advised players not to drink champagne from the same bottle when celebrating a great triumph; to swap communal baths for showers; to use a mouthpiece when giving the kiss of life; and not to exchange shirts at the end of a game. Coaches were told to wear surgical gloves when treating a wound and to ditch the old bucket and sponge.

The Professional Footballers Association and doctors disapproved of this 1983-style approach and brought up the example of poor old Kevin Moran; Moran, a Manchester United and Republic of Ireland defender, needed mouth-to-mouth during a game and might have been in grave danger if there had been any delay. And what about the resuscitation of Swindon player Andy Rogers? The sports pages and terrace fans had a great time with this one. Even the England team was warned about the dangers of the Wembley baths, and the *Daily Mirror* treated its readers to a roll call of all the stars who had used the facility in the past: 'After the World Cup triumph of 1966, England skipper Bobby Moore and his pals took the plunge in style ... there have been three double triumphs completed in those baths – Spurs in 1961, Arsenal in 1971 and Liverpool in 1986.'

Two weeks later, more hysteria. Edwina Currie had put her foot in it many times in a short career; indeed, this soon became her trademark. Despite her vociferous support of her department's education programme, every now and then something she'd say would conspire to undermine it. In mid-February she attended a press conference in Runcorn to launch a new DHSS campaign on how best to avoid heart disease. She said that in selecting a disease to campaign against her department looked for something that killed a lot of people, caused much suffering, cost a lot of money and was preventable.

The topic of conversation soon turned to AIDS, at which point Currie strayed from her prepared statement. 'Good Christian people who wouldn't dream of misbehaving will not catch AIDS,' she said, in response to a journalist's question. 'My message to the businessmen of this country when they go abroad on business is that there is one thing above all they can take with them to stop them catching AIDS – the wife.'

'Take the wife' swiftly became the punchline to many cartoons and jokes. Less humorous was the response to her 'good Christian' comment; the *Guardian* called it 'Beating off AIDS with the Bible', though Currie claims that her intention was the reverse:

I was being sarcastic, replying to some self-righteous pratt in the newspapers going on about how the Government ought to be preaching morality. What I meant by 'good Christians' was that if he did what he said he did, and behaved himself, he wasn't going to get infected and people like him then were not my problem. But it got translated into something quite different; it never occurred to me that I would get all these letters from people thanking me for speaking out, or from angry Jews assuming that I meant that they were at risk.

There was no sarcasm detected in her voice when she implored those infected with HIV to 'never make love again. I know it's like giving someone a life sentence, but they have to stop'. Her department's promotion of condoms and of safer sex practices was ignored. At the same time, HIV positive men began placing personal ads in the columns of gay newspapers appealing for partners who were also infected.

Currie's outbursts were increasingly viewed as a liability by her department. 'The term "loose cannon" was only the half of it,' one official recalls:

On one occasion, on the day Norman Fowler's house was broken into, we had to send her to take his place at a conference for social services directors in York. We tried Jean Trumpington first and she couldn't do it. Then we tried Tony Newton and he couldn't. But Edwina's people said she could cancel her arrangements to do it. Norman, who had been apoplectic at her gaffes, sighed and said, 'OK, but no funny business.' He said that she just had to read the speech. Then he called up again later and said, 'She *does* know not to answer any questions?'

'I've always taken the view that you do much better with the electorate if you are very straight with them,' Currie says. 'What they hate is being misled.' Not everyone in her department shared her views, she says. When ministers became aware of a surgeon who had contracted HIV in South Africa and had then died after operating on about 400 British patients, Currie says that she and Tony Newton wanted to trace all these patients, offer them tests and counselling and thus handle the problem efficiently. 'The Secretary of State, John Moore, didn't,' she says. 'His instinct was to cover it up.'

During one heated meeting on the subject a note was passed around which said that because of the special facilities required for handling the surgeon's body for the cremation, one of the funeral workers had talked to the press. 'By the end of that meeting we had proper arrangements. Every single patient would be given full information.' (A hotline was set up. About a quarter of his patients wanted tests; it is believed none were HIV positive.)

The potential problem of infected health-care workers was raised during *AIDS Help!*, part of a week-long series of television programmes on all channels in March 1987. Norman Fowler had been meeting the chairmen of the BBC and ITV since December, and the culmination of these efforts probably did as much to alert people to the dangers of AIDS as the paid-for campaign. There were regular documentary features, short information bulletins and what amounted to an AIDS revue, in which government ministers mingled with alternative comedians. Sir Donald Acheson claims he was the first person in the world to mention anal sex on daytime television.

Everyone seemed to be putting condoms everywhere: on fingers, cucumbers and especially bananas. Jonathan Grimshaw, 32, a co-founder of the Body Positive support group and one of the very few openly infected (but well) men in the country, soon became TV's Mr HIV. He recalls being on a show with agony aunt Claire Rayner in which she attempted in vain to place a condom 'on a phallus she'd been sent by one of her fans. She was wearing a rayon dress, which soon became covered in KY Jelly. She couldn't get the thing on, and we had to do two or three takes'.

Norman Fowler agreed to appear on another show in the same week. As the programme was intended to appeal to a young audience, the producers had asked him to appear as informal as possible. It was agreed that he should wear a sweater. On the morning of the inter-view (to be filmed in his office), the Secretary of State was struck by indecision. 'He came into the office with three jumpers,' one official recalls, 'and said "Which one do you think?" We pointed to one and he said, "*That?* That's my gardening jumper!"'

He wore his gardening jumper and the interview went fine. But at the end the television people pulled a fast one. They explained to him that they had already lined up a large number of celebrities who agreed to say the word 'condom' straight to camera. It was what they called 'condom normalization'. Would he do the same? 'Just the one word?' he asked. Just so. Fowler said he wasn't sure; he'd been around long enough to know how even one word – especially one word – could be used to make you look foolish. He consulted his private office. They said it would look a bit mean if he refused. He asked a press officer, who got a guarantee that the word would not be used for any other purpose than this one broadcast.

'Just the one word?' Fowler asked again, and said it: 'Condom.' He did it again from another angle, perched on the side of his desk: 'Condom!' Then the Secretary of State, in his gardening jumper and a nervous smile, turned to the television crew and his staff and asked, 'Was that all right?'

At the end of the government's unprecedented campaign and atten-dant media attention, there remained one big question: what next? Increasingly, money was being allocated to voluntary organizations and to the NHS, but how best should spending be co-ordinated? And how to develop and maintain interest in the public education campaigns? Ministers thought for a while and then acted true to form. They formed a couple of quangos.

On 1 April 1987 the Health Education Authority was to replace the Health Education Council. The HEA would have an enhanced and strengthened role and take over all responsibility for the DHSS AIDS campaigns. Its quasi-autonomous status would, in theory, leave it free to criticize the government's health education policies and to research and develop new campaigns. It would, however, have to submit all its plans to ministers before proceeding.

The other body, announced in May, was the National AIDS Trust, an independent charitable organization intended to co-ordinate the voluntary sector. The administration of the NAT would be financed by the government; it would receive grants for distribution as it saw fit as well as raising its own money and providing advice and information. Its first director was to be Margaret Jay, the well-connected television journalist, its founding chairman Sir Austin Bide, president of Glaxo Holdings and a member of the AIDS sub-committee at the Medical Research Council. A fundraising committee was chaired by Robert Maxwell, who pledged to raise £50 million to combat 'this scourge which has to be tackled'. At a press conference in a lavishly furnished room in Lancaster House a sweating Maxwell announced that he hoped Elizabeth Taylor would become involved.

Norman Fowler was also at the press conference. In a statement he seemed happy to be washing his hands of the affair: 'With the launch of the Trust today, my part in the operation is complete ... after today the burden falls on Sir Austin Bide, Mr Robert Maxwell and the others concerned ... I wish the Trust Godspeed.' Fowler pledged £500,000 to the new organization. Maxwell saw the television cameras and seized his chance. He said he was distressed: 'I had hoped that he would announce a million, and then I was going to double it.' He then challenged Fowler to change his mind on the spot. Fowler said: 'I will certainly consider it.'

'Of course it was mostly bluff,' Margaret Jay recalled later. 'We did get a million, though where this money came from I now shudder to think.'

Jay had been involved with this sort of thing before, and was not always popular. A year earlier, in May 1986, the UK AIDS Foundation was formed, amid some fanfare, to promote medical research, advance education, help those infected and act as a sort of overseeing body for voluntary organizations. This was no mean task given the great differences of opinion between the voluntary groups, but the Foundation was supported by the great and the good (all the usual doctors and officials), counting Sir Richard Attenborough, Sir Gerard Vaughan and Margaret Jay among its trustees, and for the first few months it made some gentle progress. Its first director, Roger Newton, with 30 years' health-care experience behind him, declared on his appointment, 'People are nervous. Facts beat fear. One of our jobs is to give people the facts!'

The fact was, two things had happened to alienate the Terrence Higgins Trust. Sir Gerard, a former health minister, suggested in a personal capacity that all people coming into Britain from various countries should be tested for the virus. And then Margaret Jay was involved in a Thames Television *This Week* programme which brought up the possibility of all infected people carrying identity tags. All of this ran counter to the philosophy of the trust and when it pulled out the organization never recovered. By the time Norman Fowler announced the new National AIDS Trust, the UK AIDS Foundation had already disintegrated.

Both the NAT and the HEA were predominently heterosexual organizations, aware of the way gay men were being affected by AIDS (about 75 per cent of all cases), but determined to concentrate most resources on the wider community (the HEA ran several other health promotion programmes too, including smoking). And so began what many gay activists and commentators believe was a conscious attempt to 'de-gay' the epidemic. At the time, many people believed this to be a healthy thing, a way of de-stigmatizing, of diverting prejudice, of generating more financial support. Latterly, this view has become less generous.

'We [gay men] were completely written off,' says Peter Scott, the founder of the National AIDS Manual and the leader of the gay men's health education group at the Terrence Higgins Trust. 'The heterosexual approach to all this was to talk about an epidemic that may or may not happen, about what to do about the "worried well", and not noticing this huge terrible epidemic that's actually raging away. The epidemic simply wasn't real to them.'

The money that was freed up in 1987 and 1988 – for education, counselling, and community-based health-care provision – found its way from regional and local health authorities to every borough in the country, including boroughs which had no incidence of HIV. People were recruited from other sectors of local government and elsewhere, often with no experience of HIV/AIDS work. Gay men were often left in the cold, Scott contends, 'and what made it worse was that there was a sort of collaborating class of gay men who de-gayed themselves. It looked like there were gay men in positions of influence, but they were either ineffectual or totally outnumbered by people who didn't have the faintest idea about gay politics.'

Work for gay men at the Terrence Higgins Trust lost its direction at this time, not least because it too was being infected by the heterosexual bug. Scott favours an orchestra analogy: that there was once a tune being played by a small number of instruments and suddenly, crash, the whole post-modernist polytonalism erupts and drowns out the original tune.

And there was another reason. The more you expressed the 'equal opportunities' element of the virus, the more central or regional funding seemed to come your way. Raising funds for the London Lesbian and Gay Switchboard, the organization that had dealt with the British epidemic from the start and had helped pioneer concepts of safer sex, was far harder than obtaining grants for less gay-specific organizations.

When the National AIDS Helpline was established by the DHSS to deal with the thousands of calls resulting from its advertising campaigns, it recruited from the London Lesbian and Gay Switchboard and the Terrence Higgins Trust. But according to one staffer, its non-gay management had a hidden agenda.

'After Christmas I noticed that it was becoming increasingly difficult for people who were gay or from the Trust to book shifts,' says Zoe Schramm-Evans, who worked at the trust and National AIDS Helpline before writing a Ph.D. on the period. Some time after Schramm-Evans left, when the helpline was staffed by what she calls 'little ladies who walked dogs in their spare time', she talked to a former manager:

He said that they'd had specific instructions from the Department of Health, who were terrified that the *Sun* or the *Mirror* or whatever would get hold of the fact that all these poor unfortunate people who had become alarmed by what the government had said were being counselled by 'undesirables'. The fact that these people might be able to give better advice or be more sympathetic didn't come into it.

In March 1988 Margaret Thatcher tackled the problem of AIDS at Prime Minister's Questions. She said, 'I think we got it just about right.'

David Owen, the SDP leader, and other opposition MPs disagreed. He particularly objected to the government's refusal to invest more resources in combating the risk to drug users. The Advisory Council on the Misuse of Drugs had recently recommended that the needle exchange scheme be expanded, and that condoms should be made available free to addicts. Dr Owen called government policy 'appallingly short sighted'.

'I do not agree,' the Prime Minister said. 'You are well aware of the large amounts of money that have been spent on warning people about the dangers of the behaviour which they assume. We have tried to get over to them an excellent educational policy and tried to make very good extra facilities available. A large amount of money has been put into extra research.'

Some observers perceived an air of conclusion, of finality, in her voice and indeed she hardly ever mentioned the subject of AIDS publicly again. But if she really thought that the problem had been adequately dealt with, she might have been taken aback by the short-term predictions contained in the Cox Report of November 1988. Sir David Cox chaired a Working Group established by the Chief Medical Officers of England and Wales. Its estimates presented the most reliable forecasts yet available. Between 10,000 and 30,000 AIDS cases were expected between 1987 and 1992; the 'recommended basis for planning' was 13,000 cases. By the end of 1992 between 7,500 and 17,000 people were expected to have died from AIDS-related illnesses. Assuming that no treatment emerged that would significantly prolong the lives of people with AIDS, the number of people living with AIDS at any particular time was expected to rise from the present level of about 1,350 to a recommended basis for planning of over 5,000 by the end of 1992. These figures, which did not include Scottish cases, related only to those reported to the Communicable Disease Surveillance Centre. Adjustments for under-reporting would increase them by at least 20 per cent.

At the end of the report came a glimmer of hope. The group made no predictions about future numbers of HIV infections (noting that these depended on unforeseeable changes in behaviour), but it did acknowledge that the rate of increase in new AIDS cases was slowing, probably as a result of behavioural changes in the gay community. It stressed that 'it would be a gross error to regard even the lower predictions as grounds for complacency'. The future spread of AIDS now hung in the balance: complacency could undo it all, but renewed vigorous commitment might ensure that Britain could avoid the magnitude of the crisis already facing France and Italy, where four times as many people were already infected.

Unless, of course, the British figures were wrong. In March 1988 Dr Anna McCormick of the Communicable Disease Surveillance Centre told a London conference on the global impact of AIDS that she and her colleagues had found many more deaths that might have been associated with HIV and AIDS that were not reported as such. At that time there had been 749 official AIDS deaths, but there was now a suggestion that there might have been an extra 597 deaths, all in men aged 15 to 54. A definition of cancer or pneumonia, rather than AIDS, might have been put on death certificates, perhaps in order to save the embarrassment of families, or just out of ignorance. 'They may not have been diagnosed as having AIDS, or they may not have met the official clinical definition,' Dr McCormick explained. 'Some of those excess deaths may not have been AIDS, but I don't know any other reason why the mortality rate among single men is going up.'

As 1988 wore on, the Whitelaw Committee began to meet less frequently, about once a month rather than once a week. Increasingly, the principal battles were judged to have been won: the panic was over, the blood supply was secure, the British people had been educated, warned not to die of ignorance. And so the debate moved on and other complex issues emerged: funding and accountability, the possibility of mass screening, the availability of free condoms, compensation to haemophiliacs, infection in prisons, civil rights and employment law. And there was one issue that came up at almost every meeting, something that could never be solved by either poster campaign or government bill: the search for a treatment, vaccine or cure.

CHAPTER 7: Suitable Treatment

I explained how the AIDS virus can infect the central nervous system. We had some pictures on the stand of the brain of an AIDS patient. The brain was normal when the patient was first infected with the disease but a year later his brain was shrunken as a result of the infection. The Queen was very interested. Above all she was interested in treatment and the prospects of a cure. That is what are all most interested in.

Professor Jangu Banatvala of St Thomas's Hospital on the Queen's visit to the Royal College of Pathologists, February 1987

A man goes to the doctor and says, 'My wife's not well, please examine her.' The doctor looks her over and tells her husband, 'Terrible news – she's either got Alzheimer's or AIDS.' The husband asks, 'Well how do I tell?' The doctor says, 'Drive her out to the woods about five miles from here and leave her. If she finds her way back, don't fuck her.'

Popular joke in the late 1980s

In 1986, gay British men added another holiday destination to their list of Amsterdam, San Francisco, New York and Ibiza. It was Mexico. Tijuana wasn't actually much of a holiday, more of a last resort. It was the place you'd go for unlicensed AIDS drugs.

Members of the self-help groups Body Positive and Frontliners had obtained a 20-page document from Project Inform in San Francisco that told adventurous drug tourists all they needed to know. Prepared from unofficial, anecdotal sources, it became a sort of underground bible, a Baedecker of alternative treatment culture.

The drugs most in demand in 1986 were isoprinosine and ribavirin. Isoprinosine was widely available in some countries as a treatment for herpes or flu and was believed to stimulate certain functions of the immune system. The anti-viral ribavirin was a stronger drug, with a side effect of anaemia often reported in users. Used in combination, people with AIDS or AIDS-related complex (ARC) reported fewer opportunistic infections, fewer night sweats, less weight loss and an improvement of T-cell ratios; others didn't live long enough to report their findings. This was the problem – no one knew for sure: without strictly controlled clinical trials, any reported benefits of these drugs were circumstantial and highly individualistic. But if you were dying and you or a friend were able to make it to Mexico to get treatments your local doctor had never even heard of, then it was probably a risk worth taking.

But where, exactly, did you go? Your new guide had it covered. 'Take interstate 5 going south from San Diego. If questioned at the border, describe yourself as a tourist.' Once you found your way to the centre of town, you should look for large store signs indicating 'Farmacia'. 'Some Farmacias may offer a substitute if they are out of stock. The only substitution you should allow is pranosine as a replacement for isoprinosine, since they are the same drug. Get the drug you came for, or go to another store.' And once you had them, once the Mexican pharmacists had served yet another grateful frail foreign customer in the biggest upsurge in trade that anyone in the business could remember, how did you get the goods through customs? Small quantities for personal use were legal (about 200 tablets, but these wouldn't last more than a few weeks). And what if you were part of a buyers' club, bulk shopping for friends? 'Dress all-American casual – customs agents will feel right at home. Wear your least noticeable earrings, or none at all. Leather gear can also be kept at home or at least kept under your clothing. Dress up: carry a camera, wear green polyester golf slacks, clip-on sunglasses, and a pressed short-sleeve shirt with pens in the pocket.' Alternatively, bring a 'blouse and skirt-wearing woman or a child'. The best trick was to double up the number of pills in each packet and hide abnormal quantities under the seats or inside your spare tyre.

If you didn't end up in jail, you had to be careful with dosage, as you wouldn't be getting a label with your pills. A good average for isoprinosine was six 500 mg tablets every 24 hours. Some people took twice as much. How much was safe? No one knew. Did it really do you any good? No one knew. Was it really worth travelling to South Africa, as some British people with HIV had done, to obtain a workable copy of AL721, an anti-viral compound made from egg yolks which could be spread on toast? No one knew for sure. But until the beginning of 1987 this unlicensed, untested, under the dashboard stuff was all you could get.

In April 1987, a full-page advertisement appeared in the medical trade press. 'Wellcome are pleased to announce the introduction of the first HIV-specific treatment for serious manifestations of Acquired Immunodeficiency Syndrome and AIDS-related complex.' The drug was called Retrovir, zidovudine or azidothymidine, but everyone already knew it as AZT.

Few modern treatments were greeted with such acclaim or such hopes. Before AZT, all AIDS symptoms were treated illness by illness – if you had PCP you'd get pentamidine, if you had KS maybe you'd have chemotherapy – but here at last was a drug to treat the whole syndrome, little white and blue capsules, three to be taken every four hours. The advert listed the possible toxic side effects (bone marrow deficiency, renal complications, nausea, headache, rash, insomnia, anorexia and five others), but these would be risks worth taking. AZT wasn't a cure, but it was probably the only chance: trials had shown that it prolonged life, made you better at least for a short while and in that while – who knows? – maybe something else would come along, maybe a cure would be found.

When Norman Fowler granted a product licence for AZT on 4 March (a few weeks ahead of the granting of a licence in the United States), doctors who had been powerless for so long against a syndrome about which they knew so little at last had something they could give their patients, and on the NHS too.

Their patients had already known about it for too long. At the beginning of October 1985, the Wellcome Foundation stuck out a press release: Compound S, as it was then known (or BW A509U), had shown 'sufficient promise to be taken forward to Phase 1 clinical trials'. This meant that it would be tested in 19 patients for the first time, to determine levels of dosage and toxicity. A week before, a conference in Minneapolis had been told that laboratory tests showed the compound to hinder multiplication of HTLV-III. Early animal studies also indicated that it was 'of sufficiently low toxicity to be considered for use in man'. No one at Wellcome actually used the word 'breakthrough', but that was undoubtedly the message. Almost a dozen other compounds had been tested by various companies thus far; none had been shown to have benefit in people with AIDS. Several other treatments were undergoing trials, almost all in America. These were the drugs people crossed the globe for: ribavirin was being tested by ICN, isoprinosine by Newport, HPA-23 by the people at Rhone-Poulenc. At St Stephen's Hospital, London, they were looking at Astra's foscarnet. None of these had the impetus or the progress of AZT; AZT had been put on the fast track; it had to work, because it was the best science could do. The release of the drug was nicely timed, too: the first report of the human use of AZT coincided with the flotation of Wellcome shares on the London stock market.

In 1964, Jerome Horwitz was working in his laboratory at the Michigan Cancer Foundation when he had what he hoped was a brilliant idea. At 45, Dr Horwitz was the foundation's director of chemistry, and although not in the scientific premier league, was a respected local researcher with his own thriving laboratory. He had spent much of the previous decade doing what many of the world's leading scientists had done: working on a cure, or at the very least an effective treatment, for cancer.

He developed a theoretical solution: what was needed was a chemical that would insert a 'phoney' compound into the DNA 'building block' of a cell to interrupt the DNA chain and prevent its replication. After years of research, Dr Horwitz came up with azidothymidine (AZT).

He tried his new compound on leukaemic mice, but it had no effect. Horwitz didn't know why, but AZT didn't work. He remembers: 'AZT was a terrible disappointment ... we dumped it on the junkpile, I didn't keep the notebooks.' Horwitz never became famous. 'But we were certainly on the cutting edge. When the pharmacologist said, "Look Dr Horwitz, your compounds are not effective against leukaemias and I see no future for them", that was like a blow to the solar plexus. We had great hopes. I remember one of my students saying at the time that we had a great series of compounds just waiting for a disease to treat.'

One of these compounds remained 'on the shelf', occasionally tried by other researchers but always found to be useless. There was no reason to patent it. But 20 years later, Burroughs Wellcome brought it back to life.

The Wellcome group was founded in London by two Americans in 1880. Its first significant achievement was the creation of the tablet: previously most medication had been administered in powder form. In the 1930s the group was split into two distinct parts: the Wellcome Trust, a large charity which devoted its income to scientific research and the maintenance of an institute and library concerned with the history of medicine; and the Wellcome Foundation Ltd, a profit-making pharmaceuticals company that was called Burroughs Wellcome in the United States. In the course of its research, Wellcome employees won five Nobel prizes.

By 1980, Wellcome had specialized in the treatment of viruses for more than 15 years, and its anti-viral drugs accounted for the bulk of its income. In that year, David Barry, a leading researcher at Burroughs Wellcome in the US, noticed that demand for its drug Septra – a drug that Wellcome had helped to develop a few years earlier to combat PCP – was suddenly on the increase. It had been in demand previously mainly from doctors treating children with leukaemia; the demand from young gay men was something else entirely. Two years later, another new Wellcome drug, Zovirax, was in great demand among the same group of people. Zovirax was an anti-herpes treatment. Barry was disturbed by the sudden demand for these two drugs and the subsequent classification of AIDS and HTLV-III, but if any company was ideally equipped to conduct research into combating a new virus, it was Wellcome.

In purely cynical terms, any scientist could see that AIDS presented what was potentially a career-making race to the Nobel prize. Millions might be made from a successful treatment.

According to Wellcome's own three-page account, its research into HIV began in June 1984. During mass testing of scores of anti-viral compounds, a substance known at first only as Compound S was found to inhibit viruses in animal cells. Compound S was AZT, a resynthesized version of what Horwitz had made 20 years before (Wellcome credits Horwitz in its account, but spells his name wrong). Its main ingredient was thymidine, derived from herring sperm.

In November 1984, according to the Wellcome account, the company sent samples of AZT to Duke University in North Carolina, the Food and Drug Administration (FDA) and the National Cancer Institute for independent testing. Within a few weeks the results confirmed what Wellcome already believed: the stuff worked against HIV in test tubes under laboratory conditions. Wellcome had already progressed further than Horwitz, but they would soon discover that the real test – its effect on infected patients – was fraught with danger.

But first there is another account of the development of AZT to consider. A US government official named Sam Broder believes he has far more claim to being 'Mr AZT' than anyone at Burroughs Wellcome. Broder, the director of the National Cancer Institute, claims that Burroughs Wellcome showed little interest in developing an anti-AIDS drug. Towards the end of 1984, Broder went on a tour of pharmaceuticals companies, imploring them to send any possible anti-viral compounds to his lab for testing in safe conditions. 'I went to one prestigious company, hat in hand,' he told the American business writer Bruce Nussbaum. 'I got about one minute and thirty seconds of a high-ranking officer's time. It was very disappointing for me. It was emblematic of the issue. There was no real interest in it.'

Broder then went to Burroughs Wellcome. He says: 'They made it clear that on the basis of 3,000 patients, there was no way they could practically get involved.' Broder says he then became abrasive: 'As I left, I said, "You know, we're going to have more than 3,000 cases. It is going to be commercially viable for you".'

Whoever pushed who, the drug came through. When Broder found that the AZT sent to him by Burroughs Wellcome in November 1984 worked against the virus, he assured the company that every effort would be made to get this great new drug to dying patients as soon as possible. The FDA's stringent testing requirements mean that most new drugs take between eight and ten years to pass from development to the marketplace. AZT was pushed through in just 20 months.

This could have been the early history of almost any drug; the difference is that during what would normally have been an eight-year test period, for six of those years the drug was already on the market. The National Cancer Institute had previously tried one other therapy, Bayer's suramin, which proved to be toxic in early tests; AZT appeared to be far less poisonous. And so AZT became an all-or-bust thing. But could any drug live up to the boundless hopes pinned to it?

This is how AZT is supposed to work against the virus. HIV enters body cells, usually T4 white blood cells that play a crucial role in the orchestration of the body's immune system. HIV is one of a group of viruses known as retroviruses, which means that, unlike most living things that store their genetic information as DNA, HIV stores it as RNA. Before HIV can replicate, it must convert its RNA code to DNA by use of a special enzyme called reverse transcriptase. It is during this conversion process that AZT works. When AZT enters the body, it is transformed into a molecule that closely resembles one of the building blocks of DNA. During the process of HIV conversion, this molecule is incorporated mistakenly into the DNA. The addition of this 'phoney' molecule makes the addition of further building blocks impossible and halts replication of the virus. Because DNA drills itself into human cells, to get rid of it you must rid every cell of its DNA if the virus is present. It is a non-discriminatory process, a form of chemotherapy. It worked fine under a microscope.

The early clinical tests were in two phases. The first examined whether AZT could be tolerated in the body at all and whether it entered the brain, crossing the 'blood-brain barrier'; this was important, because a common AIDS symptom is dementia. The first AIDS patient was injected with AZT in July 1985. This test concluded that the blood-brain barrier was crossed and that although levels of toxicity were detected, these were deemed to be safe.

The second phase of the tests, the final hurdle to the granting of a licence for mass production, soon became a shambles. It was set up seven months later to establish whether AZT would combat AIDS. This test, overseen by the Food and Drug Administration, involved 282 patients, all of them already ill with AIDS or ARC. It was to be a placebo test, conducted over 24 weeks, a 'double-blind' study in which neither patient nor doctor knew whether the capsules being taken were AZT or starch. Before the tests could begin, Wellcome had to produce large quantities of AZT and found it couldn't do it: it had run out of herring sperm. Finally, Wellcome bought it in bulk from another company.

At a press conference after the tests in September 1986, Wellcome reported that they had been a considerable success, such a success that the 24-week trial had been halted after 16 weeks for 'ethical' reasons. Mortality rates for people taking AZT were remarkably lower than those taking the placebo; there had been 19 deaths in the placebo group of 137 people, but only one in the AZT group of 145. Those on AZT also had a decreased number of opportunistic infections and showed improvement in weight gain and T4 cell counts. Wellcome agreed with gay activists who lobbied that if AZT was effective, then dying people should be taken off the placebo at once.

And so Wellcome geared up for mass production: at a capital cost of £17 million, additional plants were announced for Dartford, Kent, and Greenville, Tennessee. In October 1986, stock market analysts reckoned that annual sales of AZT could reach $12–$15 million; by February 1987, with a price for 100 capsules (just over a week's supply) set at $188 and £143, those forecasts had been increased more than tenfold. United States sales alone were predicted to reach $150–$200 million in the year ending August 1988. After this price announcement, the company's shares rose by about 20 per cent to £3.74.

Robert Windom, United States Assistant Health Secretary, said that 'treatment with AZT prolongs survival of persons with AIDS'. The results were 'exciting'. T. E. Haigler, the president of Burroughs

Wellcome, said that it was 'difficult to think of an achievement in the history of our company as meaningful to us as bringing Retrovir to patients with HIV disease'. (In fact, AZT was only licensed to treat those people who had full-blown AIDS or AIDS-related complex, not those who were HIV positive but asymptomatic; but many well people with HIV believed it would stave off illness, and soon took it as well.)

In a memorandum submitted to the Expert Advisory Group on AIDS, the Department of Health noted that there were suggestions that a month's course of AZT might prevent the establishment of infection following a 'needlestick' injury (accidental injection with a contaminated syringe). 'Some doctors are so concerned about infection they are said to be dosing themselves with zidovudine all the time ... Most UK experts are sceptical of this use.'

Some years later, interviewed in the Wellcome in-house magazine, David Barry would say that 'the staff at Wellcome can tell our children, grandchildren and great-grandchildren that we were there, that we made a difference'. When it was shown that AZT worked, 'we ... first had a frenzied, cheerful celebration, and then a very quiet one. The longer we considered the global implications, the greater the accomplishment we realised Wellcome had made in the control of the HIV epidemic'.

To ensure all patients had a shot at the drug, Wellcome then marketed like crazy. AZT was championed at every conference; every prescribing doctor was bombarded with bumph. In October 1987, Abigail Zuger, an American doctor from the University of Chicago, wrote to the *New England Journal of Medicine*: 'Of all the unsolicited material I have received from pharmaceutical companies this year, the most lavish has been the small package ... from Burroughs Wellcome Co.' It was a videocassette extolling the virtues of AZT, the third missive she had received within four months. She wondered about the cost of producing and shipping these things, the high cost of AZT and whether they weren't perhaps related. We were not dealing with a new brand of paracetamol here. 'In this tenuous climate, to launch Retrovir with the usual costly marketing glitz seems to me to be a particularly unfortunate gesture.' A Wellcome person replied that, yes, there was some cost in doing the videos, but this must be weighed against the even higher costs to doctors and patients 'that could result from inadequate or inappropriate information'. The question of inadequate information would soon rebound.

A few months after AZT was made available, a reporter working on the gay newspaper *New York Native* obtained some of the early AZT trial documents through the Freedom of Information Act. These suggested that many rules had been broken. The trial had been 'unblinded' within weeks: some patients claimed they could tell what they were taking by taste; others were so keen to have AZT that they pooled their treatment with other patients to increase their chances of receiving the drug. The documents showed that almost half the AZT patients had received numerous blood transfusions in the course of the trial because of damage to their bone marrow and immune systems; and that a few had had to be taken off AZT altogether.

What happened after the trial ended suggested something more alarming. After 16 weeks, one AZT patient was dead, compared to 19 placebo patients; a week later two more patients on AZT had died, compared to four more on the placebo. The ratio had switched from 19:1 to 23:3, which suggested AZT might only be effective for a very limited time. If the trial had continued, the ratio might have narrowed even more. The tests would probably still have shown that AZT had some benefits for very ill patients, but many now consider it alarming that a new drug was licensed with so much left to prove.

People at Wellcome now put it down to the mood and force of the times. Professor Trevor Jones, director of research at Wellcome, who has been involved in the development of AZT from the beginning, acknowledges that the trials were subject to extraordinary pressures:

> Much of these accusations [about the breakdown of trial protocol] took place, not at that stage, but later on, when the drug was showing benefit in a less sick population. All sorts of things we heard stories about, and some of them I think we can confirm from our data. Two patients would go to their doctor, get their treatments, and rather than risk the uncertainty [of receiving the placebo] they'd put the two together, mix them and divide them by half. We know this, because people who were supposed to be on the placebo already had drug levels in them.

Much of the pressure came from people with HIV and AIDS and their carers, who insisted the drug be released immediately. There was no point having treatment on the market in ten years, when hundreds of thousands would be dead.

There were other allegations into the way Wellcome conducted its trials. The *New York Times* claimed that the company had been refusing to supply AZT 'for some clinical trials deemed crucial by top government scientists'. One of these scientists was Dr Anthony Fauci, director of the National Institute of Allergy and Infectious Diseases, who was quoted as saying 'one of our real frustrations is that Burroughs Wellcome literally has complete control over what does or does not get done' in AZT trials. Dr David Barry responded with the claim that this was initially the case for the good of patients: there was very limited supply, and it was judged far better to give the drug to those who needed it urgently, rather than use all supplies on clinical trials.

Burroughs Wellcome and many other independent research institutions would spend each subsequent year trying to supplement their data on AZT, trying to find out all the things that would normally be known about a drug before it hit the market. In these later years AZT was to become for many people the symbol of all that was wrong with AIDS research. Once AZT was shown to have worked, at least for a limited time, almost all available funds were channelled to support its development and many other potential treatments were swept aside. AZT was unstoppable, despite the doubts: if you were ill and dying you wanted to believe. After all the despair and uncertainty, people in authority were saying, 'Take this, it'll do you good.' No wonder Martin Sherwood, a Wellcome spokesman, could claim shortly after AZT's launch, that 'In terms of the emotive quality of the demand, there's never been a drug like it.'

Michael Cottrell, a 23-year-old gay man, was one of the first to take AZT in Britain in 1986, before it was widely available. Cottrell says he took AZT for several months, during which time he suffered severe side effects: chronic headaches and nausea, debilitating muscle fatigue. Cottrell felt much worse on AZT than he did off it, but he persevered because it seemed AZT was the only anti-AIDS drug there was:

I had recently been diagnosed HIV positive and I went into a panic. I thought I was going to die. I remembered something about this drug coming from America and everyone clamouring to get it. I was perfectly healthy. My boyfriend's blood count was quite low and he was prescribed it at St Stephen's Hospital and I took it too. Intuitively, I didn't think it was doing me any good. I was prescribed it three times over a period of three years, and I took it out of fear. I was first prescribed 1,200 mg a day, and then 500 mg, but

I still felt bad, even on the lower dose. I had nausea and headaches and muscle fatigue.

Cottrell took it every four hours, which meant he had to have a bleeper that woke him at three or four o'clock every morning. (People joked that the real AIDS money lay in making these bleepers; in New York in the late 1980s, opera performances were punctuated by bleeps.) Cottrell stopped taking AZT after a few weeks, but then he got scared and began taking it once more. 'I got my drugs every two weeks – a big plastic bagful. I felt that I was carrying my life around in that bag.' After his lover died of an AIDS-related illness, Cottrell stopped taking for good; he still has packets of AZT at home and has become an obsessive anti-Wellcome campaigner.

Rudolf Nureyev began taking AZT in 1988, five years before his death. 'AZT was just beginning to be used in France,' said Michel Canesi, his doctor:

I didn't want to give it to him straight away, because I was worried that the side effects would hamper him [Nureyev was still dancing at this time]. Rudi lost his temper and said: 'I want this medicine.' I replied that there hadn't been long enough to judge the results. But I had to give in and prescribe it – he was so insistent. But he didn't take it regularly. He went off every time with tons of drugs, and every time I went to see him I found unused packets all over the place.

The film maker Derek Jarman, who was diagnosed HIV positive in 1986, described a happier scenario. 'It works,' he said:

It holds everything up. It stops the virus replicating. At the beginning they gave people much too massive doses, which affected us physically. I had no recognizable toxic side effects from it.

I was invited by my doctor to make up my mind whether I took the drug or not, so I rang up various people in America and the general advice was to take it – and this was advice from quite radical people, not people in with the Wellcome Foundation. I came off it because my doctor said that my [T4] count was down. We've never discussed it since. He just suddenly said, 'I think you've had enough AZT, Derek,' and I very much trust him, he's a brilliant doctor. The whole thing is so complicated, because I took a lot of

other drugs as well. I had to have suppressants for TB, toxoplasmosis and PCP. And then obviously if I got an infection there was flu-
conazole and all of that area. And then at a certain point they added
hydrocortisone and fludrocortisone to keep my energy up. My feeling about AZT is that I'm glad I took it, even though I can't prove
to you that it did anything. You can say that if it helps someone
psychologically then it must be doing some good. I think the doctors generally feel that it does some good. But how do you know?

At St Stephen's Hospital in south-west London, the frequent use of
AZT had other effects. Haematologists noticed that during 1987 their
HIV positive patients required a very large number of blood transfusions. This was due partly to the ever expanding caseload of patients
ill with AIDS, but partly to the introduction of AZT. About a quarter
of the people treated with the drug developed severe anaemia. During
the ten months to October 1987, 53 positive patients were transfused,
requiring 314 units of blood. Of these 53, 31 were receiving AZT, and
they accounted for 213 of the blood units used. This coincided with a
shortage of blood for transfusion in the south-west Thames region,
and led St Stephen's staff to write to the *BMJ*, suggesting that unless
the number of blood donors increased to meet current demands, it
might be necessary to restrict the use of this new treatment.

Financially, Wellcome plc has done extremely well out of AZT. As
the only big earner to have been launched by the company in the past
decade, the continued success of AZT soon became crucial to its
growth. Share performance has been directly linked to the sales of the
drug and the results of new trials. From a value of £3.74 in February
1987, the share price almost doubled to £7.24 in November 1989;
year-on-year pre-tax profits were up 28 per cent to £283m. In early
1993, the share price would reach 810p; the previous year's pre-tax
profits were logged at £505m.

The first Jerome Horwitz heard of AZT's use against HIV was
when he read about it in the *Wall Street Journal*. Burroughs Wellcome
established a chair in his name at the Michigan Cancer Foundation,
but he has received no financial reward.

'My wife sits across from me at the breakfast table and reminds me
of all the money that Burroughs Wellcome has got from it and I
haven't got a dime. I keep telling her about the legacy I'm leaving.
But I wouldn't be being absolutely straight with you if I hadn't
thought that I should have gotten something out of it.'

At the end of the 1980s, with profits high and sales soaring, Wellcome would face a barrage of protests from gay activists. What began in America soon spread to Britain: offices were picketed, conferences invaded. At first Wellcome defended its pricing on the grounds that AZT took $80m to develop and produce (later revised to $30m), but it soon bowed to pressure (and its economies of scale) and cut the price. The recommended dosage was also reduced for medical reasons, which meant many more people could tolerate its toxicity. In 1988 an annual course of treatment cost about £4,100. In that year the Department of Health AIDS Unit noted in a confidential document that 'wider use of the drug with asymptomatic HIV infected people and the increasing numbers of ARC/AIDS cases will increase the total bill to the NHS dramatically ... with more people with AIDS surviving longer, the pressures of AIDS-related demands on the NHS will become acute – particularly in London'.

'People say we're purely acting out of commercial interests, but it is not in our commercial interests to do anything else but get this drug right,' says Professor Jones. 'We wanted to show people that we are working night and day, weekdays and weekends to try to develop better medicines. Otherwise we look like ogres and robber barons all the time. That's the whole history of our business; if you've got a problem with a product, you must, you must, you must tell people.'

Staff at Wellcome feel that they have been shabbily treated by the media and wrongly accused of self-interest. David Barry found it 'very distressing' to read his papers or watch television news not knowing whether his company would be criticized. Didn't people realize what they were up against?

'The number of people who have shown aggression against us concerns us no end,' says Trevor Jones:

Normally the company tries to distance itself from the patient-physician interaction – it must do: the day-to-day therapy of the patient is not our responsibility. But [in 1990] we started to open our labs to people with HIV and their carers, contrary to the advice of my security and other colleagues. You then realize the uncertainty and the frustrations involved in that act of taking a tablet for the very first time. When people with HIV came through the door of the lab I could almost touch their anger. But I realized that the anger was not really about Wellcome or me, but about their mortality. They were frustrated, and saying, "Please, please what can I do?" These were genuine *cris de coeur*.'

Professor Jones is one of the few pharmaceutical industry representatives on Britain's Medical Controls Agency. Wellcome has clearly selected its spokesman with care. Wellcome's PR machine is an impressive force and much money is spent on convincing the media of AZT's worth. Its in-house magazines talk of the extra 400,000 productive years of life it has made possible through the drug, about how many thorough and independent studies have stressed AZT's efficacy.

Clearly, the criticism hurts. 'I don't take too kindly to people saying, "Oh, you don't want to listen to Wellcome, because they would say that, wouldn't they?"' Jones says. 'You can't hide anything in this business, because otherwise who will trust us when we develop another drug? You have to believe that the integrity of science is good.'

In 1988, full of integrity, Wellcome agreed to the longest and most thorough investigation into AZT yet. It was an independent trial, conducted by British and French researchers, and called Concorde. In many ways it was the ultimate test for the drug: a test not of the drug's efficacy in those already unwell with full-blown AIDS, or AIDS-related complex, but in asymptomatics, those people who had tested positive for HIV antibodies but had not yet become unwell. Would AZT slow the onset of disease? A Dutch study suggested that it did and immediately increased demand for the drug. But doctors were cautious; the results were inconclusive, the study involved just 18 men and lasted six months.

The Concorde trial would last several years and involve over 1,700. If this too showed that AZT delayed the onset of the disease, it would provide new hope to patients and even more millions to Wellcome. In fact, when the results emerged, the effects on Wellcome and hundreds of thousands of patients would be devastating. But that wouldn't be for five years, until 1993. There would be plenty of other disappointments before then.

The MRC Books a Wake-up Call

When Britain's top virologists, bacteriologists, haematologists, immunologists and molecular biologists gathered each month at the Medical Research Council's fine offices near Regent's Park, they walked in fabled footsteps. It was a humbling experience every time you saw the plaque near the door: in 1916 the discovery of the cause of rickets, in 1933 the nailing of the flu virus, in 1953 the double helix of DNA, in 1956 the link between smoking and cancer, in 1987 the role of cholesterol in heart attacks – some of modern science's all-time greatest hits, and the MRC had helped create them all. Ah, progress. Made you proud to be British.

The Medical Research Committee, later the Medical Research Council, began life in 1913 to tackle tuberculosis. A century ago life expectancy was about 45 years; infectious disease was the major cause of death at all ages, and TB claimed 75,000 people each year. The MRC was established partly as a cost-cutting venture; David Lloyd George, Chancellor of the Exchequer, believed it might be cheaper to find a treatment or cure than pay out the sickness and disability benefits promised under the 1911 National Insurance Act.

The MRC gradually took on all forms of disease, all forms of treatment and research patterns. Cancer and heart disease, the biggest killers in the West, now account for the bulk of its efforts and the majority of its expenditure; since the Second World War, most serious infections have tumbled in the face of antibiotics and immunization.

What was the MRC doing about AIDS? A little, but not much, not in the first years. By June 1986, it had funded 12 projects, most of them important but basic things: investigations into the immunology, epidemiology and aetiology of AIDS, blood-screening projects, a study of the biology of HTLV-III infection in Zambia. Most of these studies lasted a few years and cost anything from £3,500 to £160,000. Some of the findings were very useful, some inconclusive. But it was all small-scale, unambitious stuff. For some clinicians who were seeing an ever increasing number of sick patients, the MRC seemed woefully uncommitted to fighting this new virus: apparently there was no urgency; certainly there was very little money.

Money came predominantly from the Department of Education and Science, with special allocations provided by the Health Departments of England, Scotland and Wales, and was distributed by the MRC as it saw fit. Any researcher submitting a grant application faced an elaborate approval system: grants committees, systems boards, cell boards, neurosciences boards, boards that took months to approve anything. Applications would be sent back for redrafting, for cost-cutting. The period from when an application was submitted to when it was first reviewed could take five months. Occasionally, by the time a grant was approved, the science had already moved on to make it redundant, or a similar study had already been announced in the United States. America seemed to be doing so much so fast and Britain so little.

Several early projects were funded not by the MRC, but by grants from pharmaceuticals companies, Wellcome included. The main problem was that the people who knew most about this virus were not the people giving out the money, but the people applying for it.

In February 1987 the MRC Working Party on AIDS gathered for its first full meeting for four months. The doctors were presented with a 14-page document outlining, in mostly glowing terms, what the MRC saw as its contribution to AIDS research thus far. It was 'a remarkable tribute to modern science that so much has been learnt ... British scientists have contributed to the achievements which have already been made'. One achievement, the development of the leading antibody test by Dr Richard Tedder and colleagues at the Middlesex, without which, the document noted, 'we would have to buy French or American products', was not an advance to which the MRC had contributed.

The MRC report recognized that 'much remains to be discovered', about the history and future course of the virus, and much research had to be channelled into finding effective treatments or vaccines. To this end, the MRC was to step up its activities.

Until the end of 1986 the organization had muddled through on existing grants from the Department of Education and Science. Subsequently an MRC official would claim that 'there was an argument from government, when we were bidding for extra money in the early years that, "Oh we don't need to do very much, because the Americans are doing it all".' The DES tells a different story: it says that the MRC had not judged AIDS of sufficient importance ever to ask officially for more money. But just before Christmas, Virginia Bottomley, MP for Surrey South West, lobbed a helpful funding question to her colleague Kenneth Baker, Secretary of State for Education and Science. She wanted to know what was being done with regards to AIDS research. He answered: 'The Government have had urgent discussions with the Medical Research Council on immediate and longer-term aspects of research into AIDS. The MRC requested an increase in their grant in aid of £1 million a year for work that can be put in hand straightaway, and we have agreed.'

Seven weeks later, Dr Jonathan Weber, a research scientist who began his work at St Mary's before joining the Chester Beatty Laboratories at the Institute of Cancer Research, explained why this additional £1 million would be quite inadequate. The amount was piteously small compared to the funds being spent on AIDS in the United States, or indeed on other life-threatening conditions, and it was being given to an incompetent organization. The MRC, an institution not known to welcome public criticism, had never received such a devastating onslaught as the one Dr Weber submitted as a memorandum for the House of Commons Social Services Committee.

'There is no "plan" for research into AIDS in the UK,' he wrote. 'The MRC has decided to lead from behind. At present, the municipality of committees which now exist can only react to AIDS; they cannot enact research, or coordinate the direction of scientists in this country.'

Weber stated that our spending and commitment lagged behind not only the United States, but also France, Sweden, West Germany, Holland, Belgium and Italy. It was not too late to make a difference, he said. Britain had the expertise and the brilliance, and it shouldn't let the rest of the world make the running in the vain hope that results could be simply bought when a breakthrough arrived. He had a proposal: the establishment of a scientific management team, superseding all existing committees, to co-opt many scientists and direct research. It would need £20 million over the next five years. If this approach, or something like it, was not adopted, then Britain would fall even further behind in this field and 'would then resemble, for example, Spain in terms of the ability of our scientists to conduct research'. He concluded: 'The control of this disease ultimately lies with basic science, exactly as did the control of syphilis and gonorrhoea. If we neglect our research now, we will pay the penalty later.'

Weber was not alone in his criticisms. Professor Anthony Coxon, director of the Social Research Unit at University College, Cardiff, laid the groundwork for a national study on behavioural change as a result of AIDS: the number of partners, patterns of high-risk activity, the use of condoms and so on. This would seem to be an important study; Professor Coxon claims it took four years of concerted effort to get funding.

Of course, this kind of thing may not be the MRC's fault. Its defence lies in the fact that its hands were tied by lack of money and that anyway there was not an abundance of fully realized applications. 'It's not as if we were being swamped every week,' says Dr Jane Cope, chief administrator of the MRC's AIDS Secretariat. Some of the applications were incompetent or redundant; others were from inexperienced clinicians.

One might expect a certain amount of bitterness from those researchers who felt poorly treated by the MRC, but the frustrations run deeper than this. Some of those doctors engaging with the MRC as part of its Working Party felt they were mere window dressing; a front, says Tony Pinching, the group's scientific secretary, 'increasingly there to be shown that the MRC was doing something about AIDS … because we had a working party, therefore we were doing something'. The group wrote regular reports for the central MRC systems board. It gave detailed advice and accounts of the work going on elsewhere, and provided a feel of what opportunities existed for particular aspects of research in the UK. Initially there was a strong purpose to the group, which was a useful talking shop; the Department of Health gathered much important information from it. 'But when we submitted our third report [in 1986] we had the distinct impression that we were not having much impact other than as a political exercise,' Tony Pinching says. 'Our reports were received, they said thank you and that was about it. There was a sense that we were just talking into thin air.'

Professor Pinching had a personal grievance too and still feels betrayed. Before climbing the podium at a mid-1980s press conference at which the MRC would discuss its contribution so far, Pinching says he was called aside by Sir James Gowans, the MRC's secretary. Sir James said they must present a unified and optimistic picture: to this end it was important to agree that no grant applications had been turned down purely on financial grounds. For Pinching, who was about to address the assembled journalists on current and proposed immunological research, this was good news, meaning, he assumed, that the £50,000 he had recently applied for to lengthen the scope of an ongoing project at St Mary's would soon be forthcoming; the scientific element of it had already been approved, and it was now just a question of money. So he towed the line at the press conference, only to find just days later that his supplementary application had been turned down.

In February 1987, with reported cases of HIV infection at over 5,000, a detailed report from the MRC was set before the members of the cabinet committee on AIDS. This had an entirely new sense of urgency about it and a new direction. It suggested that a massive injection of funds was now needed. To date £700,000 had been spent on AIDS research; the proposed new budgets presented quite a contrast: £2.5 million in the first year; £5m in the second, £7m in the third, and £10m per year after five years. This was real back-of-the-envelope stuff: the budget was no more detailed than 'Preparation of six viral proteins: £1m' and 'chemical synthesis of peptides as potential vaccines: £0.4m'.

The underlying theme of the report was that scientific research should now be given the sort of impetus recently given to public education. Further, if Britain did not wish to turn its eyes from the potential scale of the global epidemic, then it had a responsibility towards not just its own people, but also those beyond its shores; British science was still ideally placed to lead the world.

The report acknowledged that the needs of AIDS had to be balanced against the claims of other diseases – cancer, heart disease, mental illness – but noted that 'many of these have powerful lobbies'; at this stage very little money was being donated publicly for AIDS research.

The new policy had two prongs: to develop a vaccine and to develop new strategies for anti-viral chemotherapy (more drugs which worked like AZT). The vaccine programme was receiving inadequate attention elsewhere, the report claimed. Private companies were unwilling to invest because of high development costs coupled with an uncertain market and a high litigation risk. The 'market' for a vaccine was an intriguing concept. It was envisaged that first use would be by 'health professionals, spouses of infected individuals and members of the armed forces'. A much wider use of the vaccine was foreseen in Africa, although whether or not any developing country could afford it was another question.

But why not leave it to the Americans after all? The US Public Health Service was due to spend $415m on AIDS in 1987, most of it on research. The MRC was no longer impressed with this: there were gaps in the programme, it argued, and it had received reports that there might be a lack of appropriate expertise amongst US scientists. Europe, by contrast, was ideally poised to make advances; some had already been noted at the Institut Pasteur in Paris and the Tropical Diseases Institute in Antwerp. In Glasgow, a team led by Professor William Jarrett had developed a vaccine against a virus from the same family as HIV – the cat leukaemia virus. This was now ready for commercial exploitation and there were hopes that a key factor in the vaccine – an extract from the bark of Brazilian oak trees that had been used by Amazonian Indians as a treatment for wounds – might be modified for use in an AIDS vaccine.

Vaccines act by mimicking an infectious agent and stimulating the immune system to resist a particular infection, predominantly through producing antibodies and in this case cytotoxic T-lymphocytes. Inevitably there were endless safety problems. Any vaccine must be sufficiently similar to a virus to be effective, but sufficiently different not to cause disease. Viral vaccines could consist of modified live viruses, killed viruses or virus components. This system had been established for decades. The specific problems with HIV seemed to be infinite, however. HIV had a variety of mutating strains (there was RF, BH-10, ARV-2 and countless others); later it would be shown that the DNA sequence can even change within a single person during the course of infection. No virus had ever posed a dilemma like this: because so much still had to be learnt about the molecular biology, about the way the virus spread from cell to cell, about the role of macrophages (large scavenging cells), and about the proteins which determine the structure and activity of the virus, it was not just the goalposts that were moving, but the pitch, the shape of the ball, the members of the teams. And there were some very practical problems. Mice and rabbits could be used for initial studies, but subsequent tests were best conducted on chimpanzees, the only suitable animal model found to be infectable with the virus; animal rights protesters had already invaded labs in the United States. And how could you recruit participants for human trials, even using artificially simulated portions of the virus?

As for developing effective anti-viral drugs, high levels of toxicity seemed unavoidable. Help was sought from strange quarters: Dr Max Perutz, chairman of the MRC's anti-virals committee, expressed hopes that an extract from an Australian chestnut might have some effect in reducing the toxicity of AZT. When AZT was later joined by other anti-virals dideoxycytidine (ddC) and dideoxyinosine (ddI), it became clear that these too could have devastating side effects on the nervous system and the pancreas. The process of infection was found to be far more complex than was originally believed. It was thought that HIV caused the destruction of T4 'helper' cells simply by infecting them. Then it was found that even in patients in the latter stages of AIDS (those who had very low T4 counts), the proportion of those cells that was producing HIV was small – about one in 40. The complexities continued to multiply; the nearer the mountain came, the taller it looked.

But when the MRC laid its new proposals before the cabinet committee in February 1987, there was much optimism. The key to it was the suggestion that the MRC should direct research centrally (it was called the AIDS Directed Programme) and that scientists from different disciplines should collaborate. 'We were pushing the research in a certain direction,' says Dr Jane Cope, who administered the AIDS Directed Programme, 'and if people bid for funds for work that wasn't within the confines of what we wanted, then we wouldn't fund it. To that extent the scientists were being constrained.'

Industrial sponsorship was also sought in return for agreements on commercial exploitation, and deals were struck with Wellcome, Glaxo and others to fund various strands of academic research.

Only a few weeks after the MRC report, the Whitelaw Committee provided almost everything it had asked for. It received £14.5m over three years and the new directed programme got underway. The old peer review system was swept aside in favour of another specialist fast-track AIDS review board which met nine times a year and could give the green light to projects within weeks.

This was a great improvement, but some grievances remained from the AIDS Working Party. This group was not consulted in the formation of the new plans, thus confirming earlier suspicions that the members were being used as a political exercise. Money was now distributed freely to many people who had not been involved directly in AIDS work before, 'not until the money came in', as one Working Party member perceived it. Professor Pinching and several others were taken off the committees for a while, or removed themselves.

'At that time, in '87, there were very few people working in AIDS research in this country,' says Professor Alan Stone, a molecular biologist who has worked at the MRC since 1975 and became head of its AIDS programme in 1990. 'The amount of funding we needed was guesswork, because until we knew we had some money we couldn't really encourage people to get into this in a big way, and the sums were basically worked out on the best available evidence. I think at the time the difficulty of dealing with the AIDS problem was underestimated.'

Epidemiological studies and other non-therapeutic research were to continue very much as before, with much less money, and no fast track, although there was a new system of special project grants which could be speeded through if thought fit. This was called the Strategic Programme, although there was no strategy. 'It doesn't actually mean anything,' Dr Cope said of the name, 'but it sounds better than the non-directed programme, which people were calling it, which made it sound terribly negative.'

So this was a new dawn. Money was rolling out of the MRC headquarters as if, suddenly, there was a serious epidemic to deal with. Twenty-six grants were issued in the first few months, for crucial work in most areas. In November 1987, with 1,170 reported cases of AIDS in the UK (another 7,000 were HIV positive) and about 16,000 AIDS cases reported in Europe, almost all the scientists working on these new projects met in London to compare notes. Perhaps there would be a vaccine, which would place their names alongside the creators of vaccines for smallpox, typhoid or cholera. There was talk of this happening within five years. Subsequently, one of the doctors likened the process to a giant jigsaw puzzle, where each piece added was essential, but very modest. No one could see the picture unless they stood back. And when they did, many years later, they found that mostly they had been filling in sky.

Camouflage

At the end of 1987, Sheila Dutch walked around west London trying to drum up local support for a project called the London Lighthouse. The Lighthouse was to be a beautifully designed building on the site of an old school in Lancaster Road, just down from Portobello market; on its completion, AIDS care would have come of age. Part hospice, part alternative treatment centre, the Lighthouse would treat people with AIDS and HIV in an environment of support and spiritual nourishment. Detractors would later mock its New Age mentality, its karmic properties, but they were in no doubt that this was a novel approach to treatment and a complementary service to acute hospital care and AZT.

Local residents did not want an AIDS hospice in their area, and as Sheila Dutch toured the neighbouring estates to explain the building site, she encountered much opposition: we do not want these degenerates here; this disease is not our problem. They were right of course: it wasn't their problem, though its transmission might still have been their fear. When Dutch visited a local flower shop, they didn't want to know. 'Now of course they love the place, and it's their biggest client.'

The Lighthouse was largely the vision of Christopher Spence. An eloquent gay man, Spence had worked as private secretary to Selwyn Lloyd, the Speaker of the House of Commons, and subsequently as a management consultant and in community care and bereavement projects. In 1985, two of his friends died of AIDS. One, Frank Wilson, he helped nurse to the end, and it was a bitter experience. AIDS care at the Hammersmith Hospital was appalling. This was still the time of 'barrier' nursing, when not just surgical masks but galoshes were worn for everyday care. Few could bring themselves to treat his friend as human; domiciliary care services for the dying operated by the Paddington and North Kensington health district specifically excluded people with AIDS.

And so Spence had stumbled across a glaring need, a gap in the care market. In 1986, after working with other groups on various support services, his dream began in earnest: the aim was to 'guide people safely home' by providing a continuum of care for an increasing number of men, women and children. This would include the provision of counselling for those with asymptomatic HIV, through to providing an environment where the terminally ill could die with dignity. It was envisaged the project would cost £2.5m. It was hoped that it would be duplicated in other urban areas as the disease spread.

And soon the stories started, that corpses would be displayed in glass cases outside, that the surrounding air would be contaminated. As a deep crater was being dug for the liftshaft, one local resident standing at the gate said to another, 'There you are, you see, that's the pit they're digging to throw the bodies into.' Shortly after he had applied for planning permission, Spence left his house across the road to find a skull and crossbones nailed to his front door alongside the words 'AIDS death house'.

The response from funders was more positive. The Lighthouse was presented as a well-articulated proposal in a vacuum; for the regional health authority with no formulated response to a looming crisis, it was an attractive proposition. But it was a costly one, and the early meetings with the Department of Health were not fruitful. The plan was for statutory services to match pound for pound what could be raised in the independent sector, and so Spence and his colleagues sat down with civil servants at the DHSS in 1986 and asked for £1m, half of the cost of the capital project. One official looked at Spence over the top of his glasses and said, 'Really, Mr Spence, we were looking at something more in the order of £10,000.'

'They prevaricated and prevaricated, partly to see whether you're fundable and whether you're going to stay the course,' Spence says. 'They wouldn't commit even to £10,000 until May 1987. Mrs Thatcher called a general election, and I rang the department and said, "Unless the government commits significant capital funding to this project, I am going to have to call my building programme to a halt and that is not going to look very good for you during the campaign."' He says he got a commitment within 24 hours.

At the beginning of 1988, the trick worked again. During boom time, the project cost had inevitably rocketed and the project had expanded. The total bill was now £4.85m and Spence needed more money. Enter the world health ministers for a Westminster summit; how could the government hosting the conference be seen to deny more money to a flagship project?

The first floor of the building opened in July 1988, the 23-bed residential unit in September 1988 and Princess Margaret rolled up two months later to cut the cake. She said she had never opened a place like this – such splendour, such warmth. She meant this kindly, but others took a less charitable view: 'The Lighthouse is a heartbreak hotel where half the guests sign in to die,' one newspaper reported in a piece entitled 'Inside the AIDS Hilton'. The article gasped at the mineral water in the fridges, the original art on the wall, the lovingly polished floor and geometric print curtains in the Ian McKellen room. Here was disease Conran style, where every Swedish bed 'had pine headboards with luxurious duvets or cool, cream cotton sheets'. Goodness, this place was nicer than the reporter's own house, and Paul Getty, Dustin Hoffman, Simon Callow, Joan Collins, Sheila Hancock and Frances de la Tour had all given or raised money for it.

There was a series of open days, at which doctors and other health workers were invited to tour the building, hear of its history, ask some questions. At one, a genito-urinary consultant raised his hand: 'I'm a consultant in genito-urinary medicine in Derby, and I don't want to sound a sour note, because I'm all for good patient care and people dying with dignity, but really this is ridiculous, completely ludicrous, such an over the top, luxurious place.'

Spence rose to do his value-for-money, comparative cost bit, when another NHS employee got in first. He said: 'The main emotion I have to contend with in going round this place is envy. I'm envious because I know that every patient I treat in the NHS deserves this quality of care and I know they don't get it.'

All the health ministers have been on a tour and all have pledged support. It would not be until 1993 that Virginia Bottomley would reduce the project's funding for the first time. It is now part of Lighthouse folklore that on one visit in the early 1990s she turned to a departmental colleague and said, 'If I see one more gay man sitting on a Heal's chair I will scream.'

Sheila Dutch has herself been instrumental in establishing a new form of AIDS care. Many grateful letters mark her achievements. One of them reads:

Dear Sheila,
I met you briefly in June last year when my partner went to you for advice on camouflaging the KS lesions on his face. Your time you spent with him made such a difference to the quality of his life. His old confidence, and enjoyment in going to work, and meeting people returned. Also it gave him the confidence to stop the chemotherapy, which until that time was the only hope he had been given for dealing with the KS, despite its side-effects.
He died just before Christmas, on the 23rd, but was still going out and living his life until two weeks prior to this. In fact his last trip out was to dinner at the Ritz on 9 December. None of this would have been possible without your help and advice.
Not long ago he reordered the products he used but never needed them. Rather than return them to the pharmacist or the manufacturer who have already profited once from them, I'm hoping that they may be of use to you.

Dutch was 57 when she joined the London Lighthouse as a volunteer. A middle-class woman from a small village near Tunbridge Wells, Kent, she'd been having some marital problems and decided to live in London and find something useful to do, something a long way from the building company she ran with her husband.

When she read about plans for the Lighthouse in the local paper, she was terrified of AIDS. 'I certainly didn't mind answering the phone, but I didn't want anything to do with anyone who was ill.' When she met her first person with AIDS she had to turn her face. She did the books, ran the café, unaware she was working with people who were HIV positive. Her attitude was 'Let's help these poor victims.'

Then she got a part-time job on the residential unit, administration mainly, looking after the stock and assisting the nurses. 'I found that an awful lot of gay men are desperately looking for a mother or an aunt, so I got very close to some of the younger men. One boy in particular, he wouldn't go to have a blood test unless I was holding his hand. And their mothers would often confide in me, talking about little Johnny as a baby. Lots of crying.'

One day she was talking to a man who said, 'My ex-partner's coming over from Paris, he wants to take me to tea at the Inn on the Park, but I can't go.' Why not? 'Because I've got this mark.' There was a spot on his face no bigger than the moles on her face, Dutch says. She was just about to say, 'Oh don't be so stupid', when she remembered that her mother had said exactly the same thing to her when she was 19 and had discovered a spot on her face on the eve of a big date.

She put some of her make-up on him, which gave him enough confidence to go out. She attended a course for burns and prosthesis camouflage and began to help three or four new people at the Lighthouse each month.

At home up the road, she gets out a red toolbox with her powders and creams and demonstrates on a blemish on her hand. 'Forget the word make-up. You should see it as a damaged portrait painting. It's not slapping powder over anyone's face, what you do is paint things out. There are tricks: I've found you can hide the dark KS with a light mauve.'

She will see someone for an hour. She gives them a mirror and makes them watch, and teaches them to apply the camouflage themselves. It has transformed people's lives; people hold down their jobs, go to supermarkets without feeling freakish.

'What is so frightening about KS is not recognizing yourself,' Dutch says. 'Also, when you get KS, that's it, you can't tell yourself you've cheated the virus. It's a death sentence. It's like being rediagnosed.'

One man she knows can't bear to see himself without camouflage. 'He takes it off in bed in the dark and tries to apply it without a mirror. He felt that in the morning when he put it on the disease got better, and in the evening when he took it off, it got worse.'

Chapter 8: The Church Has AIDS

The fear of disease is a happy restraint to men. If men were more healthy,
'tis a great chance they would be less righteous.
Edmund Massey, speaking at St Andrew's Church, Holborn, London, July 1722

People with HIV and AIDS have been told that they are responsible for
this disease; that they have brought it on themselves; that they are to
blame. People with HIV are not immune to these messages. It is easy,
unless one is very strong, to fall into the trap of saying to oneself, 'I got
this disease because I am gay, or because I got addicted to drugs ...
because I sinned, if you like ... perhaps I do deserve to die.' I wonder if
you can imagine how exhausting it is to resist all those negative messages
and how difficult to find, in that avalanche of emotional and spiritual violence, a calm place for a moment of self-affirmation and self-forgiveness.
Jonathan Grimshaw, director of Body Positive, addressing a Consultation organized
by the British Council of Churches and Free Church Federal Council, 1988

The first funeral I took was of a young doctor in 1984. You didn't
mention AIDS, only cancer or pneumonia. I kept in touch with his
lover and I took *his* funeral in 1993.

The second funeral I took was much worse. I got a call from a distraught young man in south London and went down to see him. His
lover had died, and the parents hadn't been helpful. They lived in the
Isle of Wight, and they had known for some time that their son was
ill, but they wouldn't take him home as they feared that their neighbours would discover what was wrong with him. The parents said
they wouldn't be at the London funeral, but they would go to
Guildford Cathedral and say their prayers at 11 o'clock, the exact
same time that the service was taking place. It was almost symbolic,
that they would go half way. I was so appalled by all of this. I had led
a rather sheltered life, had never been persecuted or oppressed, but I
suddenly discovered that there was this group of people who were
either being pushed out or hidden away.

*Malcolm Johnson, 57, gay, worked for 18 years as Rector of St Botolph's
Church, Aldgate, in the City of London. Much of his time was spent with
the homeless, but he also established a counselling service for gay men and*

lesbians in an attempt to help them find an equilibrium between their religion and their sexuality. He was once briefly married: 'an awful mistake'. He has been with his male partner for 25 years. He believes the Church of England remains 'hopelessly closety'; he runs a support group for about 450 gay priests and believes few of them are celibate. He is a sober, conservative man, far from the sitcom 'hip vicar'. He now works at the Royal Foundation of St Catherine, a retreat and conference centre in London's Docklands.

I was right in the middle of it when AIDS started. I was terrified first of all that I was going to catch it. I remember going on holiday in 1983 thinking 'that was it'. I still haven't gone for a test, so I don't know if I've got the virus or not. My partner is still feeling healthy too. Until I get the symptoms I'm not sure I could handle the knowledge.

There was a friend of mine, the chaplain of Chelmsford Prison, who died [in January 1985]. That upset me and my partner terribly. It was all over the front pages of the tabloids. He died very quickly. We knew he was ill and suspected it was AIDS, but it was heavily hidden. I'm not sure that he ever knew. He was Australian, and his parents came to England to find out he was gay and that he had AIDS all in one hour. The funeral was very quiet, there was no memorial service, and it was all left very unsatisfactorily. I think that was the thing that made the Christian Church realize that AIDS isn't just a thing that happens to other people.

I realized I had to find out more about what was going on and so I went to America. I went to Massachusetts, Connecticut and New York, and talked to doctors and hospital chaplains about what could be done; of course people weren't expected to live long at all. In New York I went to the General Theological Seminary where people were talking about whether it was God's punishment. Then later on holiday I went to Los Angeles where our two closest friends were HIV positive and that upset us a great deal. They subsequently died.

When I got back we formed a thing called the Minister's Group, fifteen or twenty of us who were working with young people. We had the first conference for Christian ministers at King's College in 1986 in London – evangelical ministers, Catholic ministers were all there. The Bishop of Edinburgh chaired it and at the end of the day he said that he had learnt a lot from the day. He told me that up until then he thought that rimming and frottage were West Country solicitors.

We then asked William Swing, the Bishop of California, to come over. He'd been a very homophobic priest from Virginia, but then he moved to San Francisco and saw at first hand the suffering that was going on. Not one of the churches that he looked after was free of AIDS. He met with the Bishop of London, Graham Leonard, and they talked about what happens when a priest is infected. To their credit they listened and asked questions and decided they would help in getting the priest early retirement. They published guidelines on how to deal with it and deal with the media. There were several clergy of course who were infected.

From about 1987 I've been most impressed with what the Church of England has done. The Mildmay Mission Hospital, for instance, which comes from the evangelical side, from a group of Christians who would not condone any genital acts between men or between women, they went straight into the field by offering their hospital. The cynics would say that it would have closed had AIDS not come along, but I think that's unkind, because the Mildmay governors immediately saw human suffering and thought they must get involved. I think overall the Church come out of this with credit.

People now no longer see it as God's judgement. I don't think I've heard that argument in the Christian Church in the last five years, that this is the punishment for an 'intrinsically disordered way of life', as it says in the Catholic Encyclopaedia. Only the nutcases believe that now. There was a very good debate in the General Synod in 1987 when the Archbishop of Canterbury, Robert Runcie, said that the bedside of a dying man is not the place to sort out your theology of sexuality. The leadership came right from the top, although it took until 1987 for that to happen.

I tend to get to know people a lot more now. I get calls from people who say, 'Will you take my partner's funeral?' I say, 'Yes of course, when is it?' and they say, 'Oh, he's only just been diagnosed.' It's good now not just to get wheeled in to take the service at the end.

The best funerals are always the simplest and most sincere, those are the ones I find most upsetting. Actually very few people think about how upset the minister might be. Recently I took the funeral of a young potter, and the church was packed with lots of people from the arts, including Gilbert and George, and it was an overpowering occasion. One has to be professional and not cry, or not show that you are too distraught. But if you do weep, I don't think you should be upset about it, but I don't think it's very good practice really. At that funeral before I went in the priest of the church put his arms round me and said, 'I will just say a prayer for you, because you need support,' and that was a very moving thing.

Malcolm Johnson spoke in the General Synod debate on AIDS in November 1987, the first and only time the subject has been discussed by the governing body of the Anglican Church. It was a level-headed afternoon, full of concern and pity. 'Whatever we conclude about judgement,' said the Bishop of Gloucester, John Yates, in the opening address, 'the primary need is to show the face of love and compassion.'

The debate was suffused with traditional theology. Few doubted that adherence to the Church's teachings on chastity and fidelity would halt the spread of AIDS through sexual intercourse. 'The challenge of the Churches is to find ways of doing that positively and attractively, rather than negatively and judgementally,' the Rt. Revd Yates maintained.

Timothy Royle, also from Gloucester, was the first to point the finger. The root cause of so many deaths was plain: plain wrongdoing. The fundamentalist's language of homophobia has a tang all of its own: Royle objected to 'the physical misuse of bodily passages or functions ... that is the corruption of the created purpose, and it must be wrong'. The Terrence Higgins Trust had produced a safer sex leaflet which described practices that were 'clearly a perversion ... if, as Christians, we believe that our bodies are temples of the Holy Spirit, we must be corrupting and desecrating them by such actions as described in the leaflet. Why can we not say so?' His words would be reinforced in the following day's debate on homosexuality and the Church, led by Tony Higton, the rector of Hawkwell, Essex, who had claimed previously that he knew of at least 20 gay clergymen with AIDS. How did he come by this figure? He knew of a specialist who was treating them all.

Malcolm Johnson rose to his feet: there was talk of fidelity in the heterosexual world, so why not in the homosexual world? Gay relationships could be 'spiritual, emotional, mental and physical', he said, suggesting that one way to avoid promiscuity was to encourage gay people to make deep long-term relationships, 'not out of fear, but out of love'.

Several Anglican Church organizations issued guidelines on AIDS and pastoral care, as well as more detailed advice on the use of condoms and the chalice. For Margaret Thatcher, the Church's moral guidance did not go nearly far enough. Her health ministers believed it was not the job of government to take a moral stance, so the Prime Minister looked instead to the Church, but told *Woman's Own* magazine that she found it wanting. Indeed, if the Church had done more, her government might have needed to do less: 'Churches are your great institutions ... when the authority of those institutions is undermined because they haven't been forthright, it is then that people turn too much to the State.'

Some clergy may have been too forthright even for Mrs Thatcher. Robert Simpson, a vicar from Barmston, Humberside, vowed to take his 18-year-old son Chris to a mountain and shoot him if he developed AIDS. 'Chris would not get closer to me than six yards. He would be a dead man,' the Revd Simpson told the *Sun*. 'And that would go for the rest of my family as well as strangers.' He feared that in six years' time, more than a million people would have AIDS in Britain. Family would be against family; gun law would prevail. What did young Chris feel about it all? 'I don't think I would like Dad to shoot me ... Sometimes I think he would like to shoot me whether I had AIDS or not.'

The Revd Simpson said he would ban practising gays from taking communion lest they infect the chalice wine. This was a common concern. In January 1987 churchgoers at King's College Chapel, Cambridge, were urged not to drink from the chalice, but instead to take bread and dip the edge of it into the wine before consumption. This was compassion with a twist: 'Carriers of the disease are more vulnerable to infection than anyone else,' explained chaplain Stephen Coles; the request was thus more to protect them than other people. 'It will allow them to take full communion without picking up the germs of other worshippers.'

More novel concern was shown by the Venerable Bazil March, Archdeacon of Northampton, who proposed that all brides and grooms should take an HIV test before marriage. 'It would be a little like having a car MOT,' he reasoned. 'Marriage is all about love, and love is about being open with each other. So why not have the tests?' Sex, in this equation, was not a premarital option. As the *Church Times* editorial noted with some relief, 'we are witnessing the end of the era when sex outside marriage seemed to incur no dangers'; for so long it was considered inconceivable that a 'puritan' morality would find favour again.

This effect was welcomed equally by leaders of other faiths.

Addressing the Union of Jewish Students in London in 1987, the Chief Rabbi, Sir Immanuel Jakobovits, found that 'the black cloud of this scourge may have its silver lining, challenging us to restore the respect for marriage'. The Chief Rabbi offered the students some clear guidelines: AIDS was not divine vengeance and the reproof of saying someone deserved it was 'utterly un-Jewish'. None the less, the current devastation was 'a consequence of a form of life that is morally unacceptable, and utterly repugnant'.

The Liberal and Reform wings of the faith took a less dogmatic line, as did the Jewish AIDS Trust, a group established in 1988 to provide a non-judgemental service of education, counselling and financial support. No issue divided the community like condoms. Although some progressives advocated their use on health grounds, more orthodox Jews regarded any form of barrier contraceptives as being against Jewish law.

The Chief Rabbi believed that condoms might encourage, rather than limit, the spread of AIDS: they provided a false sense of security, were not entirely reliable and 'in the end, when the moment of temptation comes, the lovers at the height of their passion will forget'. Roman Catholic bishops, speaking in Dublin, used a similar line when they rejected condom use in 1987; it would only encourage promiscuity. It was 'moral disorder' that led to AIDS and its containment thus had an easy solution. Less easy, perhaps, would be the containment of the news that one of its own priests had become infected.

*

I was ordained quite late, at 31. I chose not to work in the local church, and I had been working as a Catholic missionary in East Africa for just over eight years when I became ill. I'd had malaria and different things, but that's par for the course. This time I got very sick. I had to be driven to the hospital, and I had malaria, pneumonia, and I was coughing blood that night.

John White, 48, was born in Larne, a coastal town 20 miles from Belfast. He trained as a nurse in Antrim and worked in the civil service in Belfast before joining the Church as a member of the Kiltegan missionary order. He has short, grey/white hair and a full beard. His soft voice is punctuated by a dry cough.

After two weeks I was well enough to go to Nairobi. Back in 1986, people still knew very little about AIDS; what I knew was mostly

from *Newsweek* and *Time* and the *Guardian Weekly*. As a gay man, I
knew that in the past I could have been at risk. In Uganda they were
talking about 'Slim', but in Kenya people weren't talking about it as a
big thing and the doctor who saw me in Nairobi had probably never
seen a case of AIDS before. He said it was unlikely I had it, but said
he'd give me a test to reassure me. When I went back for the results
three weeks later he said I was 'slightly positive', which was an interesting thing I thought, a bit like being slightly pregnant. He said he'd
ask an American friend to do a different version of the test. It was
positive again.

I went back up country and decided to come home. The news to
me meant that I'd probably very soon become very ill in horrible ways
and face all sorts of prejudice no matter where I was, but certainly in
Africa. I thought I'd be dead within a year, so I came home really to
face the illness and die. I told my regional director and my bishop
that I probably had a terminal condition, but not what it was. I spent
a month at the mission preparing to come back.

I came via London, and went to the Hospital for Tropical Diseases.
I had no idea that HIV was treated at STD clinics – that sort of
information was far too practical to reach me in Africa. I also felt that
hospital would be a good cover. I spent three weeks in London,
became retested, and the woman doctor was from Northern Ireland,
not very far from where I lived. Obviously I was very nervous about
confidentiality.

I then went to see my boss of my order in the Republic. He was
very sympathetic and very concerned, but very ignorant. He learnt
from me. The question was what to do, because I was still quite well
at that time.

I went on a renewal course run by the Church for returning missionaries. They were really into all that stuff – getting back in touch
with your feelings. When you go into the Church you're supposed to
deny that you have feelings and needs and repress all this stuff and be
above it. I got sick during the course and began to pass blood. It was
just outside Dublin and I had to find a sympathetic doctor; the whole
idea of finding that one sympathetic doctor now seems like an age
away, but that's what it was like in 1986. I found this well-known
Jewish chap and he put me in St James' Hospital, which was well-
meaning, but really awful, treating people in the corridor, putting
huge warning stickers on the outside of my file. I hadn't told anyone
on the course and I still hadn't told my family, so I had no visitors.

With all the people I had told – my superiors, doctors – you almost end up supporting them, they're so stunned and you end up telling them everything you know about it, and I couldn't face going through that with my family just yet. I spent Christmas with them and then left for London. I wanted to remain as anonymous as I could. With my family I still had the feeling that it might be over very soon and they wouldn't have to know until the end. Looking back it was crazy, but lots of people get locked into that.

I hadn't really come to terms with my sexuality. I had a sort of dual life, and although I didn't deny the fact that I was gay, I was able to shut it down for long periods. I didn't have relationships within the Church. But on a personal level that dual life has a devastating effect.

I got a new short-term job as a chaplain at a big hospital in Slough, near Heathrow, and then I applied for a posting in the Westminster diocese. I told my Superior General that I believed they should know what they're getting, but he said, 'No, they wouldn't be able to handle it.' That's very much the Church attitude: 'Don't tell us and we won't have to deal with it.' The downside of that is that you live and deal with it all yourself and then die with it yourself. It's actually a very uncaring attitude. He said that if I was an alcoholic, as a lot of missionaries are, they wouldn't want to know, and that can actually be a lot more devastating for the parish.

I fell ill again, with horrendous dysentery. In America I think I would have got an AIDS diagnosis for that, but not over here, and that makes a great psychological difference. But by this time I had decided that I had to be open about it in the Church and let people know, for them as well as me. I saw several bishops, who were all very good on tea and sympathy. I was always advised to keep quiet. Eventually the cardinal called a meeting of the area bishops to discuss my case and eventually I was told there was no job for me.

The order kept my salary going, but basically I was advised to go somewhere and be looked after. They were trying to shoo me away, keep me hidden. So disempowering. The cardinal never asked to see me, which I think is a fine example of pastoral care. The Catholic Church would never have any trouble giving you what you wanted financially, but there was no way it could deal with the fact that AIDS was a reality in its ranks. It's different if it happens amongst lay people; they could deal with it because it's them and us. And it's not as if I was the first. Other priests had already had AIDS and died, but they'd covered it up. There was a case recently of a man practically being taken back to Ireland under cover of darkness to die.

The whole issue of sexuality never came into it either, because that would have been much too much for them. All they knew was that it was HIV, and they have presumed that it was related to gay sex, or just sex, or Africa or mosquito bites, or blood transfusion, but I never said anything to them. So at least they didn't discriminate on that basis – they just discriminated across the board. And I was never a threat to them, I was never as outspoken as I am now. So I felt huge rejection. The irony was that in December 1987 the Christmas message from the Pope was 'look after your sons and daughters with AIDS'. People were saying, 'Isn't it wonderful that he said that', but I thought it was really dreadful that he had to say it in the first place, saying it to the wonderfully caring 'love in action' Church? Wasn't that an awful indictment of Christianity?

When I told my family in 1988 the reactions were very mixed. At that point they didn't even know I was gay. My parents were both dead, but I have eight sisters and a brother, all married with lots of kids, that sort of thing. It varied from as good as you could expect to quite bad. There was no outright objection, but I was very sensitive to the little things, things like 'We love you *anyway*.' They accepted it so long as nobody else knew. The real facing for them was when other people found out. I did a local television broadcast and that was quite hard for them I think. By the time of the Vatican incident they'd just about got used to it.

The Vatican Conference on AIDS was this huge hyped thing, about a thousand delegates from eighty-six countries. This was the only conference on AIDS they ever had, in this newly built mod-cons conference centre within the Vatican. You got simultaneous translations, huge portfolios, special postage stamps. There were a lot of medical people there, including Robert Gallo and Luc Montagnier [the co-discoverers of HIV] and a lot of people with experience of the developing world. Mother Theresa of Calcutta was supposed to be there, but she got sick and didn't come, which a lot of us were quite happy about.

But there were no AIDS organizations invited, no women speakers and no chance to liaise or really meet up with people. The way the Vatican does conferences is really something else, so controlled and so manipulated. The addresses had titles like 'Is AIDS a Divine Punishment?' and 'AIDS as a Problem of the Family and Society'.

The opening address was from Cardinal O'Connor, Archbishop of New York, which really set the tone. The closing address was from the Pope. [The conference was entitled 'To Live: Why?']

I was working with a group called Catholic AIDS Link, an organization set up by a former priest and a few others, an unofficial information group. Before the conference we wrote in very sweet terms saying, 'Wouldn't it be great if there was someone with HIV or AIDS addressing the conference?' We got a stinger of a letter back telling us to mind our own business.

A few weeks before, I took part in a march down Oxford Street with about sixty or seventy others from the Church, collecting signatures for a petition to be sent to the Archbishop of Canterbury and Cardinal Hume – a sort of AIDS awareness thing. Normally it's impossible to get a route through Oxford Street on a Saturday, but the police said, 'Oh it's only priests and sisters, no problem!' We were going to call it Walk for Life or something abysmal, which sounded like anti-abortion, but it was then decided we had to get the words Church and AIDS in the title, so we ended up with 'The Church Has AIDS', the Church in this sense meaning the people of God, not the institution or buildings. We did this big banner and this big banner somehow made it into my suitcase for the Vatican conference. I thought that if I was supposed to sit there while they were coming out with this whole 'wrath of God' thing, then I might not be able to stand it. I really hoped the banner would stay at the bottom of my case.

The first morning of the conference arrived and the hall was so packed they needed overflow rooms. O'Connor spoke, and there were some good bits in it, like how he held a woman's hand on Christmas Day who was dying of AIDS, good/nauseating stuff like that, but the rest of it was pretty awful, about how scientists and other health officials were fooling people and had no moral standards because they told people with AIDS to use condoms. Then we had the Pope's personal adviser on moral issues. He stressed that prophylactics were an absolute no-go area. He said that if a married man discovered he was HIV positive, there were only two alternatives: they could either live together celibately as brother and sister, or they could risk the virus. That was it. You couldn't ask questions afterwards and there was no time for any discussion or opposing views. The overriding messages were simply that drug users were criminals, that homosexuals were deviants and that they had chosen to have these lifestyles and therefore these were the risks they took. Some people even expressed the attitude that AIDS would take care of a lot of the problems they had in the Church.

Before the end of the morning I couldn't take any more, so I went back to my little *pensione*. I got the banner and put it inside my cardigan. Then I put on the Roman collar. I went back into the conference hall where Montagnier was finishing his speech. I decided that I wasn't going to wait until the end of the conference, because it could have backfired if I'd done anything during the Pope.

I was absolutely terrified, really shaking. I sat on the steps near the podium. I waited until Montagnier had finished, and when the guy got ready to introduce the next speaker I moved forward, held up the banner and I wasn't going to say anything, but at the last minute decided I would. I said in a loud voice, 'I am living with AIDS, and people with AIDS have no voice at this conference.' The security guys hustled me out and threw people out of the way; the Reuter guy complained later that he had been thrown aside. They hustled me down into the lift and into a car which took me to the Vatican police station.

They found an elderly American nun to translate. They tried to prove first that I wasn't a priest, that I wasn't an official delegate. They took my banner and my security pass. After a while I asked if I was under arrest and they said no, so I asked to leave. They escorted me back to the cobblestones outside, and people were pouring out from the conference for lunch and loads of people came up to me and most were very supportive. I think I was talking to people there in the square for about five hours until it got very cold. Jonathan Mann [the director of the World Health Organization's Global Programme on AIDS] came up to me, and it became clear I wasn't the only one who felt like this. One German doctor wanted to give me his pass, but they clearly would have recognized me. The next morning, the Italian press were full of it, saying that the very people that the conference was designed to help weren't being given a voice and I got a call at my *pensione* from the Archbishop, saying I could come back in but I had to promise not to speak. I refused to make any promise, but I did stay quiet; I was tagged by security guys the whole time. Then there was this big face-saving exercise – cardinals couldn't embrace me quickly enough, especially if there was a camera close by.

Father White became famous for a while. Time *magazine ran a story entitled 'AIDS Ruckus In the Vatican';* Capital Gay *reported 'Priest Sets Rome On Fire'. Suddenly many more officials in the Church wanted to meet him. His health has remained fairly stable; some chest problems, a low T-cell count. He shuns antibiotics in favour of acupuncture and homeopathy, and maintains an active life. He has worked at the London Lighthouse for many years, first as a volunteer and most recently as a pastoral care co-ordinator. He has been in therapy for the last seven years, a process he describes as his 'lifeline', and has himself trained as a psychotherapist; he takes private clients one day a week. He is in a steady relationship.*

I don't think things have changed that much. If my situation was to happen again today I think it would be handled a bit more skilfully, but I think this would be based on the hassle they'd avoid, rather than on a great change in attitudes. They have become more aware of potential problems. But I have no doubt that similar things go on, with abysmal ignorance still. A bishop contacted me at the Lighthouse with a question: he said, 'I have a young priest who has just discovered he has AIDS and I want to know where can I send him?' Where could he send him to do what – treatment, counselling? He was basically saying, 'How can I ease him out of the picture?' I heard later that they had sent him to nuns in Dublin to take care of him. But you're not always ill. Of course with that sort of attitude you will be ill. Thankfully some individual people and groups connected with Churches are responding with care and concern, even if the institutional Churches are not.

I'm still a Catholic, though I'm thinking of leaving my order. I don't like the phrase 'lapsed Catholic'. I see myself more as a recovering Catholic.

CHAPTER 9: Protest

Jobs for the Boys

In 1987, the British airline Dan Air got into a spot of bother with the Sex Discrimination Act. This was a small affair, but it was a symptom of a growing trend and occurred at a time when discrimination against those with HIV and AIDS was common practice among employers. Some of this was prejudice, some plain confusion: what measures should a company take to protect its workforce and customers? Was an employee obliged to declare his or her HIV status? Should all employees be subjected to tests?

High in the sky, Dan Air thought it had found a satisfactory solution to these problems. Dan Air Services Ltd was established in 1953; by the mid-1980s its three thousand staff handled more charter business than any other British independent airline; additionally, more than one million passengers a year were carried on scheduled services. A core of about 470 cabin staff were employed on a permanent basis, with another 450 recruited for the summer. The strange thing was that not one of these was male.

Enter the Equal Opportunities Commission, which had been empowered to carry out formal investigations under the Sex Discrimination Act of 1975. Dan Air directors conceded that there were no men, but said that this had been the case for 30 years and it was reluctant to change successful business practice. Besides, surveys had shown that its customers liked things that way. And no, it would not change its policy.

Digging deeper, the EOC found other motives. Dan Air and its parent company, Davies Newman Holdings plc, were worried about AIDS. In mid-1985, representatives stated that they believed their policy was justified by the Health and Safety at Work Act of 1974, which obliged companies to protect their workforce and customers. Dan Air consulted legal counsel, who produced the following observations (as summarized in the EOC's formal investigation report): 1) AIDS mainly affects homosexuals. 2) A large proportion of men (up to 30 per cent) who are attracted to cabin staff work are homosexual. 3) Cabin staff are sexually promiscuous. 4) AIDS is principally transmitted by sexual intercourse. 5) AIDS can be transmitted by blood and saliva and could therefore be transmitted to or from passengers when staff cut themselves at work or when passengers required artificial resuscitation.

Dan Air stated that additional expert medical opinion would be produced to support its case, but none was forthcoming. Claims that HIV could be transmitted through saliva were based on scant and unsubstantiated reports; the belief that up to 30 per cent of men attracted to cabin staff work were gay and that these men were highly promiscuous appears to have its roots in either prejudice or wishful thinking.

The EOC visited the airline offices in 1986. It was established that it did not advertise for cabin crew, but relied upon direct applications; on an average month it would receive about 400 from women and about 40 from men. Men who telephoned first were discouraged from applying, but were not told directly that the airline did not employ men as cabin staff. No man was ever offered an interview, but male applicants were told that all posts were filled and to try again in the future. Dan Air also held careers talks in schools, but only to girls.

With regard to possible infection with HIV, Dan Air claimed that staff cut themselves on flights at least 30 times a day. When the EOC examined the accident book for reports of cuts or grazes, only 16 cases were found for the whole of 1985.

EOC called in some medical experts to advise on the case. Professor Pinching and Professor Geddes (an infectious diseases specialist at the University of Birmingham) found Dan Air's case to be, in the EOC's word, 'groundless'. There was no risk to passengers or crew and the virus could not be transmitted via food.

Dan Air was thus issued with a non-discrimination notice. The company did not challenge the findings of unlawful acts and undertook to remedy the situation; it acknowledged that the threat of HIV infection was no longer a recruitment issue.

But HIV continued to be an issue for many other companies, including other airlines. In 1990 all applicants for aircraft jobs with British Airways were obliged to take an HIV test; a spokesman explained that anyone who was antibody positive 'will not be fit enough to do the work'. The pharmaceuticals company SmithKline Beecham has also defended its HIV test at recruitment: a leading health care company 'cannot afford to have someone with a compromised immunological system working in high-risk sections handling animals or working with ionising radiation'. Screening existed 'as much to protect the employee as the employer'. This did not quite tally with the refusal to grant permanent employment to a gay HIV positive computer operative in April 1990. A 34-year-old man had been with Beecham's for three months when, according to a company spokesman, he was refused a staff job 'because it was not certain how many days off sick he would demand'. In the same year a woman with the virus was suspended from her job with the Torbay Health Authority a few days into her employment; her husband had recently died from AIDS and her loss of work drove her to the brink of suicide.

Legal protection was limited to existing legislation, notably the Employment Protection (Consolidation) Act of 1978 and the Sex Discrimination and Race Relations Acts. Kenneth Clarke, the employment minister, had said at the launch of his department's booklet 'AIDS and Employment' in 1986 that any attempt by an employer to dismiss or otherwise discriminate against an infected employee (or someone who was suspected of being infected) would be dealt with harshly by a tribunal. 'We are very anxious not to have people made outcasts at their place of work,' he said. 'There is generally no obligation on individuals to disclose their infection ... anything which can be interpreted as an inquisition into an employee's personal lifestyle should be avoided.' Recruitment programmes which included HIV tests were to be 'discouraged', although they were not prohibited by statute.

And so things remained, with employers defining their own definitions of risk and safety. Many large companies behaved creditably: Marks and Spencer and the Post Office issued detailed 'good practice' guidelines to its staff; even British Telecom, whose engineers had once refused to repair telephones at the Terrence Higgins Trust for fear of catching HIV from the wires, sent a personal letter and Health Education Authority information booklet to its staff.

In 1989 there were attempts to introduce specific HIV/AIDS provisions into the new Employment Act. Baroness Turner of Camden, one of the Equal Opportunities Commissioners who had investigated Dan Air, led the Labour motion in the Lords and reported that the Terrence Higgins Trust dealt with about a hundred cases of alleged employment discrimination every year. Baroness Seear, for the Liberal Democrats, said that where unfair discrimination was found by a tribunal, it very rarely resulted in reinstatement. But the motion failed by a large majority after Lord Strathclyde, Under-Secretary for

Employment, claimed that existing legislation was sufficient and that most employers heeded the government's advice to treat people with AIDS fairly.

Protection and legislation in Britain largely compared favourably to that of other countries; a useful comparison came at immigration and border controls. In 1988, Diana Walford, the senior principal medical officer at the DHSS, wrote to all domestic port medical inspectors with advice on what to do when the immigration service suspected that a person seeking entry to the UK was HIV positive. 'The diagnosis of AIDS should not in itself be considered justification for a recommendation on public health grounds to withhold leave to enter the UK,' she wrote. However, if the medical officer regarded it likely that during the passenger's stay in the UK he or she would require medical treatment, 'he should provide an estimate of the cost of such treatment in order to enable the immigration service to decide whether the passenger has the means to meet these costs'. When two American men were subsequently deported, financial grounds were cited; customs officials claimed that AIDS itself was not the reason.

In 1990 it was estimated that at least 35 of the World Health Organization member states had policies restricting those who were HIV positive from entering their country. In China, all foreigners staying longer than one year were tested; those found to be HIV positive during a shorter stay were deported. In India all foreign students were tested and African students with HIV had been deported. In South Africa all applicants for work permits were tested. In most Soviet states all foreign students were tested and anyone else could be tested at will.

In the United States, where AIDS was classified for immigration purposes as 'contagious', entry policies almost caused a boycott of the 1990 World AIDS Conference in San Francisco. Foreigners who had tested positive would not be allowed entry without a medical waiver valid for only 30 days and requiring approval by the Immigration and Naturalization Service in Washington. Entry would have to be seen to provide the United States with some benefit and would not be granted solely for tourism. If a waiver was granted, the traveller's passport would be stamped. Jim Wilson, onetime international liaison officer with the Terrence Higgins Trust, was one of many refused entry. 'I know exactly how HIV is transmitted, probably better than most people and certainly better than the immigration officers,' he said. 'I am not going to run the risk of travelling somewhere if I don't feel fit enough, and I'm not going to be this "threat to public safety".' The San Francisco conference went ahead, but the conference to be hosted by Harvard University and scheduled for Boston in 1992 was switched to Amsterdam when a boycott by angry delegates seemed inevitable. Announcing the switch, Dr Jonathan Mann, newly appointed director of the International AIDS Center at Harvard, said that it was 'an extremely serious matter when America's oldest university has to leave the country to host a conference about a pandemic'.

From the beginning of 1987, many young unmarried men encountered discrimination of another sort, discrimination associated with home ownership and insurance. With mortgages requiring life insurance, many people found that either they could not afford heavily hiked premiums or, worse, were refused coverage altogether. If you had AIDS or were HIV positive, life insurance was out of the question, but there were now any number of new reasons why you might be judged a bad risk or uninsurable.

In 1986 10.5 million life insurance policies involving £7.25m in new premiums were taken out in the UK. The Government Actuary estimated in 1987 that within a few years mortality rates could double for men aged between 15 and 50. To protect existing policy holders and to keep down premiums for the majority of new applicants, insurance companies would do everything they could to avoid taking on those with HIV infection or those they considered at high risk of acquiring it. Essentially, this was sound business practice; how they went about it, however, caused distress and controversy.

By 1987, most application forms for new life insurance policies included two standard questions agreed by the Association of British Insurers (ABI), the body that represented 425 companies. It read: 'Have you ever (a) been counselled or medically advised in connection with AIDS or any sexually transmitted disease? (b) had an AIDS blood test – if so, please give details, dates and results'.

These questions, which hardly changed in subsequent years, raised many problems: people might be discouraged from seeking advice and treatment for HIV infections and other STDs, or from going for a test; many people at very low risk might have already been tested (blood donors and those involved in surveillance and screening programmes), and fear of close scrutiny by insurance companies might lead to their withdrawal in the future. The line of inquiry appeared to run directly counter to the government's awareness campaign which encouraged many of the 'worried well' to seek advice and screening lest they pass on the virus; of the three million who attended STD clinics in the last five years, clearly only very few would be at risk from HIV infection.

Inevitably, there were other problems of discrimination, and one Abbey Life spokesman addressed the issue with almost boastful candour: 'If applicants say they are practising bisexuals or homosexuals we will only quote if they test negative and can show they are in a stable relationship, but will put an extra loading on their policy because they are proven to be an extra risk.' Premiums to certain 'at risk' groups often doubled (not only gay men, but people from African communities, haemophiliacs and those who had used intravenous drugs) and they faced intrusive scrutiny of their private life.

The questions would come in tiers. You went to a building society, filled out some basics. You'd be sent another form a few days later: were you gay or bisexual? Had you ever had a test, shot drugs, lived in Africa or slept with anyone who was high risk? If you answered yes to any of these, yet another form would demand to know how promiscuous you were and whether you had anal sex. By the time this third form arrived, your premium was likely to be astronomical or your policy days away from being cancelled. Several companies admitted that any acknowledgement of promiscuity would be sufficient to refuse an application, but there were more subtle reasons for rejection too: one AIDS specialist at St Stephen's Hospital was asked by Victory International Specialist Reinsurers 'whether certain professions indicate a greater risk of homosexuality', to which he replied in his report: 'The answer is yes. However I am on dangerous ground, as to name certain professions would result in a howl of protest from the heterosexual members of those professions. I feel I need not name these professions, as everyone is probably aware, but one that comes most strongly to mind is "designer".'

In 1988 the Institute of Actuaries estimated that the death toll from AIDS could reach 100,000, and stated that at least £1 billion had been set aside to cover claims from people who developed AIDS under existing policies. The deputy actuary at the Prudential said: 'This figure is based solely on our estimate of what is likely to happen as long as AIDS remains confined to the homosexual community. If it moves into the heterosexual community then all bets are off.'

Many peculiar insurance practices were introduced in the late 1980s.

177

In November 1987 the Institute of Actuaries issued advice that any policy worth more than £50,000 should only be issued if applicants first agreed to a blood test, either by their GP or a private agency; in most cases there would be no counselling and people might receive the results of their tests from insurers rather than health-care workers. This was not intended as a discriminatory policy; single women applicants would often require testing too. In February 1988 the Association of British Insurers called for HIV tests for all men applying for policies worth over £150,000, but some companies said they were testing for much lower amounts. Zurich Insurance, for example, tested all single men under 35 years for policies worth more than £75,000, and all single men over 35 for sums of £50,000.

Connells, an estate agency in Leighton Buzzard, cynically tried to drum up trade with a new advertisement headlined 'AIDS Warning' which read: 'The future looks bleak for all of us who will want or need life insurance in the coming years'. The Advertising Standards Authority regarded this as irresponsible; a senior partner of the estate agency said he regretted the tone of the advertisement, but not its substance.

Fear worked the other way too. After a period in which it was next to impossible to get insurance against HIV infection, it was inevitable that a company would offer a policy offering specialist HIV cover. While in 1990 the Prudential Assurance Company announced a new clause in its permanent health insurance policies that cancelled benefits if individuals subsequently became infected with HIV, the Lifeshield Foundation and Lloyd's underwriters developed a package providing cash benefits from £25,000 to £75,000 on *proof* of infection. Premiums ranged from £25 a year to £100 for those perceived to be at higher risk, and policies were aimed at groups rather than individuals – health staff, police, teachers. Anyone applying would have to declare that they had not engaged in homosexual acts or intravenous drug abuse. The BMA greeted the package with scepticism, saying that the best insurance was still education. The Terrence Higgins Trust said that people could 'buy an awful lot of condoms for £25'.

In 1991 the Department of Health commissioned a survey on AIDS and life insurance. During its many discussions with the Association of British Insurers the department had voiced its concerns about the effect the questions on insurance proposal forms were having on people's willingness to test and participate in epidemiological studies and drug and vaccine trials. The 1991 survey confirmed that these concerns were not without foundation. The British Market Research Bureau interviewed over 500 adults aged between 20 and 35, and 100 HIV/AIDS specialists (doctors, charity workers, helpline volunteers). Asked about the questions concerning HIV counselling and testing, 80 per cent of specialists and 48 per cent of young adults agreed that 'they put people off applying for life insurance'; 74 per cent of specialists and 38 per cent of young adults agreed that they 'put people off seeking advice about HIV testing'; and 88 per cent of specialists and 35 per cent of young adults agreed that they 'put people off having an HIV test'. One STD doctor responded: 'I don't think there's any question that on a significant scale [the questions] prevent people from coming to see us in the first place to discuss the issues. Amongst those who do come to discuss the issues … it is one of the major factors which influence the decision not to test.'

Ivan Massow says things have hardly improved in the intervening years. Massow, a 26-year-old gay man, has become something of a star in the worlds of insurance and investment, not least because of his practice of offering free financial services to those with HIV.

'Gay men receive the same prejudiced treatment as the early days,' he says. 'Single women are also being sent lifestyle forms and asked to go for tests now. Some companies have begun to realize they've made a mistake and have begun to compensate; among gay men and other high-risk groups they now look for evidence of a long-term relationship and a commitment to absolutely safe sex.'

In July 1994, the ABI issued a new recommendation to its members: in future they should ask applicants only if they have tested positive for HIV/AIDS or if they are receiving treatment, not whether they have had a test. The ABI explained that payouts for AIDS-related deaths had been lower than expected.

Massow believes that for most companies the 'pink pound' represents business they feel they can still afford to lose, business they find morally unattractive. 'In many of the conversations I've had with underwriters at other companies, many people have displayed pride in their moral stance. They feel they're "helping to keep homosexuals and therefore this virus at bay".'

Massow has set up schemes with several major building societies whereby he can get his clients mortgages without the need for life insurance. About 10 per cent of his clients are HIV positive; his company discusses their employment and social security rights and guides them towards companies that would pay out to a male partner after death. 'We see a lot of people who come to us in panic straight after a diagnosis, and we have to slow them down, to explain they've probably got years ahead to sort themselves out. We now have several clients who have been positive for more than ten years. A lot now even take out pension schemes.'

The best approach is a direct one, he says; clients tend to be less nervous if you ask them early on: 'Have you tested, what was the result, what's your T-cell count?'

Massow has a lot of discussions with gay men about whether they should test. A personal choice, he says; he himself has tested regularly:

When you deal with HIV so often, it seems that everyone in the world is HIV positive. I just can't believe I'm negative. I've tested three times, once every eighteen months or so. It's worrying that there are more and more cases being classified where positive men swear they have never had anal intercourse, only oral sex. I have one client who says he's had only safe sex for the past five years, and he's been absolutely careful and very aware. He's had tests every six months for the past few years and always came up negative, but the last one he came up positive.

Active

On a Tuesday evening in mid-January 1989, about a hundred people gathered at the London Lesbian and Gay Centre in central London for the first British meeting of Act-Up, the AIDS Coalition to Unleash Power. A chaotic meeting, a loud clash of egos and factions, but a broadly agreed common purpose: Act-Up would be an ad hoc pressure group 'dedicated to improving public debate, combating intolerance, government complacency, bureaucratic incompetence and media hysteria in as embarrassing, effective and graphic way as possible'. In practice this meant a series of jarring 'zaps', hellraising protests loaded with slogans and placards intended to disrupt office life or stop the traffic.

The London meeting was inspired by the organization formed in the United States in 1987 by writer Larry Kramer. Kramer had warned his audience in Greenwich Village that most of them would probably die unless they forced the medical establishment to speed up drug trials and treatments. 'If what you're hearing doesn't rouse you to anger, fury, rage and action, gay men will have no future here on earth.' Act-Up did much to alter the previously genteel relationship between patient groups and researchers and policy makers, and its efforts hastened the release of AZT and reduced its price.

It took two years for grassroots AIDS activism to spread to Britain (there were soon groups in Edinburgh, Manchester, Leeds, Norwich and elsewhere), not least because of the existence of the NHS and the far smaller number of cases. In 1988 the gay movement had protested widely but unsuccessfully against Section 28, and many of the most vociferous campaigning voices – Derek Jarman, Jimmy Somerville, Peter Tatchell, Duncan Campbell and Simon Watney – now diverted their attentions to help shape the earliest Act-Up protests.

'The demos were empowering and fun and reminiscent of the first gay lib demos that I'd been on back in the early seventies,' says Tim Clark, a member for the first year:

But as for actually achieving anything I was not at all sure. Partly Act-Up was a counterbalance to what we saw as the apologists – the mainstream of the THT and London Lighthouse, who we felt were too much in bed with the drug companies and the government and to an extent relied on the government for financial support so they couldn't voice the dissatisfactions in the way that we could.

Act-Up lived or died by its column inches. Protests had to be forceful, simple and witty, and cause as much mayhem as possible. A few arrests never went amiss. Inspired by American colleagues, the first zap took place at the Wellcome AGM at Park Lane's Grosvenor House Hotel. Simple stuff: the meeting was 'a gathering of AIDS profiteers' who made toxic drugs and charged the earth. This soon became an annual Act-Up hit: protests with placards outside and a few activists who had bought one share each inside, shouting questions at Sir Alfred Shepperd, the chairman. But Wellcome executives were baffled: who *were* these ungrateful people? Had their company not done everything it could to benefit those with HIV and AIDS, certainly more than any other pharmaceuticals firm? Was it not these very same activists who had celebrated when AZT was rushed through a couple of years earlier?

The next protest took place outside Pentonville Prison and involved helium-filled condoms. When Home Office minister Douglas Hogg refused to sanction new research into drug-taking and homosexuality in prisons, Act-Up members floated safe-sex literature attached to condoms over Pentonville walls, whereupon they were probably punctured and binned by staff. A few weeks later, in protest at the refusal to supply clean needles or condoms to inmates, they were back again, chucking over condoms and needle-use guidelines. The police threatened to arrest demonstrators for chanting 'Pentonville Prisoners' Pricks Deserve Attention', but relented when the word 'prick' was changed to 'penis'.

In August 1989 three members from Act-Up disguised as couriers chained themselves to the turnstiles at the *Daily Mail* offices in Kensington, and 30 others picketed outside, in protest at columnist George Gale's recent tirade on gay men and AIDS. For Gale, no fan of sugar-coating, 'the message to be learned ... is that active homosexuals are potentially murderers and that the act of buggery kills'. The spread of AIDS 'will never be halted by teaching youngsters the alleged delights of condoms. Any resulting promiscuity will actually assist the disease to be spread'. No arrests at the protest, but a little noise. Several *Mail* staff expressed sympathy with the activists, but the managing editor said they would have no effect: 'Gale writes what he wants'.

More grief at *Melody Maker* a year later. A review of an Elton John record, the proceeds of which were due to go to the Terrence Higgins Trust, concentrated little on the music. Instead it asked, 'Who the fuck is this bloke Higgins, and why are we supposed to give him our money?' The 'idea' behind the review, the magazine explained later, was to make people question the role of charity records. Reading on, it appeared to be little more than a coarse wind-up. 'Pop stars are queuing up to lob cash at the git and what's he ever done? Who exactly is this man who, without recourse even to a personal appeal, has for so long extracted from us so much of our dosh?' The piece ended, 'Well Tezza, you can pull the wool over Elton's eyes, he's famous for his generosity and dopiness. But don't come the spiv with us. Get a job, man. Get a life.' So Act-Up legged it up to the *Melody Maker* offices and met the editor. Letters appeared and an apology.

One of the protesters was Jimmy Somerville, the gay singer who had come to prominence with Bronksi Beat and the Communards. Somerville's presence lent a little glamour, if not legitimacy, at least for the tabloids. Act-Up events got a little more coverage when Somerville was dragged along the streets by men in uniform. In October 1989 he and nine others were carried away from Australia House on Aldwych after protesting over the new laws for immigrants which required them to take an HIV test before entering the country. Taken to Bow Street police station, the ten were charged with obstruction and then searched with rubber gloves. Five were found guilty and sentenced to six months conditional discharge and a £20 fine. A Sergeant Alan Smythe told the court how one of the protesters was 'a man I recognized to be a pop star'. It made four national papers and the BBC television news.

'It was great for a while,' Somerville says,

> especially because there was no tradition of that sort of behaviour in this country and you felt you were doing something worthwhile. For me it got to the point where I felt that my presence was distracting from the reason for being there, and there came a point when others in Act-Up didn't want to have this 'celebrity' representing them or picking up all the attention.

For a while there were other protests, other arrests, almost every week: Whitehall brought to a standstill during a 'die-in' outside the DSS to highlight inadequate disability benefit; Westminster Bridge blocked over the demise of the Health Education Authority's AIDS unit; the Virgin Megastore in Oxford Street picketed over its stocking of a Guns n' Roses album which contained homophobic lyrics; Middlesex Hospital picketed when a delay to two planned trials of the drug ddI was announced; and Texaco headquarters picketed every week in protest at the company's policy to HIV-test all prospective staff.

But by the autumn of 1990 Act-Up had all but burnt out. 'The factionalization was ridiculous,' Somerville says. 'We were still a relatively small group of thirty to fifty people, and yet some people felt we had to have a women's section, and this section and that section, and it got taken over by the extreme left as these things always tend to do.' Rob Archer and Rae Bos, the two founder members, left because they regretted that other members had forged too many links with external non-AIDS groups, at the expense of those concerned directly with the epidemic.

But Somerville eventually left for other reasons. Act-Up was far from universally supported by the gay community, and collections in bars and clubs often yielded little: 'We were seen as troublemakers, giving gays and AIDS work a bad name,' Tim Clark says. So Somerville and some friends embarked on a small-scale national fundraising and campaigning tour, which raised a little under £12,000. 'Shortly after it finished it was found that the treasurer had been lying, and the Act-Up accounts were examined in depth and all these irregularities came to light.' In September 1990 the treasurer was convicted of nine counts of theft at Snaresbrook Crown Court; money went on her car, computer and personal debts.

'I decided I would never put my name to an organization like that again, I would only act on my own,' Somerville says. 'I can't tell you how defeated I felt when I found out about the money. It was such a betrayal. I cried that day.'

CHAPTER 10: Really at Risk?

They filed into the chamber and by 9.34 a.m. they were ready. David Mellor shuffled his speech and announced that this was the first time since November 1986 that the House had had the chance for a full debate on AIDS. It was 13 January 1989, a Friday; the day was important, because most members had already sloped back to their constituencies, or were consulting train timetables and weather reports. Mellor, who had become Minister of State at the Department of Health after a stint at the Foreign Office (and before that had been at the Home Office dealing with the drugs problem), looked around the Commons and weighed up another defining political and personal moment. No Thatcher, no cabinet, hardly any front-bench opposition; in fact, fewer than 30 MPs had shown up for what Mellor and Fowler and the Chief Medical Officer were still claiming was potentially the most serious health problem the country had faced since the war.

It was an illuminating morning, bereft of the fever, prejudice and ignorance that had attended the first debate. The disapprovers now disapproved in absentia; the crusty right and family values brigade would keep their seething for the lobbies and for devastating amendments to legislation. Today was really a mid-term report: the government reported that it had done well (the awareness campaigns, the research and treatment funding) and would continue to do better. Today's proceedings would attempt to answer some key questions: were we all really at risk of HIV? Could anyone genuinely claim to know the true scale of the problem?

Mellor's speech was most significant for its commitment to new and greater spending. £25 million had been spent in the last financial year, almost £62 million was available this year and nearly £130 million would be provided next year. The government expected that of this new money £68 million would be spent on the treatment and care of those already infected, while about £50 million would go towards local prevention initiatives, genito-urinary medical services and drugs-related services. North West Thames regional health authority would continue to receive the largest sum – about £36 million – to meet the greatest demand of AIDS cases (almost 800 to date). He promised further grants to the voluntary sector, details of which emerged in the next eight months: the Terrence Higgins Trust was to get £450,000 each year for two years; London Lighthouse £300,000 each year for three; the National AIDS Trust received two one-off payments totalling £355,000; Mildmay Mission Hospital got £256,000. Smaller organizations providing community support and self-help such as Frontliners, Body Positive, the south London Landmark and the Christian-based charity AIDS Care Education and Training (ACET) each received grants of about £50,000. And so the fight against AIDS went on, along Whitehall and beyond. It was a convincing display, although Mellor's closing rhetoric did not quite have the inspiring ring to it he may have hoped for. 'If two years ago the message was "Don't Die of Ignorance", today our message is "Now you know the facts, act upon them".'

The most vocal dissent came from Harriet Harman, shadow health minister, who none the less seemed wary of turning AIDS into an issue ravaged by hard-line party politics. But she wanted much more money, not least in Scotland, and stressed that basic provisions such as housing were still inadequate. But she supported the wide-sweep heterosexual approach – that familiar straight line that declared that everyone was at risk.

Alan Williams, Labour MP for Carmarthen, put it more bluntly, suggesting that 'when the history of this chapter is written, it will be seen that, as with many environmental problems, our action was too little too late'. Then he quoted Tony Benn, who had mentioned in a parliamentary Labour Party meeting that AIDS was a greater threat than the Red Army. It was a throwaway remark, but Williams gave it greater currency: Britain spent £20 billion annually on defence, but only £7 million on AIDS research. Tories too believed that AIDS should be given even more priority. 'So far,' said Chris Butler, the member for Warrington South, 'the Government's approach to the disease has been sadly ad hoc and responsive, which is disastrous because the damage is done for seven to eight years ahead.' He endorsed proposals from his colleague Charles Irving (Cheltenham) that there should be a minister for AIDS, appointed specifically to develop and co-ordinate policy.

In previous weeks Mellor had made several speeches outside Parliament, all something of a dress rehearsal for today's display. At one, the inaugural lunch of the National AIDS Trust, he felt obliged to defend his department's policy against media speculation that it was misguided and overblown. The *Sun*'s 'medical adviser' had expressed the unspoken beliefs of many when he wrote of how 'the only people really at risk are promiscuous homosexuals and drug addicts. The DHSS and the BMA have drummed up hysterical campaigns designed to scare heterosexuals and put us all off sex. But the facts show that they are wrong.'

This was one of the earliest printed manifestations of a media rebellion that would later become widespread. At the NAT lunch, Mellor had to hand 'the facts' as they applied to the UK and there wasn't much he could do with them. Out of a total of 1,862 AIDS cases reported up to the end of October 1988, 1,532 were gay or bisexual men, 38 intravenous drug users and 123 haemophiliacs. There were only 69 cases of heterosexual transmission, 12 of whom had partners with the above risk factors (or had received infected transfusions), and 50 had been exposed to the virus abroad, principally in Africa. Six years since the first known case, there were only seven reports of AIDS among heterosexuals with no record of the accepted risk activities or exposure abroad. Still, Mellor said, this figure was on the increase and the larger numbers of asymptomatic heterosexual HIV infections warned of calamities to come.

Wherever he spoke, Mellor stressed that we underestimate AIDS at our peril. His conviction stemmed from his visits round the wards. These trips went with the territory for all new health ministers, but before 1986 they most often amounted to a few handshakes in the coronary unit and A & E. With AIDS you had to be seen to get closer; that was part of the deal, part of dealing with the problem. 'Honest to goodness, I could think of no more ghastly way to die,' Mellor says. 'Dying is a ghastly business however it happens, but seeing people die of AIDS was one of the most deeply traumatizing experiences that I've ever been through.'

After these visits, Mellor regarded it as 'my public duty, almost a privilege' to help those he had seen and prevent others from becoming infected. He insists that his actions were never motivated by political opportunism. 'One always has to be a bit defensive about this, because people always assume that if you're a high-profile minister all you're looking for is some winning steed to ride forward. My position on AIDS was that I'd much have preferred not to have faced this trauma.'

Mellor did preside over a difficult period, a period of uncertainty. Because of the nature of HIV and AIDS, the long incubation period of the virus limited the scope for measuring clear-cut success. Fearful for their own future, ever wary of impending reshuffles or elections, politicians are naturally uneasy about dealing with issues that have no prospect of swift resolution. In 1989, more than a year after the pronouncement of the *Sun*'s medical adviser, Mellor faced many opponents who believed that because no heterosexual epidemic had occurred, the government's response to AIDS was already overblown; God forbid it should waste more money. 'People wanted something clear cut,' Mellor says now. 'But we still don't know a lot of the answers today, so how we were supposed to know everything then I just don't know.'

Mellor listened to doctors, looked abroad and read the projections. In 1989 he did not regard AIDS as having yet reached epidemic proportions. 'The one thing Donald Acheson and I completely agreed on, and we discussed it very intensively, was that the key as to whether this would become an epidemic was plainly the extent to which it filtered out into the mainstream population.' For Mellor and Donald Acheson the key was the 'infectibility ratio': if you were HIV positive, would you, during your lifetime, infect more or less than one person on average? If it was more than one person, then the epidemic was gathering pace.

Epidemiology was one thing, but what really counted here was sexual behaviour. And no one really knew much about this. It was clear from the earliest cabinet committee meetings on AIDS that some sexual practices – gay and straight – were enough to cause palpitations in those present. And it wasn't just *what* people got up to, it was how often. And so a nationwide survey on sexual behaviour and attitudes was proposed, initially by the DHSS Chief Scientists' group and later by the department's Behavioural Change group. It was to be the biggest modern study ever conducted in Britain, and would be useful not just for dealing with AIDS, but also for other issues of sexual health. 'The whole idea was to get further into what people actually did, as against what they said they did,' Mellor says. 'We all know that human sexuality is an enormously more complicated thing than most people are prepared to acknowledge. I had always accepted that the inmates at the Coleherne [a gay leather bar in south-west London] had to be taken on their own terms. You couldn't treat them as if they were down playing tennis at the Hurlingham Club.'

The survey of sexual attitudes was in fact doomed from the first top-level discussions. It met great opposition when raised at the cabinet committee on AIDS, and when Margaret Thatcher heard of it she insisted it went no further. According to Mellor, ministers were frightened of the use to which the information gathered would be put and of what would be said about the government for getting it; others saw it as a privacy issue. It was frustrated, he believes, 'by the first glimmerings of what became a rather bizarre attitude towards family policy: that somehow you strengthen the family by denying that things exist that threaten it'.

After the DHSS split into the Department of Social Security and the Department of Health, John Moore had taken over from Lord Whitelaw as chairman of the AIDS cabinet committee in what Mellor calls a 'sweetener' for having lost some responsibility:

> John at that stage in his career was somebody who was less commit-ted to having an independent view of these matters, and rather more committed to worrying in advance of her [Thatcher] about what she would be worried about. So I had a number of meetings with him as he wrung his hands about this survey. Kenneth Baker was strongly opposed to it, so was George Younger. They feared that the results of the survey would be used like the Kinsey Report [the large post-Second World War American study], as if the gov-ernment was somehow endorsing the various practices revealed within the study, and it would be embarrassing.

By the autumn of 1989, Mellor had moved back to the Home Office and his post had been taken by Virginia Bottomley. Without the guidance of the survey (which would anyway have taken years to conduct and compile) she faced the same uncertainties in evaluating exactly what sort of problem she was dealing with. But she came on strong from the first, impressing the voluntary organizations with her compassion and enthusiasm. 'She kept on urging, "Give me the facts, not the fantasy",' one manager at the Terrence Higgins Trust recalls. 'It was like a mantra, and it became a bit of a joke. If ever her name came up in conversation, one party would always imitate her and say, "Give me the facts! Give me the facts!"'

'She saw it as something you could make a lot of headway with,' observed one official in the Department of Health, 'and she realized immediately that anything she said about AIDS would make big head-lines, whereas other issues would get scant coverage. That all changed when that boy climbed into the lion's den; then mental health was the big headline and she could run with that.'

The long incubation period of HIV could be worked to a politician's advantage too. This was no salmonella-in-eggs scare; if it was hard to be proved right, it was equally hard to be proved wrong or ridiculed from office, especially in the brief periods ministers spent at Health these days.

The way Bottomley began her tenure at the department was well illustrated by the speeches she delivered as the opening and closing addresses at a symposium held in November 1989 at the Queen Elizabeth II Conference Centre in Westminster. Hosted by the UK Health Departments and the Health Education Authority, it was an assessment of current and future spread of HIV/AIDS in the UK, and featured separate presentations on transmission through sex, through drug misuse and from mother to baby, as well as papers on the international and European situation.

Bottomley told the assembled research and health practitioners nothing new, but her faith in their work was invigorating. Notable was her observation that the more successful the campaign to curb the spread of HIV infection, the more intense would become the pressure to scale down the efforts and money spent on fighting the virus. This she would resist, aware of the long haul; but she would tailor the response according to what scientists and doctors and the statistics suggested. Four years later, as she cut grants and lowered the priority of AIDS on her agenda, doctors and scientists detected some irony in these comments.

One of the doctors speaking at the symposium was Anne Johnson, a senior lecturer in epidemiology at University College and Middlesex School of Medicine, who had done much work on what was still the most hotly contested topic – heterosexual transmission in the UK. From what we knew from transmission in the developing world and from the limited small-scale surveys conducted on sexual behaviour in Britain (which suggested that over the course of five years a sizeable proportion of the heterosexual population reported ten partners or more, and small numbers reported over a hundred), the potential for spread, especially among the young, should still be a leading priority. Johnson also noted that the small number of published partner studies showed that although some infected women had both vaginal and anal intercourse, the majority of those infected only reported vaginal intercourse.

Dr Johnson prepared a similar paper for the All-Party Parliamentary Group on AIDS which defined a clearer trend of heterosexual transmission. Up to the end of 1987, 3 per cent of reported AIDS cases were heterosexually acquired, but by 1989 this had increased to 7.9 per cent. Two hundred and one cases of heterosexually acquired AIDS would be reported in the UK by June 1990 (and almost a thousand cases of heterosexually acquired HIV infection); this was the equivalent of the total number of UK AIDS cases reported by mid-1985. Of this 201, 29 had partners with a recognized risk factor (drug user, bisexual, infected haemophiliac) and 151 had heterosexual partners abroad, predominantly in countries where heterosexual transmission is the principal mode of spread. The remaining 21 had no links to the above groups. As ever, the long period between HIV infection and AIDS diagnosis (on average eight to ten years) means that these figures were merely a reflection of those infected several years before.

Virginia Bottomley spoke again at the conference at the end of the day, and ran through what was now becoming the familiar 'no complacency' approach. She outlined the money spent – almost £43 million to date to the Medical Research Council, £44 on the public education campaign, £130 million to the NHS, £1.8 million that year to the voluntary sector – and emphasized that for future commitments, the government would be able to take careful stock of a new survey: a large-scale national anonymized screening for HIV.

There had been talk of such a study for over two years, and its opponents had repeatedly queried the ethics of testing blood that had been given for other purposes and without specific consent for an HIV test. It was intended that all blood screened would first have any identifying labels removed, but critics feared this system was open to abuse and wondered whether the temptation to trace those who tested positive would not be too great.

The MRC had spent several months setting up a viable screening system, and Bottomley announced that all obstacles had been overcome. It was to begin in January 1990, at which time hopes were expressed that it would provide a far clearer picture as to levels of infection than any voluntary named testing programme. When the first results were announced in May 1991 they suggested that the investment in public education campaigns was justified.

The results were compiled from surveys conducted at 27 ante-natal clinics and six STD clinics (they would subsequently be extended to general hospitals and new-born infants). They showed that the prevalence of HIV infection in women attending the selected ante-natal clinics in inner London was one in 500. In some it was one in 200; in others one in 1,000. Of the clinics surveyed in outer London and the South East the results ranged from one in 300 to one in 2,500. In ante-natal clinics in other parts of the country, only one test in 16,000 was positive.

Among heterosexual women attending inner London STD clinics in 1990, prevalence was one in 500. Among heterosexual men, the figure was one in 100. Among homosexual and bisexual men attending the same clinics, there was evidence of continuing transmission. The prevalence rate was one in five.

Figures from the World Health Organization helped to place the UK situation in a European context. In a league table of reported AIDS cases per million of population the UK fared relatively well, with 76 cases per million. We were ahead of Greece (41), Ireland (45), Portugal (58) and Germany (72), but behind the incidence in Belgium (82), Netherlands (104), Italy (142), Denmark (148), Spain (192) and France (235).

But a large sector of the London press increasingly maintained that the general risk of AIDS had been overblown, money had been wasted and the population made to feel even more uneasy about sex than it usually did (it claimed, with some justification, that the higher incidence of AIDS in Southern Europe was due mainly to a higher incidence of intravenous drug use and a greater influx of people from high-prevalence areas, but the lack of public health campaigns was also an issue). The newspapers had a strong, simple and popular point, because thousands of heterosexuals were not becoming infected and dying each year, as many had predicted. What they neglected to say was that it was often they who had predicted this calamity. Instead they blamed ministers on the make and the gay lobby (an undefined group which had been relatively weak in its other actions, such as persuading the government to equalize the age of consent or halting Section 28).

'Straight sex cannot give you AIDS – Official' claimed the *Sun*, as the *Daily Mail* detected a 'Phony face of the war on AIDS'.

They were both trading on remarks made by Labour peer Lord Kilbracken ('Eton and Oxford educated Lord Kilbracken' as the *Daily Express* had it, offering its seal of approval), who claimed that the risk of heterosexual transmission was 'statistically invisible'. He went on: 'I don't understand why the Government and the medical profession are doing so much to misrepresent the AIDS situation. It is ridiculous to state that "AIDS is not prejudiced" in an effort to imply we are all at risk of catching the disease.' Kilbracken's next comment would, within the space of three years, be received far more sympathetically by departmental health officials than it was at the time. 'It's insane to use that money to educate the entire community when the great majority are at negligible risk. Nearly all the funds should be aimed at high-risk categories.'

Acclaim from some newspapers, disbelief from some individuals. Lord Kilmarnock, who chaired the All-Party Parliamentary Group on AIDS of which Lord Kilbracken was a member, believed his views were 'unhelpful and misleading', and shared by a very small minority. Look at Europe, he said. Dr Gus Dalgleish, a prominent figure from the earliest days of the epidemic, branded Kilbracken's comments 'totally irresponsible. The spread of AIDS into the heterosexual population is going on very slowly, but in my opinion the disease is at one of its most dangerous phases'. The key point was that it was much too early to tell. The lengthy incubation period ensured that in 1990 it was impossible to measure whether the government's campaigns had much effect on anything; perhaps in five years' time criticisms of crying wolf might be justified.

Still, this was a healthy debate, and one that would latterly be joined enthusiastically by gay lobbying groups. (Some would find this ironic, although gay groups would argue that most newspapers were acting not with gay men's interests at heart, but out of homophobia: they believed that the newspapers' attitude was, it's *only* gay men, so we shouldn't be too worried.) But it was also possible to detect a more sinister air of dissent, the one linked to old-style hearth 'n' home family values. At the beginning of 1990, Family and Youth Concern, a coalition of moral majority groups which claimed much right-wing parliamentary support, distributed its own video to about 650 schools. *The Truth About AIDS* was presented by two teenagers who suggested that transmission of HIV through vaginal intercourse was impossible if there were no cuts. But other practices were dangerous, the teens said, even though they were seldom regarded so by the medical profession. These practices were oral sex and condom use. Of condoms they asked, 'Would you trust your life to a rubber balloon?' So what did they recommend for safer sex? Chaste sex. The 12-minute video came with a letter from Baroness Cox, a sponsor of Section 28: 'The information seemed to me to be accurate and well-balanced ... above all there is a moral message which is all too often lacking from many of the other sources.'

Once again, AIDS became an element in a wider political and ideological campaign. When the Health Education Authority bowed to moral majority pressure and withdrew a new condom campaign, it explained that 'the climate was not right'. The £2 million campaign included television advertisements with a 'condoms are cool' theme. One young lad makes fun of another for carrying condoms and then – close-up misery shot – watches in horror as he goes off with a stunner. The ads were withdrawn lest they encourage promiscuity, to be replaced by doctors in suits talking gravely. For Valerie Riches of Family and Youth Concern this was vindication of what she'd been saying for a while, that the HEA advertisements were 'crudely explicit and dangerously imprecise, boosting the profits of rubber goods manufacturers while selling young people the idea that sexual promiscuity is a normal way of life'.

At the end of 1990 the Department of Health announced a small but significant change in policy, the effect of which suggested that the British heterosexual population understood the risks of AIDS and course of transmission only too well. Sir Donald Acheson said that he now believed there might be a clinical advantage in knowing if one was HIV positive or not. Previously, it was thought there was little advantage in knowing, so long as adequate precautions were taken to limit the risk of infecting others. But now he encouraged all those who believed they might have been infected by the virus to come forward – especially those who had had anal intercourse with men, had shared injecting equipment, or had had unprotected intercourse with a person known to be at risk or in a place with a high HIV prevalence (sub-Saharan Africa, Thailand, the Caribbean or holiday resorts where there was a lot of intravenous drug use).

His appeal, coinciding as it did with the additional hoopla surrounding World AIDS Day and an AIDS storyline in *EastEnders*, helped to stretch testing services and boost calls to the helplines. Around this busy time the National AIDS Helpline reported an increase in callers from about 10,000 calls per week to 21,000. There was a considerable increase in women callers, particularly married women, and many callers appeared to have already decided they had been at risk and were considering being tested.

In London, all the clinics contacted by the Department of Health AIDS Unit reported a 'dramatic' or 'marked' increase in demands for tests in December 1990 and January 1991. At St Stephen's Hospital doctors reported that the most visible increase came from women. There were no seropositives found among these women, but one quarter of the men were positive. Many of those tested for the first time already had symptomatic disease. The Royal Free, one of the first hospitals in the country to offer a same-day testing and results service, reported that its counselling services were having trouble coping with the rise in demand. The hospital stated that although it was seeing a growing number of new symptomatic patients, most of those who used the same-day clinic were 'the worried well'.

The background to Acheson's announcement encouraging testing is significant. He had been advised that HIV positive people who presented early, even though free of symptoms, might benefit from early use of AZT and from prophylaxis against Pneumocystis carinii pneumonia. The Concorde study of the value of AZT in asymptomatics was still being conducted (and preliminary results would not emerge until 1993), but many doctors believed that it might have some early benefits in delaying the onset of AIDS.

Despite this, Acheson and the Department of Health had little good news on the treatment front. Since AZT was licensed in 1987, nothing else had appeared to extend its early hope. Virginia Bottomley and her predecessors had longed for good research news (even though new drugs would most likely take a heavy financial toll on the NHS), but there was none to announce.

When the All-Party Parliamentary Group on AIDS met in March 1991, it was clear that despite some optimism and much fighting talk, there was little evidence of advances that might soon be of use to sick patients. Dr Janet Darbyshire presented the APPGA meeting with an update on Concorde, which had by then recruited over 1,700 patients in a double-blind study (neither patients nor researchers knowing who had AZT and who had a placebo). The Concorde trial had been the subject of much opposition (not least from the Terrence Higgins Trust) for continuing with its placebo element after a similar study in America had been stopped once early results showed that asymptomatic use of AZT did delay the onset of AIDS. This trial, less vigorous than Concorde, was conducted over a far shorter timescale and left many questions unanswered. It was unclear, for example, whether survival was prolonged, what the optimum dosage was and whether there were problems with long-term toxicity.

Other, shorter, trials of other anti-retrovirals were also taking place.

The Alpha trial, which had recruited about 1,500 people with AIDS in Europe and Australia, was looking at the effects of ddI, a drug which earlier studies had shown to have a high level of side effects, including pancreatitis. There was also a trial at Great Ormond Street examining the timescale and dosage of AZT for HIV positive children.

Professor Trevor Jones, the research director at Wellcome, told the APPGA meeting that apart from AZT, which already had proven benefits, he held most hope for ddI and ddC, particularly when used in combinations. The crucial point was the life-cycle of the virus: when the virus replicated and the subsequent processes of RNA/DNA conversion. He then let rip with a list of putative anti-HIV compounds under present examination: AL-721, AZDU, Butyl DNJ, Oxyphenarsine, PMEA, Tibo derivatives, FLT, Oxymyristic acid, THA CD4, Compound Q, d4T, dextran sulphate, hypericin, Peptide T. He didn't sound over-optimistic about any of them.

Dr Geoffrey Schild, director of the MRC AIDS Directed Programme (ADP), put an enthusiastic spin on things. About 200 research projects had been funded since the ADP began in 1987 and the programme was now in its consolidation phase, during which new goals would be set and new initiatives pursued. The progress Dr Schild listed included research into HIV variability and studies of immunological structure. New vaccine design concepts had been developed and there had been encouraging news from animal vaccine studies. As far as the strategic programme went, there was good epidemiological work to report from Uganda and much good general collaboration with the United States and Europe. This sounded very nice. In practical terms advances had been steady but limited; there was no doubt now that the optimism of early scientific advance (not least following the discovery of the virus) had now slowed to the unglamorous long haul.

If there was no immediate good news on the research front, there was even less on the subject of service provision and community care. In October 1991 Virginia Bottomley received a worrying report from the National Audit Office that showed that millions of pounds of funds intended for use by regional and local health authorities for HIV/AIDS work had been misspent or misdirected. For someone who prided herself on the decentralization of health care and had talked often of the need for the efficient targeting of funds, the report must have made grim reading.

Under the AIDS (Control) Act 1987, each district health authority in England and Wales and each health board in Scotland was required to publish annual information on the numbers of HIV/AIDS patients and the services provided for them. Hospital and residential hospice care was regarded increasingly as a temporary or last-stop service for people with AIDS; the concept of care in the community, though clearly not unique for AIDS, was seldom so central to the care and prevention of disease, and funds were therefore ring-fenced to ensure that they were not spent on other things.

Many districts developed innovative services. But the reports under the AIDS (Control) Act and investigations by the Comptroller and Auditor General led the National Audit Office to the conclusion that the provisions to ensure cost-effective funding were quite inadequate. It found that 'some health authorities have used underspends to overcome deficits on other activities, without approval', and that out of the £121 million allocated in 1989–90, authorities underspent by £15 million.

The worst offender was the North West Thames region, which diverted £8.5 million of its AIDS budget of £36.9 million to capital projects, namely a hospital building programme that had been hit by the property slump reducing its income from land sales. On discovery, the region agreed to reimburse the AIDS budget over the next two years.

Management of the Oxford District Health Authority removed £600,000 from the budget of £970,000 to help overcome other financial problems. The district promised to repay the money, but in the short term agreed to borrow money from the region to be spent on AIDS services. A similar situation occurred in the North East Thames region, where management borrowed £500,000 to help offset a capital deficit.

Money underspent and returned to the regions (not least because the sudden influx of money in 1989–90 was deemed to be excessive) came to £9.2 million in the North West Thames region, £2.4 million in North East Thames, £2.8 million in the West Midlands, £2.5 million in Trent and £1.7 million in Wessex. £3.1 million was also underspent in Scotland, predominantly in Greater Glasgow. The £121 million provided by the government in this period was almost double that of the previous year.

Jimmy Glass, who worked for Hackney local authority in the North East Thames region during this period (before joining the Terrence Higgins Trust), recalls a situation where large amounts of money that nobody knew what to do with suddenly became available:

Believe me, having been a social worker for ten years, where all you ever saw was services being cut, to be put in a position where you just had money to spend and you could develop things, it was really exciting.

But I also felt professionally very guilty that I had to buy X number of washing machines to use the money up and other clients and other services couldn't get a penny. People coming from an AIDS-based background who haven't necessarily been involved in social care before don't fully appreciate what an exceptionally well-funded area, relative to other areas, AIDS had become.

Yet it was a sign of strange priorities, or at least excessive administrative zeal, that people with AIDS suffered at the hands of other general cost-cutting measures. A year before the great funding increase, the Department of Social Security had abolished special payments to people with disabilities or severe illness, replacing them with Income Support. This meant that whereas before a person with AIDS might qualify for payments for diet, laundry and heating, they now received a lump sum of £34.90 per week. This payment held firm for six months after their diagnosis, unless they could show they could 'reasonably be expected to die within six months', in which case they would receive higher benefit.

There were great discrepancies in the basic cost of health care in different districts. To treat a patient with AIDS in London's Riverside health authority cost £14,671 per year; in Oxfordshire it cost £17,000 per year, in Brighton £20,000 and in Parkside £27,000. (The first and last figures are for 1987–8, the other two for 1988–9 and 1989–90). London hospital treatment ranged from £190 a day at the Central Middlesex to £334 a day at Charing Cross.

These discrepancies, which reflected the varied priorities of management in different hospitals and authorities, did not bode well for the time when ring-fencing would be abandoned, leaving authorities to spend their funds as they saw fit; they would still have to treat the sick, but provision for long-term education and prevention was another matter. As it turned out, ring-fencing would be ditched within three years.

Perhaps this chaos, this controversy, was all inevitable. With insufficient figures, disputed projections, cancelled surveys, was it any wonder that provision for AIDS was proving to be such a haphazard affair? With the epidemic a decade old, there seemed to be as many unanswerable questions as ever.

Withdrawal

In 1986, John Campbell, a gay man of 18, was arrested for male importuning. He claimed that he was innocent, at least on that one occasion. He had worked as a high-class male prostitute in Chelsea, London, and had a list of regular 'celebrity' clients. A magistrate sent him for three weeks' remand while they gathered the evidence.

Campbell was tested for HIV on entering Chelmsford prison, standard practice for anyone identified as a drug user or gay.

After four days, police dropped the charges and Campbell was released; his test results were never announced.

A year later he was arrested again: 121 counts of prostitution, photographic evidence. 'They'd been sitting outside taking pictures of people going in and out,' Campbell says. More remand in Chelmsford pending a trial and social worker reports:

They said they would have to test me. I told them I'd already had a test. They said, 'Well that doesn't mean anything because you could have become positive since.'

And then the next day the doctor came in, asked me how I was and I said I was fine and he left the room.

The nurse came in, said, 'Are you sure you're OK?' and I went, 'Yeah, fine.' He said, 'Oh. I'll be back in a minute.' And it hit me then. I knew instantly the first test had been positive. And the doctor came back in and looked at me and said, 'I've got some bad news for you.'

Campbell was placed in a small HIV section in the prison hospital, a long corridor apart from the rest of the wing. Gay men were segregated from drug users, though they shared the same shower unit. 'When we showered we passed the heterosexuals and used to get attacked and swore at. They blamed us completely.'

Campbell says he received no apology or explanation for the failure to inform him of his first test result. He was confused about what exactly his status meant, but knew more than his 'nurses'. 'They're called nurses, but they're not really. I think they had six weeks' training. They reacted as best they could and were very compassionate, though very ignorant. They were scared of us, because they didn't know how they could get it, and we were scared of them because we didn't know what they would do to us.'

When Campbell appeared in court, he came armed with a stinging report from a prison social worker which detailed the service's failure in reporting his diagnosis; it claimed that the delay had potentially sentenced a lot of other people to infection. The magistrate agreed and let Campbell go. 'The only condition he made was that I never go in front of him or the court again for a prostitution charge without being charged with attempted murder for deliberately infecting someone with HIV.'

On release, Campbell contacted everyone he had had sex with over the last few years. Or everyone he could trace – he reckoned there were at least 300, most of them paying customers. He told them of his diagnosis and advised them to have a test. As far as he knows, only one person came up positive and they had only had sex once. This man is now dead.

During Campbell's confinement there were two other men in the gay section and six, the capacity, in the drug users' section. He believes that things have improved slightly for HIV positive prisoners; less ignorance, less segregation and better counselling facilities. Prejudice from warders and other prisoners probably remains as strong as ever. And one other thing: 'At Chelmsford they've got a bigger unit now, for more people.'

The problems of how to deal with HIV and AIDS in prisons first surfaced as a political issue in 1986 and have never gone away. The sticking points are the same: the supply – or not – of clean needles and condoms. But things have changed considerably from the earliest Home Office ostrich position, claiming there was no homosexual activity and certainly no intravenous drug use in British jails.

In January 1989 the Commons debate on AIDS aired several important issues relating to HIV in jails: key amongst these were the facts that no one really knew what was going on and that the Home Office didn't seem to mind this. First to raise the issue was Charles Irving, Conservative member for Cheltenham, who suspected AIDS was 'rampant' in prisons. He talked of how, when inmates are released, 'they will unleash the disease on an unsuspecting heterosexual population'. Next up, Chris Butler, Conservative member for Warrington South. Butler proposed compulsory testing of all inmates, because he believed that prisons were a major source of crossover between the heterosexual and homosexual populations; levels of homosexual behaviour, needle sharing and tattooing were higher than those in the outside community. He quoted figures from mass testing in Spanish jails which found 18.7 per cent of prisoners to be HIV positive; he had heard that in a new York federal prison the infection rate was as high as 40 per cent. Condoms were not the answer, he said, because they were so unreliable. Education was needed badly, but prison officers were already overstretched. Mr Butler then moved on to consider the 'defence implications' of AIDS, noting that there were few reported cases in the USSR, but a vast amount in the United States, 'our major ally ... there is the potential for military destabilisation'.

Liberal Democrat Archy Kirkwood concluded that we did not know 'what the dickens is going on in prisons', before calling on the Terrence Higgins Trust to bail out the Prison Service by providing education and an extension of its buddy system.

Tom Cox, Labour MP for Tooting, said that 'many prison inmates who suffer from AIDS are treated like the lepers of old. No one wants to know. They are put out of the way and out of sight. Although the rights of prisoners in general may be limited, if a prisoner has AIDS his rights are virtually non-existent'.

Harry Cohen, Labour member for Leyton, reported that in New York, Spain and parts of Italy condoms were readily available in prisons, and believed that the Home Office would eventually 'pay for its negligence'. In 1987, the last year for which figures were available, syringes were found at 13 prisons. Were they tested for HIV? The Home Office said they weren't. Why not, asked Cohen, before concluding that the Home Office had no wish to know the extent of the problem.

David Mellor had no response to these criticisms in his closing speech. Looking back, he says:

> There was a lot of scepticism about the distribution of free condoms, which I shared. It amounted to the kind of acceptance of activities in prisons that were actually going to run directly contrary to the maintenance of good order and discipline. And there was never the evidence with which to justify some of the assertions about the extent of drug misuse in prisons. There was only a mass of anecdotage.

His predecessor at the Department of Health, Edwina Currie, remembers:

> We were not prepared to be that helpful to prisoners. We were try-
> ing to help people who were not HIV infected to stay that way and
> in prison there was a very strong element of feeling, well, the
> prison authorities ought to be watching people's behaviour and try-
> ing to control it. To have taken steps to assist prisoners by provid-
> ing condoms and free needles would have been going much too far.
> We had enough trouble providing free needles to Scottish kids, let
> alone anybody else.

The extent of HIV and AIDS in prisons has always been difficult
to quantify; known figures are always likely to be an underestimate. In
November 1986 the *British Medical Journal* reported that there had
been about 50 cases of HIV identified in prisons, the same figure
quoted by the Home Office in May 1988 (between March 1985 and
May 1988, 166 prisoners with HIV had passed through the system).
Come June 1993, officially there would be 411 HIV positive inmates
in prisons in England and Wales. But most infections would not be
identified until prisoners fell ill; fearing prejudice and discrimination,
few inmates volunteered for tests.

Have conditions and treatment improved? Considerably. In 1986
AIDS became subject to the powerful Viral Infectivity Restrictions
(VIR) that had been established to deal with hepatitis B. VIR gave
prison medical officers discretionary control over an infected prisoner's
treatment and permitted segregation, withdrawal from work, exercise
and privileges, and isolation in hospital even if well. The guidelines
also allowed doctors to breach medical confidentiality on a 'need to
know basis'. If employed ruthlessly, VIR robbed prisoners of their
rights and, though wholly inappropriate, it served an important political function. Politicians and the officials knew something was being
done and staff (and presumably other prisoners) felt protected.

VIR was also a powerful psychological tool at a time when industrial relations in prisons had all but broken down in the mid to late
1980s, says Adam Sampson, deputy director of the Prison Reform
Trust. 'The last thing anybody wanted was to be having to ponce
around with fancy policies around HIV which would be unpopular
with governors, staff and prisoners.'

Sampson once worked as a probation officer, during which time he encountered a young HIV positive offender receiving terrible treatment at Feltham. He says that there were several reports of people being subject to VIR even though – and no doubt because – they refused to take a test. At Wandsworth a policy of segregation of untested inmates suspected of being at risk continued until 1990. At other institutions, says Sampson, 'You had people having their heads shaved because "Those bugs jump, don't they?" You had people being forced to eat off different coloured plates. A lot of scapegoating.'

VIR tended to perpetuate the problems, rather than solve them. It convinced prisoners who believed they might be HIV positive that they should not inform the authorities. HIV was seen to be punishable and VIR drove it underground. Intravenous drug users who might otherwise have admitted their habit felt obliged to conceal it, which meant you either went cold turkey or you carried on using inside, with all the attendant problems of shared needles. With drugs easier to conceal than equipment, there were many stories of needles being passed around Wandsworth for three months; in the absence of needles, Biro tubes would suffice.

In 1991 Lord Justice Woolf's report proposed that policies in respect of VIR should be subject to 'critical examination with a view to setting them aside', but VIR has never been officially withdrawn. Since about 1990 its status has become increasingly ambiguous. Doctors can still segregate prisoners, but they may just call it something different these days. Sampson believes that the low status afforded to prison doctors is partly to blame for the poor treatment of prisoners. Employed by the Home Office, full-time staff have little career structure and little reason for joining if they can get work within the NHS (in smaller jails care is often provided part-time by GPs, work that is very much secondary to their community practice, with quite different requirements). Full-time medical officers are often isolated from professional oversight, have less access to training than those working in hospitals and exercise considerable power in closed institutions. They may have split loyalties as well: they care for patients but are also part of prison management, so there may be complications over confidentiality. 'It's a recipe for disaster,' Adam Sampson concludes.

The education of prison officers and inmates about HIV has been a slow process. In 1987 a staff training video was produced by a committee of prison staff and members of the Terrence Higgins Trust and Body Positive. The 30-minute film included dramatized scenes of fights, self-mutilation and slops throwing as well as much factual information. The Home Office claimed that by April 1988, 25 per cent of staff had seen it. A survey of attitudes before and after screening suggested that, after watching the video, between 20 and 40 per cent moved in a positive direction on all scales measured except blame.

For prisoners, information filtered through gradually and later. Inmates were excluded from the distribution of the leaflet 'Don't Die of Ignorance' until the matter was raised in the Commons and rectified. They received no information relating to their own situation until a leaflet was issued in August 1987. 'AIDS: Information for People in Prison' was a straightforward document, but shirked the issues of homosexual activity and drug-taking. More effective was the video *AIDS: Inside and Out* which appeared a year later and contained testimony from HIV positive prisoners. When screened as part of an induction process, accompanied by other information produced by the THT, HEA and the Standing Conference on Drug Abuse, it formed a solid and comprehensive package; but the Prison Medical Service has acknowledged that the use of the video and supply of other material varied considerably from prison to prison; it was often a low priority beside other training needs such as control and restraint and suicide prevention.

When Jimmy Glass took over the prisons brief at the Terrence Higgins Trust in 1990, he was struck by two things: the eagerness of the Home Office to wash their hands of the problem and the commitment on behalf of a range of prison officers to equip themselves with relevant knowledge.

The THT had the run of most jails in London; staff went in as 'health promotion workers' so as not to frighten the horses, and found most inmates confused and threatened by the basics of infection, but eager to learn; some were unable to read the literature; most did not have access to the helpline number.

Inevitably, one or two progressive models of care and education stood out. By 1988 Saughton jail, outside Edinburgh, contained more people with HIV than any other prison in Britain. When the new governor, John Pearce, arrived he found his staff frightened, beleaguered and set upon a strict policy of isolation. 'It was not sensible in management terms,' he realized, ' because by locking people behind closed doors you assume everyone else is clear and you have no right to assume that.' There was another problem: 'The outcome of consistently telling people they are not worth anything is they attack the people telling them that.' By 1990 homespun educational material spoke in plain terms: don't share needles, razors and toothbrushes and don't have sex 'up the arse'. For a while the prison began to look like the THT roadshow: stickers and posters everywhere, with one of a lavatory captioned, 'Anyone who thinks you can get AIDS off it is full of shit'. Infected prisoners appreciated the counselling groups and the extended medical facilities. But some attitudes died hard: one officer-counsellor observed, 'There are a lot of staff in here who still want them put up against a wall and shot.'

At the end of 1991, the spirit of Saughton was embodied in new guidelines from the Prison Medical Service. Specialist staff from virtually all prisons in England and Wales were to have multi-disciplinary training in HIV counselling care and support (by 1994, there would be 500 care and support officers and 200 HIV counsellors). In addition, new minimum targets were set for the distribution of leaflets and screening of videos to inmates and staff.

But the two political hot cakes remained: drugs and condoms. In a letter written in March 1991, Rosemary Wool, director of the Prison Medical Service, outlined to Adam Sampson at the Prison Reform Trust the objections that still existed about the distribution of condoms. 'Ministers ... have not been convinced that making condoms available for use in prison would be appropriate or helpful,' she wrote. The reasons were twofold. Ministers believed they could not ignore the fact that to issue condoms would be to condone illegal activities: as homosexual intercourse is legal only between consenting adults in private, they regarded it highly unlikely that conditions of privacy could be said to exist in prisons. They were also worried that to make condoms available might have the opposite effect of the one intended and encourage very high-risk activity which some prisoners might not otherwise engage in.

The reasoning that prisons are a public place was based on either of two facts: that they are Crown Property, in which case the argument might apply equally to universities and a thousand other institutions; or that each cell has a spyhole. To argue the latter case you would have to show that prying warders would be shocked or corrupted by the sight of homosexual activity.

There have always been more direct political and logistical difficulties with condom distribution. If it was hard for a Home Secretary to explain to his electorate, it would be harder to explain to prisoners' wives: 'Oh, we're issuing your husband with a condom just in case he wants gay sex while he's inside.' In addition, most prisoners would find the issuing of condoms objectionable and other inmates would have a hard time picking them up from any location in the jail. One solution might be the distribution to all prisoners of a monthly hygiene pack including aspirins, soap, toothpaste and condoms, of which they could use as much or as little as they chose.

Such suggestions still fall on deaf ears. One senior psychologist from the Home Office with a responsibility for prisons told Jimmy Glass: 'If prisoners wanted condoms they'd smuggle them in, like they smuggle in drugs.' When Glass suggested that health education and safer sex practices were not necessarily top of a prisoner's agenda, the psychologist 'looked lost ... He thought the responsibility was on prisoners to take the lead'.

The extent of gay sex in jails is almost impossible to quantify, the levels of anal intercourse perhaps even harder. Most reports suggest that the vast majority of sexual activity seems to be low-level risk: some mutual masturbation, some oral. 'I think there's maybe a fantasy, perhaps a gay fantasy, that prisons are hotbeds of sex, like a nightclub behind bars, and that's nonsense,' says Glass. One argument holds that the introduction of condoms might change the profile to higher risk behaviour. It's a reasonable hypothesis, but one that is seldom heard when condoms are promoted as a public health policy in the general community.

Another widely adopted public health policy, the issue of clean needles to intravenous drug users, has seldom been viewed by ministers as even a subject worthy of debate. With detoxification with methadone unavailable in the majority of jails, mainlining prisoners receive little support either inside Parliament or out: even the Prison Reform Trust does not commit itself to the concept of needle exchange, not least because of the obvious safety hazard. Unlike condom provision, needles were not available in prisons in Europe.

In a circular issued to all prison service governors and managing medical officers in April 1991, Dr Wool acknowledged the existence of illicit drug use within prisons, and wrote that the latest research suggested that at least 12 per cent of sentenced men and 24 per cent of sentenced women were dependent on drugs at the time of their arrest. 'The morbidity amongst remand prisoners is almost certainly higher.' In 1992, there were 2,800 males imprisoned for drug offences, about the same as in the previous four years. The figure for women was 260.

For 1992 the number of addicts reported by prison medical officers (often taken as an indication of the extent of injecting drug use) was 1747, a 23 per cent increase on the previous year. The number of finds of injecting equipment has increased from 54 in 1985, to 141 in 1987, to 219 in 1992, and these only include needles and syringes connected with a prisoner or cell, not those discarded or hidden elsewhere. In a study conducted in 1991 of 452 men and women interviewed after release, 7.7 per cent of male injecting drug users and 15.5 per cent of female users were found to be positive.

The guidelines on drug users in prisons issued to governors and medical officers concentrate on creating a climate in which users would identify themselves and seek help. But without methadone (issued by doctors on a discretionary basis), withdrawal presents an unattractive proposition. It is partly in acknowledgement of this that the Home Office has permitted the distribution of THT leaflets outlining cleaning procedure for injecting equipment with soapy water. As this reduces transmission risks only marginally, bleach solutions have also been available in some prisons.

The Home Office is proud of its improvements in HIV/AIDS policy in British jails over the years, but privately officials recognize that levels of infection are as likely to increase as decrease in the foreseeable future. The novelist Will Self remembers a conversation with a former inmate at Pentonville which emphasizes the doomy cycle: somehow the drugs always get through. 'Everyone knew when a bit of tackle [heroin] came on to the landing, and everyone knew who had the fit [injecting equipment]. There was never any question of not banging up, even if there was still some claret [blood] left in the barrel.'

Compensation

By the beginning of 1987, it looked as though haemophilia was all but over as a political issue. The blood supply had been made secure, almost all haemophiliacs had been tested and the view from Westminster was clear: a terrible tragedy, great sympathy, but these things happen. Compensation hadn't been mentioned for a while, and when it was, Kenneth Clarke or Norman Fowler and all the health department underlings would make the same noises: unworkable, 'dangerous' even. And then they'd quote the findings of the 1978 Royal Commission on Civil Liability and Compensation for Personal Injury (the

Pearson Commission), which rejected the idea of establishing a no-fault scheme for medical accidents. So that was that.

But it was like it says on gravestones: not dead, just sleeping. The Pearson Commission had been far from clear cut in its recommendations; one of the arguments in favour of granting compensation, it stated, was that 'blood products may be used which contain viruses, the presence of which could not be foreseen'. It had taken quite a while to gather momentum, but in the spring of 1987 the Haemophilia Society came back fighting. The issue of compensation had always been on the agenda and there had been no shortage of angry members at the AGMs, but the collective shock of the HIV tests of 1984 and 1985 – about 1,200 haemophiliacs infected – had taken many months to get over; compensation was a long-term battle and many believed they wouldn't be around to reap any rewards.

By the beginning of 1987 about 40 men had died, often leaving families in financial difficulties. Before AIDS, haemophiliacs were unable to obtain life insurance without paying huge premiums; after it, they were denied it at any price. Those with AIDS and even the asymptomatic faced considerable problems in addition to those posed by building societies or insurance firms: discrimination at work or lack of work; the additional costs of maintaining a healthy lifestyle; pressures on providing for the future.

'It was really very simple,' says Simon Taylor, who helped spearhead the society's campaign:

The government had promised self-sufficiency and not delivered. If they had done that then the vast majority of these people would not have been infected. As it was, they were infected as a result of their medical treatment. And I think people wanted somebody to accept responsibility. People want somebody to say, 'Yes, there was a mistake, we're sorry, this shouldn't have happened.'

And so a campaign got underway. Letters went to MPs, sympathetic stories appeared in the press, people threatened to sue their district or regional health authority. Margaret Thatcher had always insisted that the correct course of redress was through the courts and it was clear she had sought advice on the matter. When the Haemophilia Society consulted a barrister about the likelihood of successful litigation, it was told that chances were remote. It would be very difficult to prove precisely who or what infected you; most people had

multiple transfusions from different products from different manufacturers, and in most cases it would be impossible to say that one particular batch from one particular manufacturer infected any one person. Then there was the state-of-the-art defence: because most
haemophiliacs were infected before AIDS was recognized (and certainly before blood products could be screened), you couldn't be protected
from something which you didn't know existed.

The earliest stage of the campaign focused on demands for a non-
means-tested weekly allowance; General Secretary David Watters
named a figure of £40 to £50, later revised to £65 to £70. The society also asked for a £27 million mortgage protection scheme to keep
up repayments when a family breadwinner dies or is too ill to work.
There was much anger at a press conference to launch the campaign.
'I see my patients become sick and in some cases die as a direct result
of NHS treatment,' said Dr Peter Jones, down from the Royal
Victoria Infirmary in Newcastle. He talked of 'widows left destitute,
their children left without the resources which you or I would like to
leave our children'. Twisting the knife, Simon Taylor said, 'I do not
believe that the government – if it is truly a caring government – will
stand by while widows and orphans are thrown out of their homes.'
With the majority of those infected expected to die within ten years,
Taylor says, 'We played on all that shamelessly.'

In November 1987 the society met John Moore, Secretary of State
for Social Services, but came away empty handed. Moore emphasized
that there were already many benefits to which haemophiliacs might
be entitled, whether HIV positive or not – sickness benefit, invalidity
benefit, mobility allowance and others. Any additional payments would
drain resources from other areas of the health service. Tony Newton
had previously told the Social Services Committee that the important
point was that haemophiliacs were suffering the unforeseen side effects
of a treatment designed to help them with their established condition;
their situation was therefore not on a par with, for example, people
who suffered side effects from a new vaccine designed to prevent a
condition from occurring, for which there did exist a method of dis-
tributing compensation.

For Edwina Currie, compensation was resisted

> because there were a lot of them and it was expensive – simple as
> that. It is not government policy to compensate people who are the
> subject of medical accidents. We looked very seriously at medical

compensation possibilities to avoid poor souls having to take cases to court. But the cost of doing it was horrendous because compensation usually in this country takes into account loss of earning power and potential length of life, so you're talking about settlements of £1 million.

Another, less public, argument received much support at the Department of Health: 'Payments [would have gone] to people who ain't going to get better, whose medical circumstances are not going to improve,' Currie says. Many of the more recent compensation cases will pay money during an individual's lifetime, rather than a lump sum. But

the practice then firmly was to give a lump sum based on a calculation, and then your haemophilia patient might die three weeks later and hey presto you've got a very wealthy family. They haven't got haemophilia, they haven't got AIDS, but they've got a million quid of public money which could have been used to help treat other patients. And on the whole that continued to be my feeling. If people are hurt inadvertently by treatment that in fact has made their lives better, it's awfully difficult to see where the legal position might lie.

But on 16 November 1987 there was a change of heart. Tony Newton told the Commons that the government would make a £10 million *ex gratia* payment to infected haemophiliacs 'in recognition of a specific and unique combination of circumstances'. The health minister emphasized that the government did not accept liability for their plight and that it would not open the door to similar claims in the future. The U-turn was the result of strong lobbying from Tory backbenchers, who argued that because the infected haemophiliacs were a small and finite group, they could be helped without opening up the floodgates. In addition, there was the gradual realization that the haemophiliacs had widespread public support. There was, however, no compensation for the small number of people who had become infected through blood transfusions; the Department of Health maintained that most had been infected abroad.

The £10m for haemophiliacs was an 'adequate and proper sum', Newton said, but opposition health spokesman Robin Cook called it 'short-changing' the haemophiliacs. The Haemophilia Society said it was pleased with the money, but the Revd Alan Tanner, its chairman, later told the annual seminar that the Macfarlane Trust, newly established to administer the grant, was unsure whether the sum would be enough or how it would distributed.

By September 1989 the trust had made 1,700 single hardship grants totalling £913,000, and 587 regular payments totalling £1,098,000. 'We realized it wasn't enough pretty soon,' says Simon Taylor. Taylor became one of the trustees of the Macfarlane Trust, but it was his experience as a public relations consultant that proved most useful to the society. Throughout the compensation campaign, much of the media liked to make a distinction between the deserving and undeserving: the *Sunday Times* titled its own bullish and decisive campaign 'The Forgotten Victims', while the *Daily Express* and others preferred 'The AIDS innocents'. 'While some people point accusing fingers at homosexuals and drug addicts,' wrote the *Express*'s medical correspondent, 'these innocent victims [haemophiliacs] stand apart. For they have led blameless lives and it could never be said that they have brought the tragedy on themselves.'

The Haemophilia Society was keen never to make this distinction itself. There was a 'swear box': every time a member said in a public capacity, 'But we're the innocent ones', they were obliged to contribute £1, which then went to the Terrence Higgins Trust. The society maintained close links with several AIDS organizations, but they kept them low key. 'Whilst we at a national level, at a campaigning level, understood the importance of working with other AIDS groups,' Simon Taylor says, 'Joe Haemophiliac out in the sticks doesn't. As far as he's concerned, one of the major reasons for his infection is that a bunch of drug users or gays was giving blood and they shouldn't have been. So when the media picked up the "innocent victims" line, we took the view that "You may well say that but we couldn't possibly comment."'

Between 1987 and 1989, about 250 individuals were granted legal aid to chance their arm in the courts. In June and July 1989 Mr Justice Ognall heard preliminary hearings in the High Court in London to establish the framework within which claims would be considered. Subsequently he would grow increasingly restless with the drawn-out course of the proceedings (which included a failed attempt by government solicitors to withhold documents on the grounds of public interest immunity) and with the scale of the tragedy that was being unravelled before him. A year later, with no settlement yet in sight, 962 haemophiliacs and their families would be taking legal action for negligence.

Towards the end of November 1989, Margaret Thatcher received a delegation of senior Tory backbenchers pressing the case for compensation and a settlement of the court actions. The group was led by Robert Key, MP for Salisbury, and included Sir Bernard Braine, Father of the House, Sir Geoffrey Johnson Smith, vice-chairman of the 1922 Committee, John Hannam, vice-chairman of the all-party disablement group, and Emma Nicholson, MP for Devon West and Torridge. 'She is seeing us because she cares,' Emma Nicholson said of Mrs Thatcher. 'She is often portrayed as someone without feelings for other people's suffering, but she is a woman of very deep feeling.' By this stage over 180 MPs had signed early day motions calling for an out-of-court settlement. A hundred and sixty-three haemophiliacs had developed full-blown AIDS and 107 were dead.

A day after the meeting, in a parliamentary written answer to Robert Key, Kenneth Clarke announced that the government would be stumping up more money for the Macfarlane Trust. Neither an out-of-court settlement nor an admission of liability, the sum of £19 million was intended to be split up equally into payments of £20,000 to each infected individual. In his statement, Mr Clarke acknowledged that the government 'shares the universal sense of shock at the unique position of haemophiliacs who have been infected by the AIDS virus'. He later said in a television interview that it was 'a very reasonable amount' but if he hoped that it would signal the end of the matter he was mistaken.

As the litigation dragged on, Clarke became increasingly isolated. The prospect of the sick and dying appearing in a High Court battle against the government would be potentially hugely damaging in the run up to an election and, although it was never admitted publicly, by October 1990 the Department of Health had already given favourable consideration to the possibility of settling out of court. Sensing victory, the Haemophilia Society placed a series of startling large-scale advertisements in the national press. These featured a young boy's face overprinted with the text, 'Heredity gave him haemophilia. Then the NHS gave him HIV'. Four newspapers ran the campaign, but the *Daily Telegraph* refused, fearing the advert could be libellous. 'We have not tried to be contentious for the sake of it,' countered John Dilworth, whose agency Standley Burridge Collings was responsible for the campaign. 'It is a true statement of fact.'

Several matters forced the government's hand. In September Mr Justice Ognall wrote to both the Department of Health and those representing the haemophiliacs to give anxious consideration to a settlement. In the handwritten statement, leaked to the *Sunday Times*, he wrote that the 'increasingly notorious' case contained unique moral and political dimensions that would only benefit from a swift conclusion. 'At best, those plaintiffs will die uncertain as to the outcome. At worst, they will be deprived of money to comfort their last days or with the knowledge (for those with dependants) that they will enjoy a measure of financial security.'

The following month, Clarke maintained his position – great tragedy ... Macfarlane Trust already established ... no one's to blame – while his officials busied themselves with guarantees and conditions of a possible settlement. 'Our NHS is greatly threatened by the increase in the number of writs that are being issued claiming compensation for allegations of medical negligence,' Clarke observed:

The American health care system is being ruined by excessive litigation and the mounting costs of compensation. It is possible to organise powerful emotional campaigns for many groups whose treatment has failed to restore good health. All medical treatment has an element of risk and involves considered judgment of those risks in the light of current scientific knowledge.

The 'powerful emotional campaign' was one which neither he nor Mrs Thatcher would have to deal with for much longer. By mid-November, William Waldegrave had become Health Secretary and he immediately faced vigorous claims for compensation from a newly formed all-party group. Setting out the group's strategy, Conservative chairman Patrick Cormack presented his party with a face saver: 'We are not asking the Government to admit legal liability – in this case we want it to quantify its moral responsibility.' So money, not blame, would be enough. In the end, it was pure expediency that decided the matter.

'There was an election coming up,' Edwina Currie says. That was the only reason for a settlement? 'Sure. Politics. There was no shift in attitude at all.'

'We just kept going until we knew there wasn't going to be any more money,' Simon Taylor says. 'The legal actions certainly acted as a good campaigning spur because it kept it in the news, but apart from one or two cases where there was negligence the vast majority didn't have a hope in hell of winning them.'

In the end it was John Major, the new Prime Minister, who sanctioned an out-of-court settlement in December 1990. In the principal agreement, accepted officially in April 1991, the government would provide an additional sum of £42 million, to be split among all infected haemophiliacs according to circumstance. Thus infants would get £21,500 each, a single adult £23,500, a married adult without dependent children £32,000 and a haemophiliac with dependent children £60,500. Infected partners and married children would receive £23,500 and unmarried infected children £21,500.

Mixed emotions among haemophiliacs: relief that it was over, but some disappointment that the figures were not higher. Towards the end of the campaign, a total of £90 million was claimed. 'To say that the clients "want" to accept this offer is perhaps too strong a word for it,' said Mark Mildred, a solicitor with Panone Napier, a firm representing more than 300 claimants. 'It is better to say that they are resigned to it.'

'That was all we were going to get so there wasn't much point in feeling pissed off about it,' Taylor says:

I think people felt a lot better because it's been a recognition, although it has not been enough to transform their financial circumstances, it isn't enough to provide for your wife and children for the rest of their days. But I know a lot of people who have done something which they would never otherwise have done and are pleased they've done it, perhaps before they become ill.

Soon there was a new campaign, on behalf of more 'forgotten victims', the non-haemophiliacs who were given HIV-infected blood by the NHS. Virginia Bottomley ruled out the possibility of compensation in January 1992, but a month later William Waldegrave agreed to payments on similar lines to those given haemophiliacs. Survivors, their dependants, and the relatives of those who had already died were to share up to £12 million. About 170 people are believed to have caught the virus through blood transfusions between 1981 and 1986; in April 1991 77 of them were known to be still alive; by January 1992 there were 37.

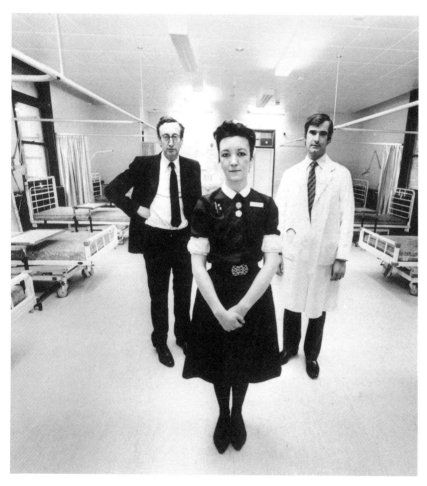

1 The Broderip Ward at the Middlesex Hospital, the first dedicated AIDS wing, before its opening in 1987. Shortly after it was opened by the Princess of Wales, it was already overcrowded. From left to right: Professor Stephen Semple, Ward Sister Jacqui Elliott and Professor Michael Adler.

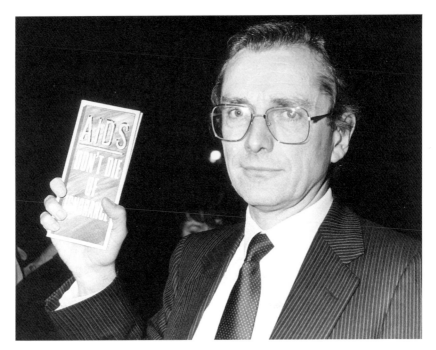

2 Social Services Secretary Norman Fowler outside 10 Downing Street in November 1986, with the leaflet which would be sent to every home in the country. He has just come from the first cabinet committee meeting on AIDS.

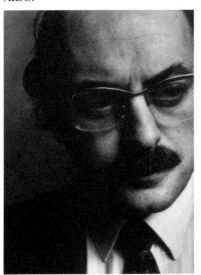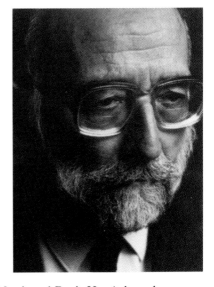

3 & 4 Professor Anthony Pinching of St Mary's and Bart's Hospitals, and Sir Donald Acheson, former Chief Medical Officer. No one would do more to educate the public about the potential epidemic.

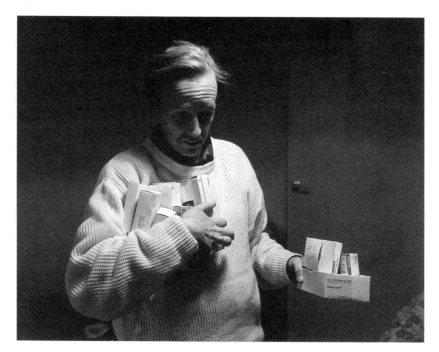

5 Vince at home on the Muirhouse Estate, Edinburgh. In one hand he carries his medication; in the other, the treatments necessary for its side effects.

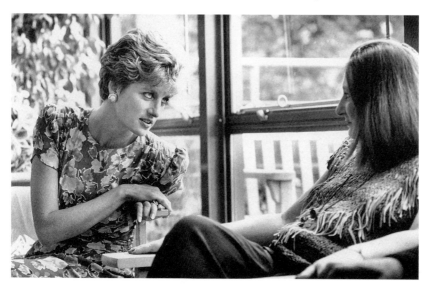

6 The Princess of Wales with Sylvia Killick, who had been diagnosed HIV positive several years before, at the London Lighthouse in 1992.

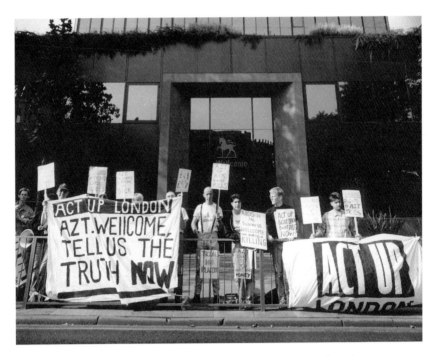

7 Members of Act Up outside Wellcome offices, protesting against the toxicity and cost of AZT. The drug, launched with a fanfare in 1987, is now the subject of suspicion and disappointment.

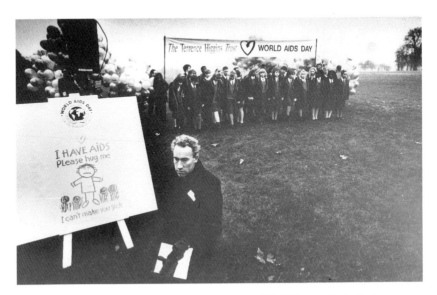

8 Simon Callow and schoolchildren mark World AIDS Day in Hyde Park on 1 December 1988. One thousand balloons were released to symbolize the number of AIDS deaths in the UK.

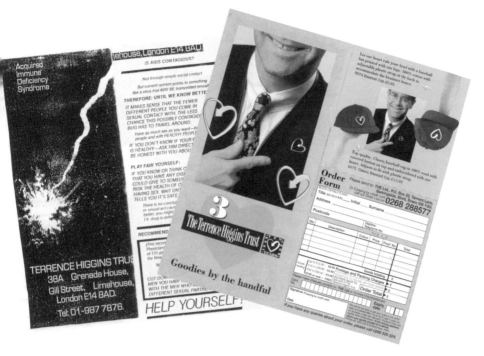

9 A decade of leaflets from the Terrence Higgins Trust. The first tentative information leaflet from 1983, and Elton John promoting the merchandising catalogue in 1993.

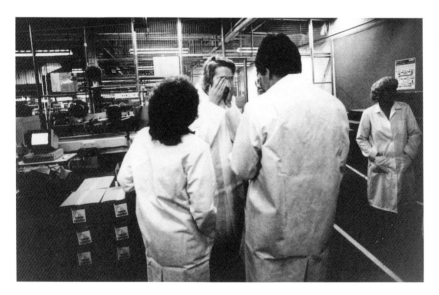

10 Virginia Bottomley, Health Minister, rubs her eyes at a condom production line in November 1991.

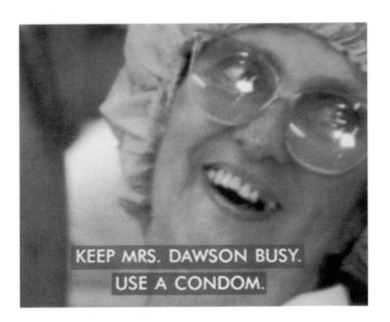

11 'We're making more of these things than ever before.' The Health Education Authority's most popular safer sex advertisement from 1991.

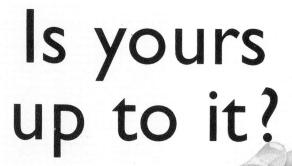

Is yours
up to it?

Not all condoms are created equal. Some are stronger than others. So if you're going to fuck, it makes sense to use one of the stronger variety. Look out for Durex Extra Strong, Mates Super Strong and HT Special.

At the very least, make sure the condom you use has a kitemark on the packet. This shows it meets certain standards. (HT Specials are German and don't have a kitemark but have passed stringent tests.)

And use a water-based lubricant like KY, never oil as this can damage a condom.

HEALTH EDUCATION AUTHORITY

YOU CAN FIND OUT MORE ABOUT SAFER SEX BY CALLING ONE OF THE FOLLOWING NUMBERS. THE NATIONAL AIDS HELPLINE ON 0800 567 123. THE TERRENCE HIGGINS TRUST ON 071 242 1010 OR LONDON LESBIAN AND GAY SWITCHBOARD ON 071 837 7324.

The HEA recognises that the above trademarks are the property of the makers or suppliers of the product.

12 A more detailed advert for the gay press. Health Ministers became alarmed at the use of the word 'fuck', and banned its use in future campaigns.

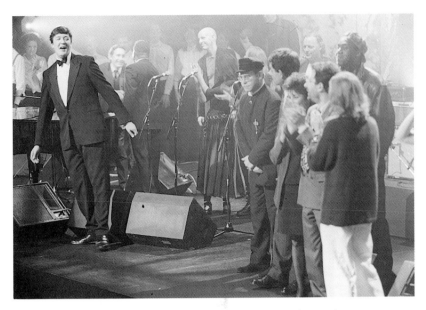

13 Stephen Fry lines up the stars for Hysteria 3. 'Not just the usual suspects being dreary and sanctimonious about AIDS.' From left to right: Elton John, Rowan Atkinson, Ruby Wax, Ben Elton and Lenny Henry.

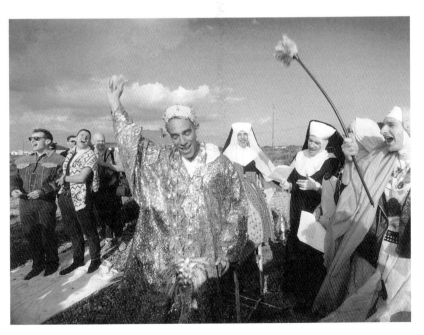

14 Derek Jarman canonized by the Sisters of Perpetual Indulgence, by his cottage in Dungeness in 1991. He called this the happiest day of his life, and at his request was buried in this robe.

CHAPTER 11: Safer Sex, Risky Sex

Not the Voice of an Actor

Had a drink in the hotel and I met this girl at the bar and we got on really well. She was the picture of health, very pretty. I suppose the little devil inside my head would have been saying, 'Go on, son.' So I suggested we went upstairs. We had a drink and Bob's your uncle. That's what it's like on holiday. I mean, I really wish that I'd taken some condoms with me, but it's easy to say that now.

Steve is 28, heterosexual and HIV positive.

STEVE: I'm from the south, in and around London.

I work in the media. I come from a traditional working-class family. Comprehensive school education, your average guy really, educated to degree level.

So I was on holiday, and I've never been specific about where because people would say, 'Oh well, I'm not going to go there so I'll be OK.' One thing I would say is that ten years prior to being infected, I'd probably gone to every major holiday spot in the world that's considered a tourist hot spot and had unprotected sex.

But before I went on this holiday I'd been steady with a girl and I hadn't had unprotected sex for months and months, basically because of the AIDS risk. I remember the campaigns in '85, the icebergs, the tombstones, it frightened the living daylights out of me. I thought herpes was bad enough.

I'd always been very conscious of STD, or VD as my father called it. At the age of thirteen, fourteen he gave me a little talk. I think there was a girlie magazine under my bed, my mother found it. So he gave me a bit of a speech that evening about pregnancies, how it could affect your life, because my mother was pregnant at an early age. And the stories that he told me, you know, a droopy dick and everything else, had always stayed with me. Unless I specifically knew a woman's contraceptive arrangements, I'd never come in her anyway, even on a casual relationship, because I never wanted to carry that burden of risk round with me.

'Steve', of course, is not really Steve. He was 31 in 1994, still fit and working in a new job. He shares a flat in north London. His voice is genuine London wide-boy, rough and slangy and jovial.

In 1987 I remember thinking that AIDS was possibly a media creation, a four-letter word that looked great in tabloid block lettering on the front page. It was the first time the papers had this cocktail of sex and death, and there had never ever been anything like it. Well they had in the last century, syphilis, but I don't think the *Sun* was around then. All of a sudden there was this new thing and it was like perfect for the eighties. It was like the come-uppance for Thatcher's Britain.

After that I think it was the general consensus amongst my friends and people I knew that it couldn't affect us because we were straight and none of us did drugs, none of us injected. We thought that if somebody got cut we might be able to pick it up, that was really the only way, or through a dodgy transfusion. I remember seeing a cartoon in *Today* I think: a young, white, heterosexual couple lying in a coffin-shaped bed and a caption with 'Bang, bang, you're dead'. I remember thinking, 'Phew, that's a bit strong. That doesn't really happen to us.'

I went to the States in '87 on holiday and I had sex, but I used condoms because I knew it was a lot more serious there. So at that point even subconsciously I was aware that it was starting to affect the heterosexual community. Back here if I slept with a foreign girl, then there was a better chance that I was going to wear a contraceptive. Where it was an English girl, not so much. I would take a few chances, but not that often.

I knew about Rock Hudson. There was all the jokes. One of them was, How do you get AIDS? Up the Hudson and over the Rockies. Those kind of things. 'The fellow down the pub's got AIDS.' 'Oh you're joking!' 'Yeah, lemonaids, cherryaids.' I think with Rock Hudson it was the gay thing more than anything else and I remember the headlines in the paper, they were putting his home up for sale and they couldn't even get half the asking price.

I remember feeling sorry for the gay community at the time. I'd had quite a few gay friends and the community had come quite a long way in the late seventies, early eighties, towards being more acceptable to society in general. And all of a sudden this was like such a kick in the teeth.

And then they had the racist element, it was all the Africans' fault, or it was a chimpanzee from Haiti, it was always some black overtone. All very racist and very homophobic.

Anyway I was on holiday. The only specifics I'll mention is that she was a white girl in an English-speaking country. As I said, she was a picture of health, I was attracted to her because she was so natural looking, no make-up, slight tan, very fresh looking, as if she'd just got out the bath. I can't even remember her name.

I was coming back from holiday, about a week later. This was in the autumn of '89, and I started feeling very unwell, headache, bit feverish, sore throat which got progressively worse quite quickly. Just altogether feeling very, very sick. I was glad to be home and seeing my family and friends because I'd been away for over a month.

I thought I'd had food poisoning or something. I went to bed, didn't sleep very well, woke up soaking. I don't sweat normally and woke up feeling so weak, my throat had got even worse. I could almost feel that I'd lost weight. But the thing that worried me was that I had red lesions all over my body.

On the recommendation of my doctor I went to the Hospital for Tropical Diseases near King's Cross. The doctor there ran a few tests, asked me if I'd had unprotected sex and I tried to skirt round the issue but couldn't really.

An hour later, they came back and said I had syphilis. There were no physical symptoms but it was in my blood. That made me feel very unclean, wanted to turn myself inside out and scrub myself with a nailbrush. Then they said, 'Well, given that you've had unprotected sex and you've caught syphilis, we think it might not be a bad idea if you have an HIV test, to make you feel better.'

Yeah, sure, no problem.

Then they left the room and I thought, 'Oh my God.'

So a counsellor came up and the counselling took the form of educating me on HIV. Only retrospectively do I know that they were almost sure that I had it, because my symptoms were so pronounced. Speaking to a doctor afterwards, he said that they'd never seen anyone with such pronounced symptoms.

But the test came back negative because it was less than three months, so that was a huge relief for me.

I was in hospital for a week, having daily injections in my arse with penicillin. I'd lost almost nine pounds in weight, I'm not exactly John Wayne anyway, so nine pounds makes a difference. They said I needed to have another test. Looking back, they were surprised it was negative.

They called me up after just under three months, just before Christmas, and said could I come up. I thought, of course I need another test, that's what it is. But when I arrived they called me into a room and said, 'We've got reason to believe that you're positive.'

They said: 'The reason we're telling you this and the reason we've asked you to come in is that it's just before Christmas and we don't want you going out making merry and then having to live knowing that you've infected someone, if that is the case.'

That was probably the worst day of my life. But not knowing, I had another test there and then. I just kept putting my head in my hands. It was like a Franz Kafka novel; it was *The Trial* and I was in it. All of a sudden somebody had told me I was going to die. I didn't have the official result yet, but as far as I was concerned I was going to die.

Now I think it's like somebody telling you you are going to be in a serious, serious car crash, probably in about ten years' time. And you've got to live those ten years knowing you're going to be in a car crash, waiting for it to happen.

My grandmother was in hospital with cancer, she died the next day. I thought, 'I just don't believe this.'

Each day got a little bit easier, and I basically conned myself. For the next three months I didn't go back to the hospital. I just told myself, they haven't called me, they haven't written to me, I must be OK. So I got to the point where although I was still worried and there were knots in my stomach when I thought about it, I was convinced I was fine. I remember joking, I fancied one of the nurses, once I get this cleared up I'm going to ask her out.

With the NHS being under resourced and the result being much more important to me than it was to them, the onus was on me to get in touch with them, and eventually I went up there, expecting them to say I was OK. I walked in to see the doctor, and he just had that look on his face. So I said, 'Have I got it, yes or no?' He said yes, and my reaction surprised me. If at any time somebody had said to me, 'Right, if they confirm that you're HIV positive, how would you react?' I would have said automatically it will crucify me, it will crucify me, but it didn't, because I'd already gone through the anguish of it. In fact there was an element of relief: I thought at least I can get on and do something about it. The only way I can describe it is a skull and crossbones being flashed before my eyes and having to make an instinctive decision, live or die, and it was live. It was 'Fuck off, I refuse to allow you to beat me.'

In that interim I'd read up a lot on it and I believed that in most cases HIV does lead to AIDS, but not in all cases. There is a heavy link between the immune system and stress levels, your emotional state, plus the mind as well. I know somebody who was diagnosed positive and immediately said he was going to die and did within six months. He just gave up.

I told my sister, but I didn't tell my parents for approximately six months. I didn't want to put them through it. I think one of the most horrific things for any parent ever to do is to bury one of their children. They've been too good to me, they taught me how to be I think a good person, and they don't deserve that.

I put myself in a situation where I went missing for a while. When I did tell them it knocked them for six, they went into a state of shock. My father works in construction, which has never been noted for its political correctness, it's not the most anti-racist area of employment, it's probably the most homophobic of areas. But he and my mother have been absolutely tremendous, genuinely supportive, not just drinking out of my cup to show me that it doesn't matter. Partly because of me, partly because of her mother, they've been to a support group.

In 1990 I got a call from a doctor saying the Health Education Authority have been on saying that they're doing a campaign.

'They're looking for a couple of straight people who'd be in a campaign that's gay, straight and drug users. Would you be interested in talking to them?'

Yeah, sure.

KATE GRIEVES: The previous campaign consisted of experts, doctors just saying 'This is our experience, this is what's happening out there.' What we learnt from that subsequently was that people couldn't translate the notions of HIV actually coming into their own locale. The classic thing: 'I've never seen a case, and it's never going to affect me.' Because HIV is so big and so scary, and so insidiously licking through society, that the majority of people just don't wish to face it.

Kate Grieves joined the HEA in 1989 after working in commercial advertising. She helped devise the 'testimonial' adverts, a series of real people

speaking in their own voices, set against a backdrop of everyday locations
– a quest for association, accessibility, empathy. She says the campaign
would have been less effective if the viewer had been able to see faces.
Steve's video was shot at a Spanish beach and bar; the focus on the beach
is of a man wearing Union Jack shorts.

KATE GRIEVES: Because it's such an uncomfortable issue, and because
it's about sex, if you see somebody on the TV and you can see their
face clearly, unless you feel that they look almost identical to you,
unless you really link with that person, or unless you find them
incredibly physically attractive and you think, 'I'd sleep with him,
absolutely no doubt, Friday night down the club, I'd have him home',
then immediately you start to rationalize all those things away. You
say, 'Oh well actually I wouldn't sleep with that person, to be honest
he's not really my type' or, 'Yeah, well she's a bit of a scrubber.'
People marginalize those people away and are frighteningly dismissive.

We tested this out to see at what level people would and wouldn't
associate with those who were purportedly HIV positive; whether it
mattered whether they were actors or not, whether their voices were
sufficient, what kind of things they had to say, was it worth having
their faces pixilated on screen. We thought pixilation might be quite
good initially but in fact it puts them in a class with rapists and IRA
terrorists, people who are outcasts of society. And the whole point is
to actually make HIV something that is very normal – not usual, but
something that can actually happen to people who have your lifestyle
or one which is very familiar to you.

I think also if we were honest we really wouldn't have got a sufficient number of people who were prepared to sit in front of the camera and to say the kind of things that we wanted to. There are people
who have done it on one-off TV programmes and that is actually
quite different from doing it in advertising where the intention is that
millions and millions of people see it again and again. For most people
it's not the general members of the public that they're worried about
finding out, it's a really close friend or an old boyfriend that they
never managed to contact.

We did five originally: Josephine, Denise, John, Mike and Paul.
Three gay men and two women. Our criteria for all our personal testimony was that everybody had been infected sexually. As an authority
we were not concerned with drugs. Needle transmission was a sort of

grey overlap area but not one that we were focusing on. We were looking for people across a broad range of experiences really.

Then the TV ones were Paul and Susan and then Steve. People just emerged. We'd had a lot of conversations and meetings with the support groups and anybody who was really involved in HIV and AIDS was flyposted. We assured them of a set of constraints, terms within which we would work and all that kind of thing. I saw quite a lot of people who came and decided it wasn't for them and I did my best to put people off because we felt quite strongly it was going to be very tough on people. With Steve the phone rang and there was a message left on my desk saying this guy wants to talk to you about HIV and AIDS advertising. And I thought, 'Oh, another media owner or journalist', and I phoned him back and he just said, 'I hear you wanna do AIDS ads, well I can do one.'

Steve came here late one afternoon and I met him with another colleague. What I would do was to run through and explain what the campaign was about and why we felt we ought to do it in this way. I also talked quite a lot about how we were anxious that anyone who participated in our commercials was very adequately protected and that nothing would be leaked from us about their identity. The people giving the testimony were always in control, they would only have one contact which would be me who would only ever know their real name and how to get hold of them and so on.

There would be a legal contract between us and the other two parties who helped us actually physically produce the ads which was BMP DDB Needham, the advertising agency, and the Central Office of Information, who helped us with the physical production.

I really tried very hard to put people off and Steve was no exception. I would say things about what a shock it is turning on the TV and suddenly hearing your own voice. Had they thought about how they might just be out with a bunch of friends who don't necessarily know their status? Or how their parents or their family, or their partner might feel about it?

And then I'd say, 'Right, go away and think about it and give me a call in a week or whatever.' Steve I think had already made up his mind and he said when we left the building, 'No, I really want to go with this.'

So we met again to really talk through what was relevant in the story. We had been looking for some time for a male heterosexual who'd been infected sexually and we had also been looking for a good testimony to put out around the summer holiday period. What we know from surveys that we do and many others have done is that the number of sexual occasions and partners increases over the summer months, basically it gets hot and people peel their clothes off, and it's cheap package holidays, sun, sea, sangría and sex.

Steve was the embodiment of it: he'd been infected holidaying abroad on a one-night stand. That was the story, absolutely perfect. And what's more, he had his own accent, which is glorious, and he sounds like a Jack the Lad, he sounds an attractive man and that was all really excellent for us.

Having talked to him more about the actual background to his story, we began to agree between us this thread of what it was that he wanted to say, because that's very important: a lot of people wanted to put a particular point across. With the help of a copywriter and an art director at BMP we drafted an outline script, and the purpose of that was so that Steve could see it and say, 'Yeah, OK, these are the kinds of things I'm happy to end up in a forty-second commercial.'

We then went into a research lab. I would chat to this person and ask them leading questions which elicited answers which would mirror the bits on the script. The first few times we did it we ended up with some four or five hours' tape. The reason for doing it was that it didn't sound stilted, so that it didn't sound like somebody was reading it. The whole point was that their stories are absolutely real and true and that they needed to sound like that. There was no dummying or faking or whatever, it was really just a question of getting it on to tape in a real way. And there were lots of emotional highs and lows. It was a very taxing thing to do for everyone concerned. We used to laugh about it, I used to say before we started, 'By the end of today you're just going to want to hit me because you're going to think this woman cannot grasp really simple things because I want you to say the same thing again and again and again.'

The images were applied over that. The imagery was very difficult to do because it couldn't be anyone or anywhere recognizable, it had to be completely and utterly normal, usual looking. We shot masses, hundreds and hundreds of feet of film for that in places, people on a beach, the atmosphere of a bar.

With Steve's commercial, the country in which we shot that has a very different attitude towards HIV and AIDS and they were very willing and keen to help us and people were incredibly accommodating in a way that we hadn't experienced here.

Then they're shown to the participant. We'd kept the participants in on every stage to make sure they were entirely happy, but if someone had actually said to us at the very end of the day, 'Actually I just can't go through with this', then undoubtedly we would have not run it.

STEVE: The ads went out in the summer of '91. First time was in between the *News at Ten*, some serious space was bought. I was very nervous on the night but funnily enough the first time I heard it, because they also did radio versions, was when I was waiting to go in to a support group meeting. I was a bit early so I was sitting in the car, listening to Capital, *The Way It Is*. That was like, I thought, 'Oh I'm going to be sick.' The whole world was going to recognize me. People who were just walking past the car would know it was me.

It was on television the next night and I felt sick. As time went on, I got quite to like it. Funnily enough I was making love one time and the television was on and my ad come on. And it was on films I was watching like *Body Heat*, which I thought was a really good space for it. One reason I did it was, if there was any denial left in me, this was going to get rid of it. Another reason was because I know that I haven't infected anyone, I know that I hadn't had unprotected sex in between having my first test and being told I was probably positive.

It lasted all summer. I was told that the AIDS hotline was usually getting calls of about a few hundred a week but during the three weeks when the ads were most intense they were getting thirty-five thousand calls. And there was a lot of people calling HEA saying, 'Is it so and so?'

So that was that: Steve was born. At the moment Steve serves a purpose because he is almost the voice of heterosexual HIV in this country. I do all these telly or radio things, now especially around World AIDS Day, and I've often said, 'Can't you find someone else?' every now and then. But I do feel a slight responsibility in getting the message across to the media and fellow carriers of the virus that it doesn't have to be 'AIDS equals death'. Fortunately someone else hasn't cornered the market, another Steve who's doom and gloom, 'Oh my God, I'm going to die.' Because what chance have you got if that person is the voice at the time? I just want other carriers to feel a sense of nobility, to hear me and think, 'Well fuck me, he sounds all right.'

It's very traumatic doing this interview because you're totally having to face up to the situation like a boxer who is admitting the day before the fight that he could get beaten. Because he knows his opponent's just as confident as he is. But if every time I do something, put myself through the trauma of it, it makes one person practise safe sex, then it's been worth it for me.

Basically I've been healthy. A couple of times I had diarrhoea and went up the hospital. I'm not the healthiest eater in the world, never have been, but I'm just really gradually eating slightly more healthily, but not in a major way. I walk a lot more, run three miles a day to keep fit. Unfortunately I smoke. I know I have to give up because I'm not really giving myself that much of a fighting chance. At the moment I can get away with it but I'm going to have to stop if I'm serious about it.

I know there will come a time when the virus will attack me and occasionally I get a bit frustrated with the wait. Come on, try me now, come on, attack me now, I'm ready, I've been ready for four years for you, what's your problem? I ain't going to be any different in five years' time as I am now, I don't think it's going to catch me off guard.

It hurts so much to see my parents wanting to tangibly, physically, help me, and there is nothing they can do. The support they give me is incredible and it's so beneficial, but because they can't physically help me it's killing them, it really is. And to see them is very painful and I wouldn't want anybody to go through that.

If somebody who thought they were too macho to put a condom on, or a girl thought that she didn't really want to upset this guy she's going to sleep with, by confronting them with the grief they could cause, they might change their minds.

I don't like having this dual personality. David Bowie and Ziggy Stardust. I have thought about just coming out as me, the real person, my face on camera, but I can't do it yet. The most important reason is to protect my family because my family work in environments that are not conducive to being HIV friendly. The second reason is that people have got used to Steve. And the longer Steve's around, please God he will be around in ten years' time, still doing interviews, there'll be people who are HIV positive thinking, 'I remember listening to him in 1991, and fuck me, he's still around.'

I hate talking about him as a third person. But I do tend to think the subject's in reasonably safe hands with me for now until someone else comes along and picks up the mantle.

The thing most people remember is the 'Bob's your uncle' bit. They used that on *Only Fools and Horses*, Rodney saying to Delboy, 'You don't want to end up like that chap on the telly, you know, Bob's your uncle.'

The De-gaying of AIDS

On St Valentine's Day 1992, Sir Donald Maitland, chairman of the Health Education Authority, received a letter of resignation. Signed by Jonathan Grimshaw and other members of an HEA advisory group, it revealed a great dissatisfaction with the safer sex promotion work the HEA was producing for gay men and the failure of the group to influence its direction. As well as Grimshaw, the group consisted of Peter Scott and Edward King, both of whom had worked extensively for the Terrence Higgins Trust and other community-based organizations, and four others who had much experience of education programmes among 'men who have sex with men' (gay men, bisexuals and men who engage in homosexual activity without acknowledging their sexuality). Their objections to the HEA were numerous, but centred on one issue: after years of trying earnestly to get to grips with gay lifestyles, to understand diverse gay sexual practices and politics, the quango simply never got it. The requirement for safer sex education became ever more sophisticated each year, but each year the 'heterosexual' advertising company employed by the HEA struggled in vain to comprehend even the basics. The advisory group met every few weeks for over two years and offered advice and objections, but they say they were ultimately ignored or overruled.

One HEA leaflet, 'Safer Sex for Gay Men', widely available in 1990, emphasizes both the unique aspects of some gay sexual activity and the communication problems inherent in defining their risk. After some sound general advice ('Be bold ... talk about condoms when your head still rules your feelings'), the leaflet breaks down into an activity checklist. Here an awkwardness enters the dialogue; the section on anal intercourse has a subheading '(often called fucking)'; the one on masturbation has the subhead '(often called wanking)'; then there's digital intercourse, '(usually called fingering)'; and of course frottage '(usually called body rubbing)'. There are also sections on fisting '(although uncommon)', in which calving gloves, properly lubricated, get a mention, and rimming (oral-anal contact), which may

225

increase the risk of developing AIDS if you are already infected by HIV.

Then there was the question of priorities. The honourable attempt to destigmatize those most at risk from AIDS had swung too far the other way. The government's earliest mass campaigns – AIDS was not a gay plague, heterosexuals got it too – were accurate enough and gays were grateful (and partly responsible) for this approach. But this observation increasingly concealed a fundamental truth, that men who have sex with men remained by far the most vulnerable group. Gay men accounted for over two-thirds of reports of new infections from the late 1980s onwards (in the North West Thames region it has been as high as 78 per cent). There were more infected women and more cases of heterosexual infection, but their numbers were very small in comparison.

And here was the problem: in the financial year 1990–91 the HEA spent £9.3 million on HIV campaigns, but only £1.7 million of this was aimed specifically at gay men. In 1991–2 this budget was cut to £700,000. By April 1992, 4,421 gay men had been diagnosed with AIDS and 10,364 had tested positive since the UK epidemic began. Sixty-nine per cent of all those who tested positive in 1991 were gay men. 'This is not an equal opportunities epidemic,' Keith Alcorn, a gay journalist and AIDS educator, wrote in *Capital Gay*. 'Things have gone so wrong largely because gay men have been written off in this epidemic ... We have had an AIDS lobby which has sought to hetero-sexualise itself.'

Alcorn believed that gay men working in the AIDS field faced a terrible compromise, either to put gay men's needs second and gain funding, or to face the possibility of having any statutory funding removed. The lack of specific services for gay and bisexual men was highlighted in a survey, published in July 1992, of 226 UK agencies with an HIV prevention remit (190 of which were NHS organiza-tions). Sixty-six per cent reported that they had not engaged in any work for gay men and only 3.5 per cent (eight agencies) said they had engaged in a 'substantial' amount of work (this meant establishing a written assessment of local requirements and employing at least a part-time worker to deal with these needs). The respondents provided many reasons for this. They believed that others were doing the work, that it was too sensitive and even illegal because of Section 28, that it was too difficult to contact gays in the local area, and that even if they did, they were suspicious about the stigma attached to the notion of

high-risk groups. Nine per cent of agencies reported that there were
no gay men locally; one district HIV prevention co-ordinator said,
'We've no homosexual community here [but] you might try district X
– they have a theatre.'

The authors of the report, which was sponsored by the North West
Thames Regional Health Authority, stressed the many reasons why it
was crucial to maintain a high level of gay and bisexual safer sex education: it was difficult to sustain changes in sexual behaviour without
substantial support and continual reinforcement of its importance; a
different focus of education was needed to help people become informal peer educators and so normalize safe-sex practices within the
community; men new to the scene had to be educated, not least young
men who believed that AIDS was a disease of the older generation
and thought they were infallible; and detailed safer sex information
was needed for those who were already HIV positive.

The HEA had produced campaigns targeted specifically at gay men
from 1989 and it had been a bumpy ride. Political correctness was an
issue here, as was the use of language; how graphic could the campaigns be? No one could take offence from the first gay press and
poster campaign, a series of shadowy, homoerotic photographs of
beautiful men by Herb Ritts, the American who had made his name
snapping Madonna. The caption read, 'They used to say masturbation
was bad for you. Now it could save your life'. It noted that the threat
of AIDS had not gone away, but that 'It's not all doom and gloom
though.' Safer sex could be fun, especially if you had it with the
Greek gods in the photos; unfortunately, few gay men could associate
with bronzed pectorals like that.

The next campaign also featured beautiful men, this time photo-
graphed by Jean Batiste Mondino. One caption held that 'They don't
have safer sex just because it's safer', and went on to list a few examples of what was meant by the phrase: masturbation, massage and so
on. The copywriter then hit top gear: 'There are plenty of others you
won't have [heard of], and half the fun is finding out new ways of
enjoying each other'. Too patronizing, alas: many men complained
that they did not take kindly to being addressed in this way.

Next up, two men in a restaurant, one of whom looks longingly at a
waiter passing the table with more coffee. The caption reads, 'If your
sex life is unprotected, so too is your relationship' and under this the
gay press reader is told: 'In the past, you may have had an HIV test
and have been given the "all-clear". Remember, however, that it

wasn't an "all-clear" to abandon safer sex in the future. And talking of the future, what about yours?' And then a line certain to infuriate anyone who hadn't been asleep for the entire past decade: 'the ever-present threat of HIV is a serious problem'.

The condom campaigns struck a more resonant note and employed stronger language. One spoke of waiting 'until your cock is hard before putting it on' and of squeezing the air out of the tip 'so there's room for the cum'. One advised that 'for anal sex you should choose the strongest condoms such as Durex Extra Strong, Mates Super Strong or HT Special'. You could use any condom for oral sex, 'although the flavoured ones taste better than most'. Health ministers even approved an HEA press ad that used the word 'fuck', though they would later regret it when the newspapers objected to the fact that the government was footing the bill for what some columnists – and not a few backbenchers – regarded as nothing but filth. There was a minor uproar, which resulted in the HEA being told never to use the word again. A campaign directed at bisexuals was judged to be more tasteful. The most widely used press advertisement featured a close up of two male hands clasping each other. On one hand there was a wedding ring. The caption read, 'If a married man has an affair, it may not be with a woman'.

And then there were some real disasters. In 1991 the authority printed for distribution in bars and clubs laminated Fact Cards that contained information on condom use, HIV testing and oral sex. The gay men's health education group at the Terrence Higgins Trust reckoned these six 'collectable' cards contained 126 factual errors, omissions or examples of confusing language. This may have been over-stating it a bit, but some of the text was plainly absurd. One attempted to evoke the effects of alcohol and drugs on safer sex: 'Back home, when the sex is all over, it may only take a few minutes before you think: I've had too much booze. Did I use a condom? Did he use a condom? Could he have got a condom on? What the hell is a condom anyway? HIV? What of it?'

Some draft campaigns were judged by the HEA gay advisory group to be so ill-conceived that they never made it into print. One of these, produced in October 1991, featured two archetypal 'clones' (moustaches, muscles) who had discarded their leather and chaps for a day in order to stand on top of a wedding cake. The punchline was: 'We vow to love, cherish and never put each other at risk'. Another featured a photograph of an elderly and effeminate man, a Quentin Crisp figure.

Designed to look suave and stylish, he only looked lonely and unhappy. The caption read, 'Practise safer sex and you could end up like this'. The text read: 'Life is there to be enjoyed. And the longer this enjoyment can continue, the better.'

'That man was everyone's worst nightmare,' says Edward King, one of those who resigned from the advisory group shortly after this campaign was proposed. 'The subtext was that he was the only gay man left alive, which is not what you would call a positive image. These were presented at a reasonably advanced stage and they were the worst AIDS education materials we had ever seen.'

King believes that the campaigns were being driven far more by the 'runaway' advertising company (BMP DDB Needham) than the HEA. 'The last campaign confirmed that everything we had tried to do had failed and that they weren't listening to anybody.'

King, who works on the National AIDS Manual and writes a column for the *Pink Paper*, believes that the HEA's prevention campaigns have improved in recent years, as have those of other regional and national agencies (indeed local groups often take their lead from the HEA). And the deficiencies of the HEA were by no means unique. Between 1990 and 1992, King was employed by the Terrence Higgins Trust as the gay men's development officer; when he joined he was astonished by the lack of new education material aimed at gays. He believes there was a simple reason for this: in its attempt to do everything, it had neglected its most important constituency.

'All the Don't Die of Ignorance stuff seemed to have a profound effect on the trust,' King says. This meant that in the effort to develop its work for young people, for women and for prisoners, nothing new for gay men was produced between 1987 and 1990, or at least nothing original. There were reprints of old material and as a stop-gap emergency in 1989 Nick Partridge, the trust's press and liaison officer, went to Amsterdam to obtain some plates of Dutch posters, translated them and printed them for British use. The message on the posters was: 'Safe Sex – Keep It Up'.

Edward King, Peter Scott, Simon Watney and other volunteers came up with a series of photo-story leaflets, each featuring a series of erotic images based on real-life situations. Thematically not that far removed from the HEA's Fact Cards (they focused on the effects of alcohol on the decision not to use a condom, on the false security of being young and on the belief that condoms don't have to be a turn-off), the leaflets revamped the notion of how, ten years into the epidemic, health prevention could be made vital and even fun. It was acknowledged that leaflets would not change people's behaviour by themselves; there was often a big gap between information and know-ledge. But they were a starting point intended to stimulate again the feeling of collective persuasion surrounding safer sex that had been crucial in limiting the epidemic in the early days.

'We recruited not amazingly good-looking models, but real people from the scene,' King says:

> We wanted people to read a leaflet, look at the photos and then look up and see one of the people in it across the bar or club they were in. We were also trying to break down the perceptions of safer sex as somehow second rate. That's always going to be an uphill struggle. Some people would argue that that's a waste of time and it would be better to acknowledge that condoms are horrible, smelly, slimy, disgusting things. But we felt that if we could turn people on with photos of safer sex, then that was good.

In order to show images as explicit as possible, the storyboards went through an elaborate system of legal checks. The THT board considered it absurd that it was illegal to show a condom being rolled on to an erect penis, but was unwilling to risk adverse publicity or a court case by battling the obscenity laws with an 'educational' defence. The accompanying text was also the most explicit yet devised: there are two main ways you can give or get HIV – by getting infected blood or semen into the bloodstream and by 'getting infected blood or cum up the arse or down the opening of the dick (by fucking or get-ting fucked). Getting cum in your mouth is thought to be very low risk'.

A million leaflets were printed and a survey conducted among more than 200 gay men found them to be the most widely known HIV prevention materials and much liked and admired. The trust had sup-ported the leaflets with a launch at a Covent Garden gallery in August 1991. There were coffee and croissants and a few journalists and health workers turned up, but Edward King detected a peculiar sub-text in the speech given by Naomi Wayne, the trust's chief executive. 'I'm paraphrasing,' he says, 'but basically she said, "We're here to launch these new gay men's leaflets, but I wouldn't want you to think we're a gay organization. I want to stress to you today all our work with women and prisoners." It was almost apologetic, as if gay men's work had to be explained away.'

A year later there was another launch, this time of a safer sex video. The idea came from the producers of the (heterosexual) *Lover's Guide*, the bestselling educational video that had the priceless asset of also being regarded as soft porn. The British Board of Film Classification was very supportive of the idea of a gay counterpart, King remembers, 'but when the rough cut was shown to them they were appalled and shocked and began getting cold feet'. After some minor editing and the addition of a voiceover and captions, BBFC confidence returned. 'There were only minor things that worried them. They'd tell us not to linger too long on the oral sex shots. There was one scene with someone lying on a bed and someone else humping him from on top and you couldn't see any more penis or anything, but they objected that it was an unorthodox sexual position that would outrage the public.' On release, the video spent several weeks at the top of the best-seller charts at Virgin and Tower Records.

In the spring of 1992 a new group announced itself to the readers of *Capital Gay*: Gay Men Fighting AIDS (GMFA). Initially the group consisted of the usual names, those disaffected by the lack of urgency that existed at other organizations. It was a campaigning group, and one which produced its own explicit safer sex material. It was outraged by the mismatch between the reality of the epidemic and the resources allocated to fighting it. It was inspired by a dream of Peter Scott's, in which he had met a friend who died in 1986. His friend said, 'So much must've been done over the last six years to protect gay men against AIDS. I imagine hardly any gay men get infected any more.'

Moral Panic Revisited

In mid-January 1994 junior health minister Julia Cumberlege approved a new safer sex advertisement designed for the national press. Unfortunately for the Health Education Authority, she disapproved of 12 other safer sex advertisements and in so doing effectively pulled the plug on a £2 million campaign.

She wrote to Lindsay Neil, director of the HEA's AIDS and sexual health programme, explaining that the bulk of the campaign was confusing and inappropriate. Neil found this astonishing, not least because officials at the Department of Health had approved the

general strategy of the campaign months before and had assured her
that everything would be fine. Perhaps there was a new moral climate
along Whitehall and at Westminster. Perhaps the decision was not un-
connected with John Major's policy of 'back to basics' and the sex
scandals that had recently embarrassed several government ministers.
Or perhaps it was just coincidence that the only strand of the campaign that had been approved was one reassuring young women that it
was OK not to have sex if they didn't feel like it.

One element of the campaign, designed for bus shelters, was intended to emphasize all the places you could now buy condoms: pubs,
supermarkets, garages. The illustrations featured heavy line drawings
of, respectively, a bottle pouring into a glass, a baguette being placed
in a paper bag and (the oldest of them all) a petrol pump being placed
in a petrol tank. These were 'confusing, didn't get the message over
very strongly and ... extremely crude,' Baroness Cumberlege says.
'We didn't feel that was something we wanted to pay for.'

Another, a large-scale press advertisement, aimed mainly at women,
featured all the brands of kite-marked condoms, including Femidom,
and the caption 'You can't try them on in the shop, so how do you
decide which are best to buy?' Despite the fact that it did not favour
one brand over another, Cumberlege feared the advertisement would
cause problems with the Monopolies and Mergers Commission which
was at that point conducting an investigation into condom production.

Then there was a series of radio and cinema advertisements, about
how to raise the issue of condom use and how young people shouldn't
have sex until they felt they were ready. Cumberlege said that she and
her officials weren't really sure exactly what they were saying:

> I think it's quite difficult for the HEA to continue year after year
> with campaigns and I do think there's a degree of fatigue and per-
> haps one does need a fresh look at it. I look at the other advertising
> on television, and I think some of it is extremely clever and I'm not
> sure we've got into that degree of sophistication with some of our
> campaigns.

Lady Cumberlege, a former chair of Brighton Health Authority,
was handed the AIDS portfolio when Virginia Bottomley became
Secretary of State in 1993. Since that time, she says, some HEA HIV
prevention campaigns tricked her into thinking they were for
Benetton. She likes the funny ones best: the Mrs Dawson campaign,

in which she says she's never been so busy on her condom production line before, and the Mr Brewster campaign, in which an elderly man talks about his sexual conquests with a reusable 'Geronimo', which he describes as 'like having a bath with your socks on'.

Indeed these and the personal testimonials have been the HEA's greatest hits, but a tracking study showed that their credibility was diminishing and their impact had lessened since 1992. Hence the need for these new campaigns. The government's Health of the Nation programme included HIV/AIDS as one of its key planks, but broadened it out also to other areas of sexual health, to other STDs and unwanted pregnancies.

In March 1993 the HEA had a new set of campaigns ready for pretesting. This was the regular process, independent researchers getting together focus groups of 16- to 34-year-olds and showing them mock-ups of potential cinema campaigns. One featured another attempt at what they called 'condom normalization' and featured a woman in a supermarket throwing condoms into her trolley alongside the baked beans. Another had a stand-up comic saying condoms don't get a laugh any more, 'so I don't use them in my act, only in my life'. The third one developed the Mrs Dawson approach and featured a technician in a condom factory filling them with water in order to emphasize their reliability.

But the results of the pretesting were surprising; the audience was ahead of the game and found the adverts tired and predictable. So the whole campaign was scrapped and Lindsay Neil went to the Department of Health to explain why a new summer campaign wouldn't be happening and why tens of thousands of pounds had to be written off.

Yet the research would be valuable in constructing future campaigns. Two strands emerged as potentially the most valuable: making condom purchase and use easier for the sexually active and supporting those who were reluctant to have penetrative sex. This resulted in the campaigns judged by Lady Cumberlege to be confusing and crude, in spite of the fact that this time pretesting showed them to be well received and effective.

'It is not in our interest to put anything up to the ministry that we don't think they're going to approve,' says Lindsay Neil, who worked in strategic education planning and at the Terrence Higgins Trust before joining the HEA in 1990. 'We were getting green lights all the way through. And I had spoken at inter-government department meetings about how difficult it was to get these messages over in a way that youngsters won't laugh you out of court. So there were a lot of different government departments who knew what it was we were trying to achieve.'

Neil says that the integrity of the HEA's campaign research has never been questioned; ultimately it is a minister's subjective taste, shaped by the political and moral climate, which will always win out. The battle only gets harder. 'We've done the easy stuff,' she says:

> People know you can go out in King's Cross and ask ten people and they'll be able to recite to you the basic information, but it is clear through unintended pregnancies and sexually transmitted diseases, as well as what we know about HIV infections, that people are not practising safe sex for a whole variety of reasons. And when you've identified what the difficulties are you've got to do something about that, not continue to give people the information they've already got.

With hindsight, some saw the ditching of the latest campaign as inevitable. The relationship between the HEA and the DoH had been deteriorating for months, not least since the announcement in May 1993 that another agency had beaten the HEA's agency and others to a tendered bid for a summer campaign warning Britons of the dangers of HIV infection abroad. Matters didn't improve two months later when the HEA pulled its own travel-safe posters showing an air stewardess holding a condom and wishing people a good holiday. Gatwick Airport refused to display it, and British Caledonian complained that the tartan jackets worn in the advertisement resembled its own.

It is impossible to measure the impact on the lives of young people of writing off a major health campaign. The financial cost, however, is more quantifiable. Tens of thousands of pounds had been spent on the aborted 1994 campaigns.

Lady Cumberlege acknowledges the waste too. 'But it seems to be reasonable that we should have some sort of influence over what we spend our money on. I think it's unsatisfactory for ministers to have to pull the plug so late on some of these things, and I think it's totally unsatisfactory for the health education authority.'

So what will happen to health education in the future?

'I can't tell you exactly,' Cumberlege said. 'But it is clearly something that concerns me a great deal.'

CHAPTER 12: Stars and Red Ribbons

Stars and Money

In the early days you heard all these jokes. Like, 'What turns fruits into vegetables?' Now of course you think you'll regret them until you go to your grave.
Ned Sherrin, broadcaster and stage producer, November 1991

It's critical to influence people who are just beginning to grope their way into their own sexuality and to rid them of the notions that my generation imbued them with – the idea that sex is OK, the idea that you shouldn't feel guilty, just rid yourself of all inhibitions and enjoy yourself. It's a wonderful notion but unfortunately it's no longer acceptable.
Bob Geldof, International AIDS Day Concert at Wembley Arena, April 1987

I think one really has to trust that the good cause will speak even through bad characters. It's just no fun to watch polemics. If you're telling a story it has to be full of all the twists and nooks and crannies that people's stories are full of. If you're really committed and you badly want to see the world change, because you believe it's very screwed up right now and people are in great danger, and you're engaged in the struggle in your own life, you can trust more that it will come across in your writing. I do think that if your politics are good enough it will come through.
Tony Kushner, writer of *Angels In America*, talking at the Cottesloe Theatre, January 1992

The unspoken logic of all fundraising now is that if you say too much about what you're actually raising money for, people won't give. You have to be very general and talk about sympathy and hugging AIDS victims and support and care. What the fuck does that mean actually? The result is that no one actually knows the specific use to which their money is being put.
Simon Watney in his role as director of the Red Hot AIDS Charitable Trust, 1994

It is November 1991. You are at home one evening and the phone rings. It is someone calling on behalf of the Terrence Higgins Trust wanting money. *More* money: they've called you because you're on the charity's 'donor base', a confidential list of those who have given

235

before. The trust is going through a rough time: a funding crisis has led to job losses. Will you help them? Do you have any chance at all of putting down the phone without donating?

You're at a disadvantage, of course. AIDS charities have caught up with other charities and the other charities have all caught up with the United States. This is direct telefundraising and the person who's called you has a script on their desk. 'Hello,' it begins. 'May I speak with Mr/Ms YOUR NAME HERE please? Good evening. My name is THEIR NAME HERE, and I'm calling on behalf of the THT. I hope you don't mind me ringing you at home, but owing to the recession we're having financial problems and as a relatively new charity we have no reserves here and this was the most effective way of reaching everyone in a short time. (Pause, wait for response.)

'First, thank you very much for your past support of the trust. It has been a big help to us. We're having a difficult time at the moment because, as you may know, the *Hysteria* telethon only raised half its goal for this year, leaving us about £60,000 short. Now we have had to reduce the staff at the trust to make ends meet.

'That's why we have to turn to people like you who we know care about the effects of AIDS.

'Freddie Mercury came forward about his illness at the last moment because he hoped it would help raise awareness and increase caring. What that tells us is that there are many more people who have AIDS that we are unaware of. And this Sunday is World AIDS Day. We really need you to join with us at this special time and give again now.'

The call goes on to describe the several ways you could give: a single gift, a standing order, a deed of covenant, cheque in the post tomorrow, credit card on the phone now.

The response is good, says Tim Bussell, the managing director of Facter Fox, the company employed by the THT to operate these appeals. Fifty or 60 per cent of all calls would yield a donation; for each person spoken to the company would get about £30 pledged; if you include covenants it may be £100 per person called.

These telephone appeals are a late-1980s thing, the obvious extension to direct mail. The THT doesn't do cold-calling, the picking of names at random from the directory or from other, more tailored lists. But it calls up its sympathetic donors every six months or so, and the Facter Fox callers, who also work for the Red Cross and Scope (formerly the Spastics Society) say it's a joy to do. 'There is no hostile response,' Tim Bussell says. 'It does morale in our phone room an awful lot of good. Young and enthusiastic people who are pleased to hear from you.'

So you know about Freddie Mercury and the trust's woes and you've got one ear still tuned to the television and you're thinking maybe, um, yes, well. This is known as an undefined objection. The caller can find it on page three and responds: 'Well Mr/Ms [Blank], I certainly understand. But when you give to support the Terrence Higgins Trust, your gift goes directly to help someone living with AIDS have a better quality of life and that may even prolong their life. Do you support our efforts? (if yes) Wonderful. Then is £20 to £30 a month difficult for you right now?'

If this is difficult, what about £10 to £15 a month? And so down the line and down the page, to a one-off payment or a polite hang-up.

You may be thinking, 'Is this person being paid to call me?' Response eight: 'Yes, I was hired to make these calls because this was the best way to reach everyone as quickly as possible. Can we count on you to help tonight by giving a covenanted standing order of £— a month? All right? (if yes, confirm address ...)'

'The typical charity donor is a woman over sixty-five,' says Tim Bussell, but this is not the profile of THT donors. Being younger, they are much more responsive to the telephone and understand bankers orders and deeds of covenants. Most of them are also close to the issue personally; this is no African drought appeal. It works the other way too; if you're not close to the epidemic, then the epidemic is all drug users and homos and you don't even want to be caught on the phone with one of these people. Homophobia is rife, Bussell says, and you forget this when you you live in the capital and work for the media. 'The change,' Bussell says, 'is that people might now not be as vocally abusive.'

There is a scripted response to the comment that the trust places too much emphasis on homosexuals. It reads: 'In fact, over half the people who used our helpline last year were heterosexuals. And as there was a 99 per cent increase in the number of heterosexuals with AIDS during 1990, we are well aware of the need to target the heterosexual population. We have a new cinema ad which is aimed exclusively at heterosexuals, and of course our work with women and babies and our educational efforts in the schools and colleges continue.'

This concern is likely to come from those who responded to the trust's appeal for Romanian babies with AIDS. This raised over

£200,000. It was a guilt and innocence thing again and the babies were innocent victims. By mid-1994, almost all of those who had given specifically for this appeal had requested that their name be removed from the trust donor base and that their evenings were not disturbed again. 'Incredibly hostile,' Bussell says. 'They didn't mind giving to AIDS babies in Romania, but they weren't going to give to a bunch of queers.'

There is one last response on the script: 'I have been diagnosed HIV positive.' 'Well then, I'm sorry to have troubled you. Since records about who is ill are kept strictly confidential, I could not have known of your situation. Our only goal tonight is to raise funds to support the work at the trust. I will not note any information you have disclosed to me. Goodbye. (End the call politely. Do not ask for funding. If the individual offers to make a gift then you may accept it.)'

By 1994, this script had been changed a little. It's a little less abrupt these days, rather more interactive, but it's just as efficient. Short-term fundraising is seen as less important than establishing a long-term relationship with the donor so that they give on a regular basis, a form of brand loyalty. The operation has become a lifeline for the trust. Statutory funding doesn't meet the cost or demand for its services; every year bucket rattling brings in less than it used to. People have AIDS fatigue. Isn't AIDS all over now? What about cancer and heart disease?

Bussell, a gay man of 28 who used to run the fundraising at CND, has himself lost a lover to AIDS and gets hacked off with this fairly fast. 'I think you get a very high media profile, which is great, but I do get fed up with those stupid old gits who write in the paper about "Why does AIDS get all the coverage?" The reason is, just have a look at that list ...' The list he refers to is included in 'Charity Trends', produced annually by the Charities Aid Foundation. This is a top 500 of who earned what from fundraising in the year 1991–2 (the last available figures). Top of the table is the Save the Children Fund, which pulled in £70,399,000; then there's the National Trust, with £65,207,000; the Royal National Lifeboat Institution, with £55,791,000; Oxfam with £53,254,000; and the Imperial Cancer Research Fund with £47,495,000. The British Heart Foundation came in at number 14, with voluntary income of £25,728,000. The Donkey Sanctuary was at 48 with £5,226,000.

The THT comes in at number 215, having raised £1,248,000 from the voluntary sector (this cost £509,000 to raise, not far off half of total income; the fundraising expenditure of the Save the Children Fund was £7,505,000, some 10 per cent). London Lighthouse is at 330 with £677,000 (which cost £116,000 to raise). Crusaid comes in at 381 with £530,000 (this cost £6,000). For the year ended 31 March 1993 the trust had raised £1,716,000, at a cost of £606,000.

In 1991–2 health and medicine charities made up 201 of the top 500, and raised over £525 million in voluntary income between them. There were 22 cancer charities in the list, which received over £177 million. The six AIDS charities between them received just over £4 million.

'I'd like to say it wasn't incredibly hard work,' says Lyndall Stein, head of fundraising at the THT:

> We have different problems to other charities – we get relatively little from trusts, and we're only beginning to get more corporate funding. We get fantastic support from schoolkids, they write all the time, and sent us £40,000 [in 1993]. Our image is upbeat, irreverent, sexy, youthful. When we've been looking for new donors, we've been really successful going to readers of literary magazines, people who are a little bit more open-minded.

The general strike rate varies: on a general 'prospect' mailing more than a one per cent response is considered good.

Then there are the events, the film premières, the comedy and rock shows. Unlike the United States, where the wealthy socialize through fundraising suppers ($3,000 a 'plate' and you get to sit on a table near Gerald Ford), Britain has a flatter approach to such things. We like sitting near celebrities too, but we demand value for money; for £25 we get a seat at the gala première of *Dracula* or *The Age of Innocence* and the stars are celebrity chefs and Bob & Paula and Miriam Margoyles.

At the première for *The Age of Innocence*, Paul Gambaccini announced another fundraising scheme, the 300 Club. Gambaccini is American, and this had a Stateside tang to it. To make up a £300,000 cut in statutory funding, the broadcaster had the idea of asking 300 people to contribute £1,000 each. Simple stuff, and a good starry response: U2 has joined the club, as has John Cleese and Angus Deayton. In June 1994 they show they care, and for some the showing is important.

But there is another list to rival the top 500 fundraisers, albeit a poor relation: the list of charities people have heard of most. The THT came in the top ten, and people mentioned Freddie Mercury and Elton John and the glamour that attends the AIDS world. At first glance it's a peculiar dichotomy: death and homophobia versus the silver cascade of show business.

The effect on the arts worlds has been devastating. In Britain, as in the United States, the response from the entertainment industries was slow, even as their colleagues began to disappear in the mid and late 1980s. Michael Cashman, the gay actor who rose to prominence as a gay character in *EastEnders*, says he was told not to get involved in AIDS work, as people would assume he was HIV positive and refuse him employment. The few fundraising benefits that did take place featured the same names who had lent their support from the beginning. The singer Jimmy Somerville declared it his 'duty', failing to comprehend how more people didn't help, and help themselves, by expressing their own grief and anger. 'There's one megastar who recently lost a boyfriend to AIDS,' Somerville says, 'and he still keeps it all inside and won't admit anything. I'm not sure that pop stars talking or singing about AIDS does an awful lot, but it must do something.'

Towards the end of the 1980s there was a slight sea change. With the epidemic shedding at least some of its stigmatism, the artistic community faced up more squarely to its profound loss and to its responsibilities. 'When I go into an AIDS centre, it's like walking into an Equity meeting,' the actress Kelly Hunter said a week after Ian Charleson's death in January 1990. 'In the theatre we are obsessed with the subject and talk about it all the time. There's always an AIDS benefit in some theatre on a Sunday.'

The American writer Michael Shnayerson found a more lyrical tilt. 'People are dying,' he wrote, 'and as they die their absence assumes a peculiar resonance, as if so many children playing in a forest vanished one by one, until the few who remained suddenly stopped to listen to the stillness, and to wonder where their friends had gone.'

So more AIDS films were scripted and we had more dance and ballet and art and rock benefits. For a while it seemed as if AIDS was becoming a hip cause. 'Five years ago it was harder for people to participate willingly,' noted Geoff Henning, director of the AIDS fundraising group Crusaid in 1991. 'Now they are actually coming forward, and it's not just the same old names.'

'I decide to do something if I can make a difference,' Stephen Fry says. He thought *Hysteria*, a large-scale comedy benefit, would make a difference to the Terrence Higgins Trust in 1987, and he produced this and two more in subsequent years.

'My inspiration for this was Michael Palin,' he says:

I turned up once at a benefit quite early in my career, for a very small charity at the Hackney Empire. I'd never met Michael Palin, so it was very exciting for me. I was chatting to him in the wings, trying not to fawn too much, and he said, 'My philosophy on these things is that if they ring up and say, "X is doing it, Y is doing it," I tend to say, "Well you don't need me then." But what these people did is say, "We're absolutely desperate, nobody's doing it," so I said all right.'

So Fry called Dawn and Jenny and Lenny and the rest of them, and in those earlier days:

It was clear that AIDS was not a sexy subject. We'd had Amnesty and Comic Relief, but this was different. A lot of people like to believe that actors attach themselves to AIDS at the expense of other illnesses that affect, for example, more children. It's not true. We've all had those complaints from people we could cynically call the anti-AIDS lobby, though perhaps the pro-AIDS lobby would be a better description.

My view on AIDS sounds rather callous in a way: shit happens. I think that the most tender and appropriate thing one can do is stop fussing about where it came from and actually cope with it, both in the terrible day-to-day way that people with the illness have to cope and cope with the education to try and halt the thing.

There is something very distasteful I think about the Larry Kramer way of talking about it [Kramer was the author of the early AIDS play *The Normal Heart*]. You know, 'It's our *holocaust*!' One doesn't want to play into the hands of the very powerful apocalyptically homophobic people who can't help but regard it with something approaching smugness; but one doesn't want to be hysterical either, like some people in the gay community, as it's so laughingly called, whom one can see so riling the rest of the world in their manner of speech about AIDS. It almost justifies some of the columnists who say, 'To hear some of the AIDS lobby, you would think they would only be satisfied when it is killing everyone and is really a heterosexual disease.' Of course this is an appalling thing to suggest, but you can't blame people for saying it, because of some people's terrible self-righteous indignation about it, as if it's someone's fault.

When the big gay or bisexual names die – Bruce Chatwin, Ian Charleson, Freddie Mercury, Rudolf Nureyev – the newspapers talk of artistic tragedy; but when heterosexual sports stars Arthur Ashe and the HIV positive Magic Johnson announced their infections the situation was a little different. Now it was a personal tragedy, and the inference was that whereas gay men infected themselves, someone else infected the sports stars; that is, someone was to blame and the finger pointed sternly at gay men.

Bizarrely, Elton John seemed to swing the same way. Initially reluctant to speak openly about being gay, or of his gay friends who died from AIDS, he threw his very vocal support behind young infected American haemophiliac Ryan White. Everyone loved Ryan. Michael Jackson visited him too – a great cause and no cloying PR aftertaste.

There was talk of Elton supporting infected gay men too and donating money behind the scenes, but publicly he did little to shift prejudice. And then suddenly in 1992 he opened up: he sold his record collection for the THT (£181,000), he modelled for the trust merchandising catalogue, he sang about AIDS and he set up his own foundation to distribute his record royalties. He talked of AIDS in the same breath as he talked about his drink and drug binges. He took an HIV test every six months and thought himself lucky to be alive.

Holly Johnson

My very first experience of AIDS, or ever hearing the word, was one night in 1983. I was living in Liverpool on the dole, but I regularly used to come to London to stay with gay friends. Part of that was going to Heaven on Saturday nights and usually taking acid or MDA or some form of recreational drugs. You had to have a moustache, of course, and I didn't, so I was a bit of the odd one out. I was the charity case from up north. Anyway, we went to Heaven one night, and there was a sign up saying, 'Tonight all the music we play will be dedicated to the memory of Patrick Cowley, who died of A. I. D. S.' People were saying, 'What's this disease? What's this AIDS? What does it mean?' One of the guys had a vague idea, because he was an air steward with British Airways and he'd heard a bit about it in America.

I've never been interested in the political aspect. We were going to have a good time, and the activists were a cliquy little bunch who really just weren't on our wavelength. As far as we were concerned, me and my friends, the activists were just the ugly queens who couldn't get laid.

Holly Johnson is in the front room of his house in Parsons Green, south-west London. On the walls are many of his own paintings, on the tables his intricately decorated heart-shaped boxes. Throughout the house, which he shares with his long-term boyfriend and manager Wolfgang Kuhle, there is little commemorating his days as a pop star, as the singer with Frankie Goes To Hollywood. He speaks with a slight drawl, heavy with camp Scouse. It is September 1993 and he is in good health.

I was particularly innocent until about the age of twenty-three. In Liverpool, the gay experiences you can have are very limited. I left home when I was about seventeen to live with a man of about twenty-two, sharing a flat with friends, and that didn't last very long, and I was quite heartbroken about that. I'd have a couple of one-night stands in a period of five years, hardly any sexual activity at all. It was the New Wave thing going on at the time, and I had bleached blond hair and it was skinhead short and I was considered a bit of a freak on the Liverpool gay scene, which was all kind of blow-dried hairdos and nice clothes. I was very much torn between the music community in Liverpool and the gay community and I never felt like I fitted in either one particularly, so I'd led a fairly innocent type of existence. I hadn't had anal sex probably until I was about twenty or twenty-one and it was a fairly kind of a ... it wasn't in a back room with a bottle of poppers up my nose, do you know what I mean? My two best friends had moved to London, Paul Rutherford and a very close friend, let's call him Jake. Paul Rutherford worked in Subway and Jake was a freelance hairdresser and he kind of married a businessman or a travel agent, and set him up in a flat and they lived together. So I used to go for weekends. Paul and Jake would say, 'We're having a fabulous time in London, they're all these fabulous men and all these wonderful drugs.' So I come to London, and here's Paul and Jake, talking about fist fucking and amyl nitrite and ethyl and MDA and crystal, these words and these experiences I'd never had. I was introduced to Jake's friends – one was an air steward, he was this seemingly successful gay man with a nice house in north London and a partner rather older than him. They really were the first gay people who I'd met who had integrated into society in a successful way, whereas everyone I knew in Liverpool who was gay was on the dole. I felt 'Oh, well, this seems fun!' They were role models for me and I thought what they were doing seemed the thing to do. This particular air steward, who I kind of had a big crush on, he was going to New York and coming home and telling about his antics in sex clubs and he won a competition for keeping a dildo up his arse longer than anyone – they used to have silly competitions like that in these sex clubs. I never slept with this guy and all of a sudden he got ill. And we didn't know what it was.

This is the beginning of the winter of '83. He got ill and lost a stone or something. And he was a big, attractive muscular man, blond. And I said, 'Oh, dear, you've been overdoing it on the drugs!' and he said, 'Oh no, I don't think it's that.' And then he got better and then he got ill again. Around about this time I was recording *Relax*, and we'd signed to ZTT, and I hadn't gone to art college, which I'd planned to do. Anyway, he got iller and iller. And the word AIDS was never said by his boyfriend. And Jake used to go round to visit him in his house and there he was, just wasting away, trying to put down this weird orange liquid medicine that they were feeding him, God knows what it was called. And then, a couple of months later, when *Relax* was a big hit, he was in St Mary's, Paddington. And he was in this little room on the top floor, I think it was isolation on the top floor, and he was very thin. He didn't have KS lesions, not externally, but he'd had things like an abscess between his legs, which is quite a common thing apparently. And he was just getting thinner and thinner. And his mind would go, he'd wander off.

He'd had a definite idea what it was, because there were even discussions like, 'Oh, they don't know how you get it, but we've heard you might get it through rimming' [oral-anal contact]. The concept was, the only reason he'd had it was because he was a regular visitor to America through his work. It might sound laughable now, but really … We all carried on, behaving exactly the same way as we had, going out to places like the Subway and copping off, etcetera, thinking if we avoided Americans, we wouldn't get it.

By April '84, he died. I'd seen this fabulous man degenerate really quickly in a matter of six months.

After that I remember Jake, who was my best friend, saying to me, 'I think this thing is going to get bigger and there is going to be lots of opportunities in helping people to deal with this.' Jake was a hairdresser and he said, 'I think I'm going to look into it, because there are definite employment possibilities for this in the future.'

He said to me one night, 'I really think that we should start assimilating in our minds that we, too, might be infected with this disease.' And I was absolutely gobsmacked when he said this, it was the most shocking statement I'd ever heard him make, and we were rather stoned and I went to the loo and I got really weak at the knees. I had a panic attack over the idea of it. And I said, 'No, no, we couldn't possibly ... we've never been to America, we've never slept with Americans.' This was the kind of denial aspect everyone was going through on the gay scene.

And then I was off on this whirlwind of Frankie Goes To Hollywood and I lost contact with a lot of my gay friends. I met Wolfgang and I really did fall madly in love with him, head over heels. And perhaps knowing about AIDS pushed me into forming a monogamous relationship. Possibly I might not have done that if I hadn't been aware of some danger lurking. But little did I know I was already infected.

I don't know for 100 per cent sure, but I'm pretty sure that I was infected as early as 1983, because I had actually been very ill, in the summer of 1983. In the summer of '83 I came down with some mysterious illness, couldn't eat for five or six days. I couldn't eat, glands, sweats, lost weight, I lay on my bed at home in Liverpool and I just couldn't move for five days and there was no one there to help me. I don't even think I had electricity in the flat at the time, I was pretty poor and on the dole, spending all my Giro on tickets to London. I had a blood test by some doctor that I'd never met before and he said to me, 'Oh, have you heard of this lifestyle-related gay disease that people like you are going through?' It took about a month [to get better]. He said, 'Your blood's OK, you've got no glandular fever.'

It was a classic situation of someone who was getting bad nutrition, on the breadline in Liverpool, taking recreational drugs, living a fairly hedonistic lifestyle, but not as hedonistic as I would have liked at the time! It was purely an every third weekend type of situation. And obviously, my immunity was weakened to a degree that I was open to pick anything up that was going, if you think about it logically, but when you're twenty-two, twenty-three, you don't really think in those terms. You think you're invincible and you're just going to have a good time.

So I met Wolfgang and kind of blanked the gay scene to quite a large degree and never went to a gay pub, never went to a gay club ever again. I was really thinking and hoping that I would escape this terrible thing. I never went out with the band. I threw myself into work and, to a sense, marriage, which is effectively what our relationship was.

The concept of safe sex eventually came out and using a condom. I thought, 'Let's do a Frankie T-shirt'. 'Frankie Says Use A Condom' was the very last Frankie T-shirt made. We were giving condoms away with *Watching the Wildlife*, one of the last Frankie singles. There was also a Durex condom ad with *The Power of Love* in the background.

I was approached by a TV producer who was doing a thing for Central Television, *Coming Soon to a Bed Near You*. I did a putting a condom on a banana sketch for them. Then there was The Party, the concert at Wembley, a fabulous night. It wasn't fashionable at all. I was amazed that George Michael did it, amazed because people weren't out to be associated with AIDS as an issue at this time. The very next year there were plans to do it again. But by this time there had been a bit more publicity about AIDS and it was becoming more and more unfashionable to be gay. People weren't volunteering for this gig. Then people who had agreed started to drop out and it was very, very strange. And George Michael had been ringing me up frantically. Then three weeks later it was the Nelson Mandela concert and that's what they were all doing. Nelson Mandela was fashionable that year, because it was going to be a worldwide televised telethon. How sickening is that? They really only jumped on the Nelson Mandela bandwagon because it's going to give them the most exposure. After that I became massively cynical about the music business and its charity possibilities.

I also got involved in another AIDS charity press call, Lynne Franks's Fashion Acts. Photo call at the Groucho Club. Some asshole journalist from the *Sun* asked, 'And have you had an AIDS test, Holly?' I was absolutely gobsmacked by the question, but the absolute truth came out my mouth, which was, 'Oh, no, I wouldn't dare, I'm too scared.' A really foolish statement for me to make, and there it was, next day, in the *Sun*: 'Holly Johnson Too Scared To Have An AIDS Test'.

246

With Wolfgang, the more we learnt about safe sex, the less we had unsafe sex, and after about a year of knowing each other we ceased to have unsafe sex. I thought, 'We've been together about three or four years now, I'd probably get away with it.'

In the mid-1980s Frankie Goes To Hollywood could lay claim to being the most successful pop group in Britain. A string of number one singles and albums, a stream of outrage. The band's notoriety began in January 1984, when the BBC banned the first single, Relax.

Relax wasn't about gay sex in any sense. The *video* was about the gay scene, because when we came to make the video I said, I'd like to portray this innocent who comes into this Babylonian place called London, and blah-de-blah. We went out and got all the leather boys we could find, all the drag queens, just people we knew from the gay scene in London, and we put them in this video. People started to write, 'Oh, it's about gay sex, it's about gay lovemaking.' There's no reference to gay lovemaking whatsoever in the lyrics. When I wrote that song, about two or three years before, I was late for rehearsal, and I was walking along the street and it just floated into my head, like a little motivational thing, 'Get to rehearsal, got to relax ...' It just came into my head, like millions of other little rhymes that had come into my head from the age of four years old. There was no thought of outraging the public morality and getting banned from the BBC. But we did have this hedonistic image, and yes there was a sense of 'Fuck the world, let's party!' We were influenced by Heaven and the gay scene that had filtered over from San Francisco, which was that attitude of 'Have a fabulous time, darling!' But I'd really given up any hedonistic life, which I'd only led for about six months in 1983. The group wanted me out there with them, posing in the nightclubs, but I was married and getting up early and I didn't touch another drug because I wanted to look fabulous on television, I no longer wanted to look a wreck the next day. I'd worked for many years in the music scene in Liverpool and got nowhere and here was my opportunity to make something of myself.

Throughout the band's brief success, Johnson became increasingly isolated from the rest of the group and increasingly unhappy with his record label, ZTT. After winning an acrimonious court case in 1988, he began a solo

247

career with MCA. But here too, he felt marginalized and misunderstood and the victim of homophobia, particularly in the United States.

I was having hell with them, working my guts off downstairs in my basement, trying to write the second album, and my health was starting to deteriorate. I was suffering from what they call ARC. I'd had no test, but I started to develop ear infections that wouldn't go away for six months, glands would start swelling in my neck and I was denying it all this time. I was suspecting, and getting more and more depressed, that I really might be ill. I came out in all kinds of eczema and didn't want to appear on television. My relationship with MCA was deteriorating and I just became a bit of a wreck [they parted company shortly afterwards]. We're in about September 1991: I was maniacally exercising every day and going on these weird nutritional binges, because I knew, essentially, that my health was failing me. Even though I was living the life of a nun, you know, I hadn't drunk, or taken drugs for years, and I was starting to get all these weird infections and weird toenail fungal things, just horrible little things.

So I started making demos and writing more songs, and I was plagued with this bloody chest infection and I gave up smoking, eventually. It was a time when record companies were dropping people left, right and centre and they weren't signing anyone. We didn't get any positive feedback from the tapes we sent to major record companies and this threw me into an even further depression. And then the bumps appeared. One little dark coloured bump here [on his cheek] and a little bump here, not coloured [points to his chest]. And then this other one on my foot, a bit purplish, but that came later. Wolfgang said, 'Oh, it's on your face, you'll have to get rid of that.' I said, 'I know, it's awful, isn't it? I don't like the look of that at all.'

So I went to a skin specialist. I'd been going to a skin specialist because of eczema. I had a biopsy done and I didn't hear for weeks and weeks. This was at a private hospital. I had very good medical insurance, that I'd been paying £30 quid a month for a couple of years. The doctor finally rings me one day: 'Oh, hello, Mr Johnson. What I've done is, I've made an appointment for you to see another doctor at the Lister Hospital tonight at six o'clock. I advise very strongly you go to see him.'

And I said, 'Well, what were the results?'

'Ah, no, he'll have all the results there when you see him.'

He wouldn't give me any information over the phone. So I go to the hospital and I knew that something was very, very wrong. The doctor says, 'You've got Kaposi's sarcoma.' I knew what Kaposi's sarcoma was by that time. I'd been getting up every morning for the last three years and inspecting my arms for these purple lesions that you read about. It was my biggest nightmare come true. He was quite gentle in the way he told me and he said, 'Now, look, it doesn't necessarily mean you've got AIDS, you must have these tests.' And he said, 'How are you fixed for money?' I said, 'I'm not a millionaire or anything, but I've got a few bob.' He said, 'Well, perhaps I'd prefer to see you [on the NHS] at the Kobler Centre [at St Stephen's Hospital] where I normally work, it's better for the facilities.'

After about half an hour he says, 'Oh, do you know about safe sex?' And I said I'd been having it for years and I'm not going to infect anyone else. I was a bit numb, I didn't have an emotional reaction, really. So I get a taxi back and told Wolfgang, who burst into tears, you know, this drama. 'I don't want to tell anyone. We mustn't tell anyone.'

I thought, 'I'm dead. I'm gone. I've got six months. Write your memoirs now.' About four or five days later, I went to the Kobler Centre in a complete state of panic. I refused to go in the daytime, I would only go when it was empty, during the evening clinic, under cover of darkness, in disguise. Just a baseball cap and a funny pair of glasses. Wolfgang walked me over there, I had to sit down in the park halfway there, in such a state of panic of going to this place, where I might be seen entering by any amount of queens, who'd know me and gossip. Eventually I walk in and I'm taken into another room by this tall, skinny, camp sort of queen, a couple of years younger than me. I said, 'Oh, my God, the press are going to get this … and they're going to kill me.' And he said, 'Yes, the propagator of sexual promiscuity has finally got his just desserts, that's what they're going to say, isn't it?' And then I was given a blood test. And the relief of leaving the building was immense.

A couple of days later, my GP rings us both up and says, 'Wolfgang is not HIV positive, but Holly is.' Of course I expected that. I was basically having a nervous breakdown, bursting into tears every couple of days, and Wolfgang would be bursting into tears, it was a very depressed time. Our secretary at that time guessed what was going on. She saw the bills from the Lister Hospital for the blood test or whatever and she was amazed that I'd had no initial counselling. She was very, very good in the way she didn't even tell her boyfriend about it. There was only three people in the world who knew. I insisted that I wouldn't tell any of my friends, basically because I didn't particularly trust any of them to keep it quiet. Wolfgang was saying I should tell my family. And I just got on the couch, and basically waited to die.

They put me on Septrin and AZT almost immediately, and my chest cleared up and I started putting on weight immediately. The KS shrunk down a bit due, they said, to the initial effect of AZT. I got downright gross for a while, because my initial reaction was, 'Get fat!' I just stuffed anything into my mouth that I could.

Knowing that one day it would become public knowledge was an extra burden for me. For years before, my biggest fear was seeing a photograph of me emaciated on the cover of the *Sun*. Which I'd seen of Ian Charleson. Then one day I got appendicitis and I didn't want to enter into a dialogue with my private insurance, because they knew who I was.

It was a shock, being in a wheelchair, in my disguise, being wheeled by a hospital porter to get a fucking scan of some kind, and I pick up my notes and it says 'This man has AIDS' on the first page. And actually reading it in black and white made me understand it was real. I got better slowly but it took me quite a while, because I was opened up from here to here, where it should have been just a little slit.

Eventually I plucked up the courage to tell my sister. She's four years older than me. We've always been very close. So I told her and she came down to visit me in hospital, and she was saying to Wolfgang, has he written a will and blah-de-blah. I'd been given a pretty low T-cell count, below twenty initially. I think it went up to ninety after three months on AZT. Then they try me out on ddI, as a supplement to AZT, and they since discovered that 60 per cent of the people with a T-cell count below fifty develop pancreatitis on ddI. I became very ill, I was admitted into hospital four or five times with bouts of pancreatitis. One particularly severe time they thought I was going to die. They were monitoring me like every two hours. I suffered from pancreatitis right from about August or September 1992, to January 1993. I was taken off ddI, and we pushed and pushed and got ddC. As well as the ddI, which is the current vogue in AIDS treatment, which is what I'm on. I've never suffered any side effects from AZT, I must say, as far as the nausea and the headaches some people talk about.

The more you learn about it, the more you know they don't know.

You go to these doctors and basically they don't know a fuck! They just don't know a fuck. Really! And they'll admit it even, if you press them. They say, 'Yes, we know a bit about treating the symptoms, but really we don't know.' And more and more you feel a bit like a guinea pig. The huge dilemma for a person with AIDS is, do I take the fucking drugs, or don't I bother? Am I going to die anyway?

It's quite an effort to educate yourself, because the more you read about it, the more psychologically you're reminded about your situation, and the more of a battle it is to stay on top of it and to remain optimistic. My experience of AIDS is different to other people's experience. They don't have to deal with schoolkids shouting 'AIDS man!' at them.

Telling people I had AIDS was like the second coming out for me. About June '92, a journalist from the *Sun* knocked on the door and said, 'We have three reports that Holly is very ill.' Wolfgang denied that I was ill and at the time I wasn't ill, and we panicked. We notified an old friend of ours, Regine Moylett [a press officer who listed U2 among her clients] and she was one of the first outsiders we told. We said, 'Look, this is the situation, I don't know what to do, they're going to get me in the end, anyway ...'

Regine said, 'When you feel ready, I know the right person to do the job, this Alan Jackson. You can even wait until a few rumours appear and do it then.' I was desperately wanting to make the announcement, but what was holding me back was I couldn't pluck up the courage to tell my mum and dad. The relationship with my mum and dad wasn't that good anyway, and ringing them up out of the blue and saying I've got AIDS is not any easy thing to tell your mother. But I did it in the end. I rang my mother up, and I burst into tears and said, 'Mother, I've got AIDS.' Perhaps it was not the kindest way to do it, but I was just in such an emotional state, it was causing a lot of friction between me and Wolfgang, because he was in the terrible position of, if I died suddenly, and I was regularly ill at this time with this pancreatitis, then he would have to be the one who'd ring them up and say, 'Holly's just died.' They reacted well, they got a train from Liverpool the very next day. They're coping with it in the only way they can cope with it. They didn't expect me, of course, to eventually go public about it.

Round about February '93, I got more weird phone calls from some journalist. By this time, I'd almost finished my book [an autobiography up to the time of his diagnosis] and I had this dilemma. I thought, I couldn't bring this book out with 'and he said I had AIDS' as the last chapter. I'd read a couple of Derek Jarman's books by then and Derek had become my kind of spiritual hero, he was like this god to me, because he was so fabulous in this way that he dealt with the media. I thought I'd love to create something positive out of this terrible thing that's happened to me. And then I started getting weird phone calls off another journalist, a freelancer who'd used to work for the *Daily Mirror*, and he was obviously a desperate man looking for a story, claiming he'd had reports from the Westminster Hospital. And we thought this was the time to make the announcement. So Regine brought Alan Jackson round and I did the interview for *The Times*.

The Sun *saw the story before* The Times *Saturday magazine appeared and scooped it by two days.*

All my worst nightmares came true. It was quite sickening, because if I'd wanted to have gone to the *Sun*, I could have given it to them in the first place and got fifteen or twenty grand for it. Then again I am proud enough not to ever go with a begging bowl to the *Sun*. I specifically did not want to earn any money out of the announcement, just for my own self-esteem, but it didn't stop people asking me in the street how much I got for it. The worst thing was explaining to my parents that they were going to get journalists knocking on their door, and they did. I didn't get doorstepped on the day of the announcement, they doorstepped my parents, which was particularly disgusting. People put letters through the door saying, 'We'd love to know what your attitude to your fabulously brave son is, and we'd love to do a piece on how you're supporting him', and really fucking sickening, leech-like overtures to them. You know, 'We had John Curry's parents' story, and we dealt with it so sensitively ...'

Nowadays we do feel rather isolated, I must admit. I don't know what the record companies' attitude towards me would be, at this point. Put it this way, none of them have rung me to say, 'Would you like to make a record?' I think that perhaps record companies would see me as a bit of a dilemma: how does one market a gay man with AIDS for public consumption? It's a rather different situation to Derek Jarman, where you're not selling Derek when you're selling his films, you're selling a film. The work I've always done is for mass consumption, not an avant garde, esoteric thing. I understand people aren't going to expect a long-term, six album scenario from me.

I definitely think that the stress involved in the music business contributed to my coming down with AIDS. Perhaps if I had led a less hard-working, more sedate life ... because there are cases of people with HIV infection who don't suffer any symptoms, aren't there?

I was quite a careerist pop star. In one sense, this AIDS diagnosis has made me view life in a very different way. I really see, faced with something like this, what a load of shit my value system was. I became lost in a kind of eighties pop star dream world. It was a nightmare really and I even ended up doing things that I wouldn't have done in a million years. At one point, when I was under pressure from MCA, I even considered going back in the fucking closet for a moment, just to help the album in America. It seems quite ridiculous. It was suggested to me that I fake a liaison with some American female pop star. I even found myself considering the option for five minutes.

It's an illustration of the depths that one can sink to, in terms of careerism. I haven't made many friends in the music business and the media. I haven't picked up any real, valuable relationships in the past ten years; in fact, I've lost valuable relationships because of my success and through AIDS. Then again, there's also the self-obsessed artist in me that enjoys media attention, that burning desire for immortality that people like me have. But I don't think I've turned into a workhorse like Derek has. I don't want to criticize him in any way, but I think he's constructed a fabulous legend of Derek Jarman in the past couple of years that perhaps wasn't there before, and he's kind of burned very brightly since his AIDS diagnosis. It seems like Derek's crammed in a whole lifetime in the past five years.

Not one single AIDS agency or company has so much as written me a letter since my announcement. It is very interesting. Before my announcement, I used to get a healthy amount of letters from Fashion Acts, and Positive this and Positive that; but I haven't had one approach, not even to say, 'Can we put your name on our letterhead?' which absolutely amazes me. Here we have someone with ten years' experience of dealing with the media, doing radio and television interviews and doing them well; I am quite good at it, I have a certain amount of charisma, and not one of them has approached me to help them in any way. I think it says a lot about the AIDS industry. It is peculiar that no one wants to use someone like me to create positive propaganda.

Because I was never like Jimmy Somerville and a political banner waver, I don't think I was particularly popular in the gay community. I think perhaps, if I'd have waved a few more banners for the gay community, that perhaps I might have been treated differently at this time. Perhaps if I'd ever walked at the beginning of a Gay Pride parade one year, or something. I have been criticized for not doing that and I've tried to make the point that every day of my life is a Gay Pride parade, when I walk down the street. Perhaps Kenny Everett's got the same dilemma. That was a very strange thing, the way three days before my *Times* announcement, they forced Kenny Everett into that situation, telling him that they were going to publish it anyway, whether he denied it or not.

I am convinced now that I do need some kind of help; I had some counselling at the Kobler Centre, but it got very political for me over there, with me falling out with certain doctors. So I have just recently sought out a place called the Red Admiral Project, which was set up by someone with a psychology degree, who used to work at the Kobler Centre. I'm also looking around for a psychotherapist, which I think I might benefit from. Because I get very angry and I get very depressed at times and I tend to take it out on Wolfgang and it's been quite a strain on our relationship. I can't stress how difficult it is for the non-HIV partner of someone with AIDS. I almost feel more sorry for him than I feel sorry for me. I tend to think he needs counselling more than I do. But counselling is a very weird thing. I want someone who's going to give me a hug and say, 'Oh, you poor thing! What's wrong, love?' I don't want someone to be this impassive brick wall that I bounce my feelings off. That's really not what I'm looking for. I'm perhaps looking for a bit of sympathy. Perhaps someone I can unload on, but someone human, rather than a trained set of responses.

Also I feel that I might be discriminated against, because people see me and think that I've got two million quid in the bank and what's he doing here? People react to me slightly differently because of who I am. There's one doctor who I got the weirdest attitude from, because I even get the feeling that he's somehow jealous of me, because I'm a well-known person, because he wants to be the saviour of the queer nation. There's a terrible ego clash there. I do have particular problems that perhaps I wouldn't have to deal with if I was an unknown person.

Several months later, in June 1994, Holly's on the phone, gossiping about how much Derek Jarman's agent will get to write his biography, about what's happening in George Michael's court case. He is in good health, painting and singing a bit, looking forward to appearing in the forthcoming Gay and Lesbian Pride concert.

I'm on this gamma-interferon trial, this double-blind study, and I go to St Bartholomew's once a month. Gamma-interferon is a cytokine, a messenger between T-cells and macrophages, something normally produced by the body, and obviously there's less in people with not many T-cells. So I'm injecting myself with that three days a week. I've only been on the trial for two months and because it's a placebo trial I don't know if I've got the real thing or not. I haven't detected any particular effect at the moment. I've been asymptomatic for quite a long time, I've been quite lucky since the initial bout of KS. They treated the five lesions with radiotherapy, so they've kind of gone really.

The record companies over here are all a bit scared off by the HIV thing. You would have thought it would all be, 'Let's get Holly's last album.' I've recorded a song, a kind of roll-call of queers past and present. There was a little snippet in the *Evening Standard* about it. A German company is supposed to be releasing it. It goes: 'Michelangelo, Leonardo da Vinci, William Shakespeare, Nijinsky/ Alexander the Great, Tchaikovsky, Bernstein, Mahler, Liberace'. That's the first verse. The punchline is, 'they're all of them queer'. I think all the British companies gagged when they heard the lyrics.

Symbolism

This ribbon, Jeremy Irons explained, fingering his lapel, has a special meaning. It means you show concern for people living with AIDS and those who care for them. Irons was speaking at the beginning of June 1991, at the Tony awards, Broadway's biggest night. This was the red ribbon's television debut, and it had a huge impact. Within months they were *de rigueur* at every awards ceremony, every tribute. And then you looked around on the street and those red loops seemed to be everywhere, the new symbol of compassion and remembrance, the new poppy, the new peace logo. And it was inevitable that soon there would be metal red ribbons and diamond-encrusted ribbons for £300 and red ribbon dinner plates and red ribbon Christmas tree baubles called 'Miracles Happen'; inevitable too, perhaps, that what began as a small community project would swiftly degenerate into a legal dispute about ownership, copyright and quality control.

The red ribbon came into being at a meeting of the Visual AIDS artists' caucus in Manhattan. In the spring of 1991 one member suggested creating a public artwork that would signify support for people living with HIV/AIDS; something simple, something everyone would understand. Someone else mentioned the Gulf War and the symbolic act of tying yellow ribbons around trees for our boys dying overseas. What about something for our boys dying at home?

What shape should the ribbon take? 'Something anybody can do, from kindergarten up,' said Patrick O'Connell, Visual AIDS' director. 'I know it looks like an A for AIDS, but it's not about that.' What colour? 'Red was the colour of passion, and so you could also make it the colour of compassion,' O'Connell said. 'Apart from Sally Jessy Raphael [American talkshow host], red is going to show up on everybody.'

After the Tonys, Visual AIDS joined forces with Broadway Cares and Equity Fights AIDS to establish the Ribbon Project and spread the message wider. Ed Asner mentioned the purpose of the ribbon on the Emmys (the television awards) but noted there was still a reluctance to wear them. Hollywood then embraced ribbons for the Oscars, the music industry for the Grammys. Maya Angelou wore one at Bill Clinton's inauguration. Even Barbara Bush wore one at the 1992 Republican Convention, or at least she did when she was in the audience. By the time she joined her husband on the podium, the ribbon had disappeared. Her office explained that she did not want 'to distract from the President's big moment'.

By the beginning of 1992 they were common currency, available at shop counters and sporting events. In Britain they were on every lapel and frock at the 1992 Baftas, and worn on stage and in the audience at the Wembley tribute to Freddie Mercury. This was the beauty of the things: costing so little, their value appeared to be priceless. Also, they looked good in almost any environment: on pop stars' jackets, on Princess Diana's jackets, even on book jackets.

But gradually eyebrows were raised and a backlash began. What did wearing the ribbon actually amount to? How quickly would it become the handy way of appeasing guilt – the way of displaying the entire extent of your AIDS activism? 'It's easy to wear a ribbon,' said Peter Tatchell, a spokesman for the gay and lesbian pressure group

STARS AND RED RIBBONS

OutRage. 'I'd much rather people worked to get legislation outlawing discrimination against people with HIV.'

Patrick O'Connell has received a special award from the Council of Fashion Designers of America. His ribbons were praised for being 'an eloquent statement of love and promise'; never before in the history of fashion had 'an accessory been so pure and meant so much'. There, they said it: fashion accessory.

O'Connell stands his ground. It's an educational tool, he says: more people are seeing the ribbon than ever before, even on postage stamps. 'They start talking when they see a ribbon – oh, what is that? And I don't think these celebrities are hypocrites. You don't sell any extra seats by talking about AIDS. One doesn't actually know who's writing the million dollar cheques, but I do see a huge amount of people throughout the country doing fundraisers, and guess what, that's what they're good at – they're not good at finding the cure for AIDS.'

The question is, how do you control the red ribbon's use? How do you control unscrupulous merchandisers with no connection to AIDS organizations? When Red Ribbon International formed as a charity in London in 1992 it thought it had a solution to this issue and set about establishing itself as the controlling body of the red ribbon in Britain and Europe. But it wasn't long before this organization was considered the biggest problem of all.

'He doesn't get it,' Patrick O'Connell says of Andrew Butterfield, Red Ribbon International's founder and director. 'He doesn't get what the Ribbon Project is all about. It's fascinating to me that he has ploughed ahead in direct conflict to the expressed wishes of the people who created the project.'

Andy Butterfield first became interested in red ribbons when his twin sister brought some over from the United States at the beginning of 1992. She had visited O'Connell in New York and believed his project could have a large impact in Britain. Butterfield had worked in design and communications, but had recently lost his job when a film company he was working for went broke. With time on his hands, he looked around for a suitable event at which to launch the red ribbon in London. With the tribute concert to Freddie Mercury, the singer who had just died with AIDS, he could not have hoped for a more perfect opportunity.

He received financial help from the charity Crusaid, assembled a group of volunteers in London and Liverpool (many of whom were in the Queen fan club) and distributed boxes of the things inside and outside the stadium. About 70,000 attended the show and about a billion watched on television in 76 countries. It was a dream launch: Butterfield remembers fans knotting them in their hair and even ticket touts seemed happy to wear them. 'All our dealings with Mr Butterfield have been extremely professional,' cooed Jim Beach, Queen manager and executor of the Freddie Mercury estate. So successful was the operation that Beach instructed his solicitors to help Butterfield's company, guiding it through the paperwork necessary to obtain charity status.

Towards the end of 1992, Butterfield's ambitions had expanded. His company, Red Ribbon International (RRI), was soon able to supply ribbons and safety pins at marginally above cost price to any organization who wanted them; it bought them at £18 per thousand and sold them at £21. The purchaser was then encouraged to distribute them in return for a donation, much as another charity would organize a flag day. Red Ribbon International would also raise its own funds in this way.

The company also set itself up as educators and would promote the ribbon at local youth groups, colleges and other institutions, often at the request of a regional health authority. The organization popped up at nightclubs, at fashion shows, at the National Union of Students annual conference and at several rock tours. 'As the awareness of the ribbon grows, thus AIDS awareness grows,' it explained in its presentation to the World Health Organization in August 1993. 'As awareness grows, the demand for education grows. The more RRI promotes the red ribbon symbol across the world, the more existing educational structures can be utilised and prejudices eliminated.'

When Patrick O'Connell heard of his intentions in New York, he was not pleased. What made Butterfield think he and a few friends could set themselves up as the representatives of someone else's project? 'It has been very painful for us to learn that an individual would choose to ignore our specific request not to attach a monetary exchange to an expression of compassion and support,' O'Connell wrote to Ian Poitier, the World AIDS Day co-ordinator at the National AIDS Trust. 'His self-appointment as the arbiter of our project is a brazen attempt at self promotion for personal profit.' He went on to explain how the ribbon was 'not intended as a fundraising tool. How can you put a price on goodwill, compassion and noble action on behalf of those in need? Reaganism/Thatcherism is not appropriate to the Ribbon Project'.

Members of the National AIDS Trust, whose brief was to co-ordinate and regulate voluntary organizations, did not object to the ribbon being used as part of a fundraising effort, but they did become alarmed when Butterfield objected to the design of their own World AIDS Day logo, which featured a ribbon placed inside a triangle. In a letter to Ceri Hutton, the NAT's head of policy, he expressed concern about 'the ease with which it could be associated with the gay Pink Triangle, once again marginalising the AIDS issue which the Red Ribbon is breaking away from'.

For Hutton there were wider issues of concern. For her, Red Ribbon International was an ineffective organization which 'ran the risk of being positively negligent'. Initially

> they didn't have any financial accountability structures, they weren't legally set up when they started ... If they had picked up the money and run off with it which they could have done, they weren't accountable to anybody, then that isn't terribly good for the AIDS sector. Also they were coming in and doing stuff, a lot of which was very duplicating, for example producing leaflets on AIDS which were badly written and badly researched compared to those which you can get from the Terrence Higgins Trust.

Then things really hotted up. In June 1993 Butterfield wrote to the National AIDS Trust informing it that he intended to obtain two trade marks for a red ribbon graphic that he and a partner had designed specifically for his company. The graphic featured a ribbon in a vertical box with two phrases along its side. The phrases for which he sought trade mark protection were 'Red Ribbon' and 'AIDS Awareness'. In his letter to the NAT he stated that he objected to the use of 'Red Ribbon graphics or resulting products which appear from sources other than Red Ribbon International itself'. He said that as a charity dependent on a symbol, his company had a duty 'to protect and monitor the symbol's development in any form. It is necessary we notify you of the legal situation regarding the symbol, and therefore set a president (sic) for preventing any possible commercial abuse'.

Butterfield was proud of his company's achievements thus far and will show a visitor many sincere letters from those grateful for its services. He is concerned about the future of the red ribbon symbol, he says. He understands symbols, for that is his job, and as a symbolist he pleads his case:

Why not actually have an image that is well-designed, has taken a lot of money and a lot of my own personal time to get this far? We've come up with a design that will go up and down [enlarge and reduce], whatever the scale, with one piece of artwork. It's no good if you actually do something that looks weak and badly designed. What I'm trying to get across to the NAT is to show how the corporate side can work for AIDS charities; you've got to take things out of the book of corporate imagery and make it work for you.

He says he's trying to be totally honest with people at the THT and NAT and Crusaid and just get everyone to work in the same direction. 'Now some of these backbiting and backstabbing things that go on just astounds me within the AIDS business. It probably happens in other area of charities as well, but it's all new to me.'

At the NAT, meanwhile, Ceri Hutton recalled that when Butterfield came to see her about his trade mark applications, he felt that his graphic 'was the most perfect thing ever to have been given to man or womankind'. In July 1993, Ian Poitier wrote back on behalf of the NAT, making the following points:

1   Any attempt to gain control of the red ribbon project was incompatible with its original aims and intentions.
2   If any rights or origination of ownership do exist they are vested in Visual AIDS.
3   It would be absurd for any organization to have control of the phrases 'red ribbon' or 'AIDS awareness', as they are in such common usage.
4   The red ribbon symbol has already been adapted for use throughout the world.
5   Other voluntary organizations would view the move to gain exclusive control of the graphic or the words with disquiet and distrust.

The letter concluded: 'These points lead us to the inescapable conclusion that your application for a trade mark is wholly inappropriate and therefore unsupportable. Accordingly we invite you to disown the application to the Registry and halt its progress.'

Solicitors came on board and a long battle ensued. The NAT found its own suppliers of ribbons and refused to lend support to RRI or agree a joint statement of aims for the symbol. Eventually RRI capitulated and withdrew its trade mark applications at the end of February

1994. For a while the two organizations worked harmoniously, and RRI continued to produce the bulk of the ribbons made in Britain and much of Europe.

But two months later it all fell apart again. In mid-April Butterfield sent a stinging letter to the AIDS Community Trust (ACT), a small voluntary group in Newcastle upon Tyne. He had received two metal badges from ACT, which he judged to be of inferior quality to those made by Red Ribbon International. Further, it appeared to him that they had been cast from badges originating from RRI.

'Two years of hard work by five volunteers and a considerable amount of development money has enabled RRI to produce a high quality product at a price that enables not-for-profit agencies to fundraise by buying at a wholesale price,' he wrote. 'We do not want to stop you producing a metal red ribbon of your own for the same purposes, but it is unacceptable that inferior products should be passed off from RRI's established and copyrighted design. I would like to reiterate that you and your manufacturers are in contravention not only of copyright law, but also the law of passing off.' He threatened legal action unless all badges were destroyed.

Two days later ACT sent Butterfield a letter of apology and promised to dispose of all existing badges. 'The metal ribbons were never passed off as official Red Ribbon International products,' wrote ACT's director:

All badges were supplied with a sticker giving AIDS Community Trust's telephone number and buyers were told that they were made locally to help our organisation raise desperately needed funds.

I wish to stress that we produced the bows in all innocence, unaware that the metal bow was not to be reproduced, and believe that we could make copies in the same way that we make our fabric ribbons.

ACT wrote a similar letter to the RRI's badge manufacturers, the Bullog Buckle Company of Somerset. Again it deeply regretted 'any offence given, which was purely unintentional and caused by our ignorance'.

At the NAT, Ian Poitier read this correspondence with disbelief. He wrote to Butterfield in early May: 'We were disturbed by the tone of your letter with its threat of legal action against an organisation

261

which we would have thought and hoped we would both wish to support wholeheartedly. We were also concerned at your view that ACT somehow owes a duty of care to RRI as to the quality of ribbon produced.' Poitier also wrote to ACT in support of their efforts.

Butterfield soon realized he had made a serious error and admitted as much to ACT. 'We consider our approach was a mistake, and apologise for the obvious distress caused to your organisation.'

Back in Manhattan, where people wear pink ribbons in support of women with breast cancer and blue ones to increase awareness of child abuse, Patrick O'Connell was considering how to sustain the power of his public artwork, how to ensure its impact wasn't deadened by AIDS fatigue and mass visibility. 'When we started the project, it would have been unthinkable that people all over the world would be wearing the ribbon, even people who have never known anyone who died of AIDS. We can't complain. There's no doubt we got something. People just love to wear them.'

PART II

Journal of a Plague Year

8 August 1993

Waiting for the lift by his fourth-floor flat, Derek Jarman says he feels
like an 80-year-old man, not only old, but lonely, missing all his
friends.

Walking along Charing Cross Road towards Chinatown he holds a
thin brown stick, too short for his needs. On this bright summer Sunday he wears black slippers, baggy blue trousers, a cardigan and a
heavy wool jacket. His polo shirt is pink, his cardigan yellow – loose,
lounging clothes that were hell to put on. Occasionally, Keith Collins,
27, his partner of seven years, will tuck in his shirt. As he reaches a
crossing he asks Keith to hold his hand.

'They're always very kind to me in here,' he says at the door of
Poons, 'they always say "Hello Derek".' And so they do. He orders
duck, rice and mineral water. His new haircut means you can see
more of his face, ruddy from drugs, dotted with small inflammations.
At 51, he is a picture of wrecked beauty. One side of his mouth turns
down, as if he's had a small stroke.

Four days ago he was in hospital, one of several recent visits, this
time to fight pneumonia. Three days ago he was with a specialist trying to save the sight in his left eye; at the moment he can't read.
Every morning and evening he is on a drip. He refers to his body as a
walking lab, pills slushing against potions in his insides. One of his
new eye drugs is called DHPG, which has the following potential side
effects: rash, fever, coma, nausea, anorexia, bleeding and 33 others.

AIDS has mapped out his life for about a year. He tested HIV positive in December 1986 and he has become increasingly ill as the years
have passed. Now his days are measured out in medication, and the
virus informs all his artistic endeavours. 'I do feel I've got some puff
in me still. At least I haven't got cancer, because that's a pretty lethal
thing. I don't know how long I've got. Every year I say, "Maybe I've
got another year", and it surprises me that I last long enough to say it
again. I'm tough physically. I got that from my father.'

Jarman distrusts the PC concept of 'living with AIDS'. 'A lot of
these slogans are ludicrous. I wish you *were* living with AIDS, but it's

the opposite, only dying, dying with AIDS. It's much better to face the facts. I'm still surviving, but I don't think I'm going to survive. It would be extraordinary if I did. God only knows what sort of state I'd be in. A sort of ruin. An AIDS ruin.' He laughs and chews his bony duck. He says it again: 'Ha, an AIDS ruin!'

I have come to talk about *Blue*, his new film. It is a remarkable work, even by his standards. For 76 minutes you sit in a cinema waiting for the action, but the only action is a blue screen. Four reels of blue, unchanging blue, altered only when your eyes play tricks, or when dust and scratches invade the print. It's a great blue, actually, rich and bright, a blue you'd be proud to have on your new Vauxhall. But still – 76 minutes?

Thank God there's an inspired soundtrack. This is structured around his illness, around his hospital diary, told in tiny fragments with music and effects. Nigel Terry, John Quentin, Tilda Swinton and Jarman himself read out grim highlights: finding a vein, night sweats, drug trials. There are also some poems, some dreamy, watery recollections and many meditations on the theme of blue: on the metaphysical, monochromatic work of the French painter Yves Klein, on bluebells in the wood, the cobalt of the sea, blue-eyed boys of yore and the blue funk of fear. It sounds like death on screen, and so it is, but it is also gripping and affirmative stuff, never self-pitying, lots of gallows humour, terrible honesty. And slowly the blue screen works on you, a spell, a canvas for your own vision.

The stewed greens arrive. 'I thought that it would turn out to be an interesting experimental film,' Jarman says, 'but it's bizarre that the film just became a film, rather than an experimental film. It's jolly difficult to make a film about illness. All those cancer films of the fifties, all rubbish. It will be very interesting to see how the *Sun* copes.'

I suggest that the film feels like an epitaph.

'Oh yes. I think it will be my last. There are no plans to do another one. It's a good end film, so I'm not too worried about that. In fact I've made quite a lot of films now, about eleven or twelve of them, and enough is enough. I don't feel shortchanged. I've done everything I can do. I'm not an unfortunate person, thank God, who thinks that if I was given a few more years I would do this and this.'

Though it is easier to see his films in Japan than it is in Britain, Jarman believes he has had a good run artistically. He made some fascinating stuff – *Sebastiane*, *Jubilee*, *The Tempest* – well before Channel 4 became the saviour of low-budget films. His more mature work,

Caravaggio, *The Last of England*, *Edward II* and *Wittgenstein*, explored issues off limits for almost all his contemporaries – religion, sin, redemption, philosophy, sex, Britain's national decline. He glorified the art of elevated home movies; some of it was a little high-flown, some of it pretentious, but it was constructed with a painter's eye and much of it was thrilling to watch.

But now he says he's broke. Once he believed that *Blue* would not be his last film, but he has been unable to raise the money to make a film of *Narrow Rooms*, the James Purdey novel. 'This is a bit of a blow, because we've been working on the scripts for about a year. I don't have any income. Suddenly ... I'll just have to paint. We sell just enough to keep me going. Someone came round the hospital last week and said, 'Are you claiming any benefits?' I said no. Like most middle-class people I really didn't think about it. She said I could get disability benefit, this and that. I may be able to get £100 a week, which would come in very useful now.'

On the way back to his flat, Jarman says he would like some sweets, anything but mints. Keith arrives back with fruit-flavour Polos and Opal Fruits, which Jarman consumes addictively for the next hour. It's a tiny, sparse flat, a real artist's lair – white walls, a couple of desks and chairs, a futon, some old dark paintings. He's been here for 15 years. His Prospect Cottage, in the shadow of Dungeness power station, the backdrop of his terrific journal 'Modern Nature' and his film *The Garden*, he sees less and less – too much apparatus to cart, too far from the wards.

Jarman settles in a high-backed armchair that all but swallows him. He asks Keith for his 'Chinese gunk', his leftover bean curd, and Keith brings it in a Styrofoam cup with some pills and a white liquid. 'Will you do me a great big favour?' Keith asks, like a mother to a four-year-old. 'You want me to take those, don't you?' Jarman asks. 'These ones are especially good,' Keith says, 'especially good after food.'

He takes them and splutters and wipes his mouth on his sleeve.

'What am I going to do with the time I've got left, eh? That's what goes through my mind now. Please God that I don't have another bout of pneumonia. I've got fed up with that after three bouts. I look at people in hospital and they're very ill, most of them, the people who are unconscious, just lying there ...'

Jarman has become a saintly figure. He has actually been canonized, albeit by the Sisters of Perpetual Indulgence, a group of men who dress as nuns. He is revered by the gay community, not least for his outspokenness and AIDS fundraising (although he lost some friends when he opposed Ian McKellen accepting a knighthood in the wake of Section 28).

'I don't feel saintly. I've always maintained that I wasn't a spokesperson, I was just talking about myself really. I've always felt a responsibility. It would be very hard to pop one's clogs without saying anything about it. I've tried to give people a feeling of what it was like. I try to keep a balance so that I'm a person who is making films, not just someone who is ill.'

Recently Jarman has campaigned against the closure of St Bartholomew's Hospital. Once again, he was really just talking about himself: 'There's a good deal of fun about the place. And I don't think you could get treatment like that anywhere else in the world. It's state of the art, both in the treatment and in the freedom you're given. "Derek, we're going to give you this, this and that." But if you were to say, "I honestly don't want these, Mark," he'd say, "It's up to you." How long do you carry on against the inevitable? Do you let it happen? There is that freedom for you to say, "end of treatment".'

There is a line in *Blue*: 'We all contemplated suicide. We hoped for euthanasia.'

'I just wanted to know what my doctor would think,' Jarman says. 'He was very, very uncommittal about it. I said that I really didn't want to end up an absolute wreck, that I'd prefer to be quietly terminated. We discussed it and he didn't really say anything apart from a tacit agreement that it might be a possibility. What's the point of hanging on grimly if it's just a few agonizing weeks? The funny thing is, if you are very unwell you don't register everything, you just come and go, half-conscious. I told one of the sisters that it's worse when you get better, when you begin to feel the pain.'

You can gauge some of Jarman's despair from his paintings. Near the door there's a small black and glass assemblage that reads, in his own scrawl: 'Dear God, Please send me to Hell, Yours sincerely, Derek Jarman. Dear God, If you insist on reincarnation, please promise me that I will be queer – tho' I heard you don't approve, I'll go down on my knees ...'

His larger, more recent, garish works exploit tabloid scares. These are called *Spread the Plague*, *Blood*, *Sick*, *Panic* and *Morphine*. According to Richard Salmon, his dealer:

He still has more energy, even when he's got tuberculosis in his stomach, pneumonia in both lungs, measles in his right foot and half blind, than anyone else who happens to be in the room. He'll run to pick up your paper if you drop it. As long as he's not in bed and half-conscious, he's remarkable. He can even make people envious of his illness, people who without the illness do one-tenth of what he does.

Salmon says his gallery receives a stream of letters from all over the world, from young people who are really in love with the idea of what Derek does and says and makes. 'This doesn't happen with other artists. In the early eighties I worked at the Marlborough Gallery and looked after Henry Moore and Francis Bacon and Barbara Hepworth and Ben Nicholson and somebody might write once in a blue moon. But with Derek he inspires a whole generation.'

'How often do you see him depressed?'

'The official answer is absolutely never, because he never uses the fact that he is ill or in a lot of pain to advance himself or seek sympathy. But I know him well enough to have occasionally seen him very depressed. I know that he can be terribly saddened by it all. He did say to me once last year, "I just wish somebody would come and put a bullet through the back of my head."'

'Personally, I keep on taking more drugs,' Jarman says. 'I take lots. I believe in conventional medicine. I don't believe in these therapies that people go off to Mexico for. I can't see that there's anything there that can help. If there was we'd know about it over here because there's such an urgent necessity. It's for the quacks. And, of course, I'm a target. I get these letters saying, "Dear Mr Jarman, Come along to our clinic in Mexico or Paris". They want me to put my name to their thing, but I won't.'

Jarman says the worst thing about his illness is the uncertainty. 'Suddenly my left eye is going, out of the blue. It makes you laugh in a way. So we'll cure this eye, no doubt. I hope we do, but I'm not that worried, except that it's going to be an absolute bind for Keith to have to look after a blind person. Another bloody nuisance. I have to say I'm very *laissez-faire* about it. I won't be the first person it's happened to. You try and make certain it doesn't win the day, you know?'

Jarman gets up from his chair and walks to his futon. 'I'll just have a little rest here.' I apologize for tiring him. He says: 'Not at all. Me and Keith wouldn't have had anything to do if you hadn't come round. Bloody things, Sundays.'

9 August 1993

At the launch of National Condom Week, Cynthia Payne has a few tips. 'Madame Cyn', once jailed for running a brothel, is 60, but understands the pressures of young life and modern living. 'I think girls should carry condoms at whatever age they need to because the risks are so great. The danger is that when people – especially young girls – are emotionally involved they can be persuaded to do almost anything for the person they love.' She presented an advice list, a top ten:

1   Use a condom.
2   Get to know your partner intimately.
3   Don't get drunk and careless.
4   Enjoy sexy movies and magazines.
5   Delight in Page Three girls.
6   Explore your own needs and desires.
7   No one-night stands.
8   Act out your fantasies.
9   Entice your lover by undressing provocatively.
10 Use aromatic oils for sensual caresses.

12 August 1993

When police were called to the Brixton flat, David Sawyer said: 'My lover has been really ill. I held his head under the water until he stopped breathing. I kept telling him I was sorry for doing it and that I love him and he would be going to heaven. I wanted to make sure he wasn't in pain any more. My purpose was to bring his pain and suffering to an end.'

His lover, Alex O'Mahoney, had AIDS; Sawyer was HIV positive. At the Old Bailey seven months later, the plea was manslaughter on the grounds of diminished responsibility. The defence held that O'Mahoney only had weeks to live and had ordered Sawyer to leave the flat so that he might make a determined bid at suicide. An argument ensued and Sawyer lost control. Patrick O'Connor, defending,

said that the strain of looking after his friend as his condition deteriorated caused Sawyer much anxiety and depression.

'The physical burden of tending to O'Mahoney was almost impossible,' O'Connor said. 'Alex had violent mood swings and outbursts of
aggression. This is a truly tragic case. Sawyer devoted his life to the
welfare of Alex. His sole object was to preserve the quality of life of
the man he killed. He has suffered incalculably himself and it is
impossible that he will reoffend.'

Mr Justice Kay said: 'No one could view this as a mercy killing
because of the substantial physical violence you used. In any event,
the court does not and will not sanction any form of mercy killing.'
He gave Sawyer 30 months in prison.

15 September 1993

The posters were going up all over town: torsos, buttocks, forearms,
all branded like cattle. The branding said 'HIV positive'; the brand
name was Benetton.

What they are, said Benetton's UK publicity director Marysia
Woroniecka, 'are metaphors for the more extensive branding practised
throughout society towards those who are different. With these
images, Oliviero Toscani [the photographer] wished to highlight not
only the channels through which HIV can be transmitted, but also the
dangers of stigmatising certain social groups and their lifestyles.'

Others, from Act-Up and OutRage, saw it differently. The campaign was prejudiced and exploitative and the activists would do a little zapping, a little privacy invasion, to register their objections.

Benetton would be ready for it; it wasn't new to this game. In 1991
it ran a poster campaign featuring colourful condoms, an attempt, the
Italian jumper company said, to demystify condoms by displaying
them in a playful way, 'like fashion items'. No hordes jammed the
phone lines on this one. A year later, something more contentious: a
new poster and press campaign featured a photograph from *Life* magazine of AIDS activist David Kirby on his death bed, surrounded by
his family. Benetton spokespeople jumped up fast and all over: it's
OK, they said, because his family are behind the idea, and it creates a
debate and increases awareness. Why should it sell any more woollies?
The company mentioned the concept of brand loyalty.

Act-Up joined forces with the London advertising agency WCRS to
create some posters of their own. WCRS, which also handled BMW

and Parker pens, donated the use of a hundred sites to display the same picture with a new caption: 'There's only one pullover this photograph should be used to sell'. Underneath this was a picture of a condom. Underneath the condom, the legend 'Silence = Death'.

'It was a highly emotive issue,' says John Campbell, who orchestrated the Act-Up campaign. 'Benetton came to an Act-Up meeting and they were absolutely ripped to shreds and left feeling very frightened.' The meeting sanctioned another wheeze: to accompany the petition signing outside Benetton shops, members would enter and engage in a mass unfolding of jumpers, 'like something in a Victoria Wood sketch. Then we'd go up to the counter with a dozen jumpers and, just as we were about to pay and they'd been run up on the tills, we'd go, "Oh, you're those people that are doing that advertising, aren't you? We don't like you." Then we'd walk out. And we used to pick the vilest colours.'

Campbell had no problem with the new branding campaign, so he didn't join a group of demonstrators from Act-Up and OutRage when they paid a visit to Benetton's London headquarters in Fulham in September 1993. One who turned up was Ben Croall, 27, who first came to the attention of the police when he was a philosophy student in Leicester and poured a carton of yoghurt over visiting Education Secretary Kenneth Baker.

To Croall, the branding images were 'feeding into the worst Nazi images. It may be fine for the chattering classes to say, "It's a good campaign because it provokes debate," but I'm sure other people looked at it and said, "Yes, that's a good idea – brand the bastards."'

The plan was to enter Benetton's HQ, make a bit of noise and leave. However:

What actually happened was that the police had got a tip off and put a man on the gate. So we constructed this manoeuvre in which one of us would go in to get an annual report and hold the gate open for the rest of us. We shouted a bit and handed out leaflets. Some of the staff were a bit frightened, but some said they agreed with us. So we got inside, and within a few minutes two vans of police officers arrived and were very heavy handed and carted nine of us off to the cells for seven hours.

27 September 1993

Some very direct marketing arrives in the post: 'On September 27th, the Terrence Higgins Trust will be launching its Catalogue IV Christmas. Hot on the heels of its latest The Catalogue 3, the Catalogue IV Christmas is a bumper 16 page edition offering a range of new and exciting Christmas gift ideas, available by mail order for a limited period only.'

Highlights include:

Betty Jackson T-shirt: 'A design with an inspirational Leaf = Life = Hope design' (£11.95 plus p&p).

Big Love Heart Brooch/Pendant: 'Big metallic heart from Pure Fabrication, with photo-etched iridescent detail will be a sure hit' (£19.99 plus p&p).

Corpi Seducenti: 'Designed in Florence, these hand-made talismen by Arista Visitatore draw their inspiration from mythology. To protect a loved one from harm, hold the sensual shape in your hand before you present it. Made of aluminium, the Idea and Alpha talismen can be used as a keyring or worn as a pendant. Complete with three rings and a leather thong' (£14.95 plus p&p).

Heart Studded Candle: 'Swoon by candle light with a long-burning, four-inch diameter candle. Studded with golden hearts, the interior burns down to leave a hollow shell in which you can place a night light' (£9.95 plus p&p).

14 October 1993

In the Great Hall at Bart's, the epidemic became the pandemic and for a while we went global and seemed very small. To mark the tenth anniversary of the Terrence Higgins Trust, Professor Jonathan Mann flew in from his Harvard AIDS Institute. Until recently, Mann led the Global Programme on AIDS at the World Health Organization (WHO) in Geneva and few people had a firmer grasp of the way a virus affects populations throughout the world. Mann possesses a

THE END OF INNOCENCE

cultured and academic air, but he speaks with the passion of the
newly converted. In fact, he's been in the AIDS business almost from
the beginning and has gained enormous respect for his insights.
Pinching and Adler and other pros are here tonight to hear his
thoughts on the future. Before he gets up to speak, I glance at the
new WHO figures.

They come in two tiers: the actual reported figures and WHO's
estimate of the real figures, taking into account under-diagnosis,
under-reporting and delays in reporting. In the first tier, there were
851,628 cumulative cases of AIDS by 31 December 1993. It was estimated that over three million cases had occurred, and that over 14
million adults and one million children had been infected with HIV
since the start of the pandemic.

Developing countries accounted for about one half of all reported
AIDS cases, although WHO estimated that well over three-quarters
of all cases occurred in these countries. Continent by continent, the
figures break down as follows:

Africa	301,861
The Americas	435,978
Asia	5,559
Oceania	4,828
Europe	103,402

The estimated distribution of total adult HIV infections at the end
of 1993 was:

Sub-Saharan Africa	9,000,000
South and South-East Asia	2,000,000
Latin America and the Caribbean	1,500,000
North America	1,000,000
Western Europe	500,000
North Africa and Middle East	75,000
Eastern Europe and Central Asia	50,000
East Asia and Pacific	25,000
Australasia	25,000

Professor Pinching said a few words, as did Nick Partridge. Then it
was Jonathan Mann. 'We have come together at a rather difficult, even
painful, moment in the history of our confrontation of AIDS,' he said.

'For despite our optimism, our honest experience and the realities of the pandemic tell us that our work is in serious difficulty.' There were several problems: current efforts – funding, scientific expertise, prevention – were insufficient to contain the global spread. But there were also the external problems, brought on by denial and complacency and encouraged by those in the media and government who wanted to minimize AIDS at every opportunity. 'We speak yet we are not heard; we warn about the future and few seem to listen.'

Calling for a new approach, he applied lyrical terminology. We were not to 'stew in our dismay'; we should rekindle and renew the 'essence' of past glories, not repeat the past's 'external facts'. We needed to fashion a new beginning.

In practical terms this meant one thing: the rooting out and eradication of discrimination. There have been many successes of the early and current policies of health education and safer sex programmes. In Britain, peer-group education amongst gay men followed by a national government-sponsored campaign has led to projections that the increase in the number of AIDS cases may soon level off. Campaigns in some other countries have had similar effects. But even in the most forward-looking countries, hundreds and thousands are becoming infected every year. Prevention and education programmes may have only kept the epidemic in check; they have certainly not destroyed it. In Africa, India and, say, Thailand, such programmes have clearly had less force and seemingly little impact.

Professor Mann reasoned that if the existing framework for such preventative work had not resulted in sufficient behavioural change over the last decade, the policy must ask why and then act on the answers. 'AIDS is really about people and society, much more than about a virus,' he suggested. Scientists had to concentrate on the virus for treatment and cure, but he believed that its containment lay in far wider issues than those considered previously. 'The critical discovery was that the spread of HIV is strongly determined by an identifiable societal risk factor ... the scope, intensity and nature of discrimination' which exists within any society.

It's quite simple. Most of us have felt discrimination on a personal level; societal discrimination is that expressed against a group – towards blacks, Jews, gays, Asians, whomever. People who are discriminated against are far less likely to receive health education adapted to their needs; their needs may go unrecognized altogether; in many countries they are likely to have less direct access to health care, counselling, testing facilities, condoms or needle exchanges. 'Ask yourself,' Mann entreated: 'who was discriminated against in my community and my country before AIDS came? And then ask yourself: are those people receiving their appropriate share of AIDS programme information, services and support?'

There is an even more fundamental link between societal discrimination, vulnerability to HIV and the capacity for HIV prevention. Women's status and rights are crucial to this equation. Poverty, despair and unemployment are key players too. 'The decision about using a condom is very different for a young person with hope for a bright future through education and a young person with little realistic expectation of a meaningful job.'

Socio-economic status may seem an unlikely determinant of HIV risk exposure, but it is an important element in more general health factors: it is hard to explain differing mortality and morbidity rates between the highest and lowest social classes in Britain in terms far removed from nutrition, housing and education factors. Mann quoted other examples, closer to his own home, where socio-economic factors were only part of the problem. Studies showed that overweight women married less often, had lower incomes and fewer years of schooling than other women – despite their families' similar socio-economic status and similar scores in academic achievement tests. In the same study shorter men were more likely to live in poverty, while other research found that taller men do better in business. (You can take these studies seriously or not; as yet there is no conflicting evidence.) There were more imponderables: among parents with college degrees, why was the child mortality rate among blacks twice that of whites? Another study of military veterans found that although they enjoyed equal access to government hospitals, whites were significantly more likely to receive angioplasty or a coronary bypass operation. With regards to AIDS, white men were more likely to receive AZT than women or blacks with the same clinical conditions.

So what should be done? The people assembled tonight at Bart's – all these health-care people and educators and managers close to burn-out – what could they do? And how could what Mann described as this global societal discrimination be changed by individuals? What was needed was participation in discussions of community, national and global priorities; we had to ask the right questions in debates about education, housing and social services reform. A little vague perhaps and rather sweeping, but the point hit home: health is too big

an issue to be left to health departments. Experience of AIDS provided an example of how even small changes – peer-group education,
condom use – could affect the growth of the epidemic and nowhere
was this more visible than in Britain. If this limited experience of success could be applied universally, and a wide-scale lessening of discrimination allowed greater access to education, then there was no
limit to the improvements this might have on global health.

Mann wrapped up his vision with some old-style soapbox rhetoric.
'History is watching,' he observed:

> In a totally unanticipated and unexpected manner, a global epidemic
> has brought us to the threshold of a new era in the history of health
> and society. At this turning point in the history of AIDS, we need
> every bit of our hard-headed realism, every bit of intellectual hon-
> esty and personal integrity – yet we need also to regain confidence
> in our insights and our dreams ... Now to the challenge ahead – to
> our inescapable responsibility, our fate, our destiny!

When the applause died down, most of us left the hall and walked
out into the darkened Bart's courtyard, where health people bristled
with urgency and doctors hurried past petitions against imminent
mergers and closures and were bleeped into wards where patients had
little time for dreams and visions.

19 October 1993

I am about to meet the Princess of Wales; nothing fancy, not exactly
an interview, though I'm hoping to squeeze in a question or two. In
fact I've paid to be able to talk to her – £50 for an intro and a handshake, which is probably good value among royal circles. In an hour,
people will pay thousands for photographs, snaps of Henry Moore's
hands, Hockney in a bathroom somewhere, Nureyev on a throne, and
my money will seem like the bargain of the night, especially if she
flirts as much as people say.

People with AIDS who have met Diana talk of being transformed,
but I'm not after healing at Christie's tonight, just a little information.
What is it with this young woman who started off all trust fund and
pony club yet has now become the princess of all compassion, the
genuine tape-cutter of choice at every new AIDS and drugs and
alcohol supermarket in town? This was the one question, if I only had

the time and money for one, that I would ask tonight: why do you do it, D?

Standing in an ante-chamber at the St James's auction rooms, 6.45 as ordered, formal evening wear and none of those brocade waistcoats or cummerbunds, I am not the only one to have forked out tonight. There are 170 other folk with their one question. Many have met Diana before, at other fund raisers, other state dinners, and if not Diana then close members of her family. Others may be distant relatives themselves, mingling with the lords and viscountesses, mostly the arty and patronly sort, the type Diana likes best. And we're all waiting, with half an hour until D time, sucking champagne, rehearsing under our breath, thinking about keeping it short and clean – so nothing about Charles and phone calls – hoping she hasn't heard it all before.

We're to meet her in a group, not a line. There are 15 groups with about 11 of us in each. Each group has a host who, having been introduced to Diana first, will introduce each of his or her charges in turn. The host of my group, 9A, is John Russell Taylor, the art critic of *The Times*. Taylor is an avocado-shaped man and is sweating a bit, like us all, but probably more than us, with the added responsibility. He is holding a crib sheet with all our names, which he runs through like a mantra. Mr Chris Malcolm from Canada, Ms Kathy Tallman and Ms Kristy Tallman, Mrs S. Cowan and Mr D. Hotz, Anders and Christine Wester, myself, and Prince Hannibal Reitano and Princess S. Reitano, if they ever show. Only twenty-five minutes now and still no sign of Hannibal. 'We're the Canadian contingent tonight,' says Mr Malcolm, a handsome managing director of the Berkshire arm of something called Continu-Fix. He's here with his partner and his partner's sister, just over on vac and no way was she going to miss something like this. As he speaks, there's a little action around the walls as the photographs up for auction tonight are taken down ready for the hammer. The friend from Canada says she will bid for the Marilyn by George Barris and maybe the Warhol as a woman by Chris Makos.

The photographs do not have an AIDS-related theme. The closest it gets is that a few of the subjects have died of AIDS-related things, like Rudolf Nureyev, and many of them have what might be called a gay sensibility. Other than that it's what you'd expect of any graciously accepted and generously donated collection – some masterworks and gelatin silver prints from Weegee, Roger Mayne, Irving Penn and

Sebastiao Salgado, alongside some snazzy celebrity stuff from Snowdon and Greg Gorman and Terry O'Neil. The cause that will draw Diana here tonight is the London Lighthouse, which aims to make up the cut from its government grant. The auction is called 'Out of Shadow'. Personally I am prepared to go to £100 for any of the prints, with the exception of Snowdon's 1988 portrait of Joan Collins in the Oliver Messel suite at the Dorchester. Alas, most of the estimates pitch even the lacklustre stuff at £300.

Diana hasn't done anything for the Terrence Higgins Trust (too political, too strident, the story goes), but she's rattled buckets everywhere else. She particularly likes the Lighthouse, the National AIDS Trust and women's centres, but given an afternoon off she'll be talking with her people about dropping in anywhere, press or no, any treatment centre, any ward, any hospice, any country.

Everyone wins, the patients more than anyone. I remember a story to please the Canadians here tonight. In 1991, on the final day of a brief visit, Diana found she had a little time on her hands and did what we expected of her: she found a hospital unit to open. The Ottawa Heart Institute had spent £250,000 on a new wing and was delighted when Diana stopped by to stroke a few hands. 'And what is wrong with you?' she asked Aileen Beaulieu, 41. Silence. Ms Beaulieu, a former patient, was now fit and well, but had been called back to the hospital 15 years after her first treatment to fill an empty bed. She had had her hair done especially for the occasion. Seven other 'fake' patients also greeted the unwary princess. Shortly after she left the hospital, her patients got changed and left too.

The Canadians liked this one, so I told them that I had also met a reforming HIV positive drug addict called Peter Stransky, who said he was distantly related to one half of the Tate & Lyle sugar people. More interesting was his claim that he too had been called back several times to meet Diana at a residential rehabilitation centre near Ladbroke Grove. Why? Because he was respectable, 'and knew how to behave and wouldn't lunge at her screaming "Give me my SCRIP!"' At his flat in Islington he showed me a photograph; there he was, chatting with Diana at a wooden table in a sunny garden. 'My third visit,' he said. 'We got on great.'

It began publicly in April 1987, when she opened the Broderip ward at the Middlesex, the first dedicated AIDS unit in the country. She wore neither gloves nor protective clothing and all the newspapers went wild over this. The *Evening Standard* spoke to a male nurse who worked on the ward and was himself HIV positive. 'We heard a lot about the Princess wearing gloves for this visit,' he said. The fact that she didn't gave 'royal approval' to the fact that it is impossible to become infected through social contact. Diana shook hands with nine patients, 'some of them on more than one occasion' as Professor Stephen Semple observed. *Today* headlined its report 'AIDS: Help Is At Hand' and expressed hope that a cure would be found within five years. When she returned four years later with Barbara Bush at the end of an economic summit, she learnt that the Broderip had been fully occupied since its opening and that a cure seemed further away than ever.

More handshakes in September 1988 at the opening of the £3.2 million Kobler outpatients centre at St Stephen's Hospital, Fulham. First in line was Philip, 35, a hotel catering manager who was sacked after his employer learnt he had AIDS two years earlier. He was at the Kobler for a blood transfusion and presented Diana with a bouquet. The *Daily Telegraph* wrote of her bringing 'laughter to relieve the suffering'. As Philip rose from his chair, still connected to tubes, Diana said: 'Don't get up. You can't get away anyway. You are very attached. You are very brave. I'm very bad with needles. It makes me feel dizzy just looking at you.' When she had gone, Philip said she hadn't made anyone feel like a leper. In fact, 'she shook hands with me twice and I didn't have to wear gloves'. The *Evening Standard* mentioned the gloves thing, but majored on an exclusive: 'A "buddy" who helps the AIDS victims revealed that when one patient said to the Princess: "I hope this won't be appearing in the *Sun*," she replied: "I never read the *Sun*." But Diana did admit that she used the newspaper for bedding for her children's pet hamsters.'

This was the pattern: a few gags, some gentle compassion, a little self-deprecation. 'I'm as thick as a plank,' she once told a young patient who offered her a game of Trivial Pursuit at a hospital in Surrey. But she knew how to play a room; Princess Anne did as much, if not more, not least in the developing world, but she didn't suit a photograph like Diana, didn't grasp the power of the held baby. Diana loved holding babies, she loved to hug. And the emotional display thrilled the hacks. 'Princess Anne doesn't pick up babies,' a 'royal watcher' lamented to *Vanity Fair* in 1989. The watcher remembered being in Bangladesh with the Queen, 'willing her to touch a baby. It makes such a good picture, but also it shows compassion. All you get is this ramrod woman with steely looks, who doesn't show any emotion. Diana's totally different from all that.' The awe has a habit of orbiting the moon: 'Probably shaking hands with an AIDS patient is the most important thing a royal's done in 200 years. She's going to shake hands with a leper in Indonesia next month.'

One key incident highlighted the great difference in approach between Diana and the Princess Royal. When Anne addressed the biggest ever gathering of world health ministers in London at the beginning of 1988 she chose to depart from her prepared speech. She claimed that AIDS was 'a classic own-goal scored by the human race against itself'. There was a 'real tragedy' to this epidemic: 'The real tragedy is the innocent victims, people who have been infected unknowingly, perhaps as a result of blood transfusion, and a few who may have been infected knowingly by sufferers seeking revenge.'

The rest of the speech was standard fare – the hope for a cure, the importance of prevention – everything you'd expect from an intelligent opening address. But it was the distinction between the guilty and innocent, the deserving and the less so, that shocked the conference, not least perhaps the ministers from African countries who had hoped that all talk of blame for the epidemic had long passed. Though publicly glossed over by summit members fearful of offending royalty, the Princess's comments were shunned by the Terrence Higgins Trust: 'What does she think,' said one staffer, 'that we sit around volunteering to be infected? It's a virus for God's sake.'

Certainly Luc Montagnier appreciated Diana's worth when he escorted her on a tour of the Institut Pasteur in November 1988. 'I was able to show the Princess the exact spot on my workbench where I first isolated the virus in 1983,' Professor Montagnier said. 'She was generally well-informed on the topic.' Charles was on the trip too, but he spent the early afternoon reviewing architecture.

Private visits are nice for the researchers and patients, but they also have a financial impact on the hospitals and charities. It is impossible to quantify the financial rewards generated by her public endorsements, by her photograph in the annual report. 'I was at the Middlesex Hospital when Diana took Barbara Bush to visit the AIDS unit,' says Jimmy Glass at the Terrence Higgins Trust,

and you can imagine, Barbara Bush must have been absolutely *delighted*; her big day out with royalty and they go to the Broderip. And I've never seen a woman more terrified. Barbara Bush stayed in the centre of the ward. No one has come close to Diana and I think her contribution has been immeasurable in terms of keeping the profile, in terms of bringing in famous names and in terms of showing sympathy that the public can relate to.

When people see Diana they see one of two things: scandal or good cause, sometimes both. 'The day after those photographs of Diana in her leotard in the gym appeared, I got a phone call from a charity up north,' Glass says. 'The woman who runs it says, "Hi, how are you, have you put your bid together?" And I said, "What bid?" "Oh," she said, "the bid for the damages Diana will get for these pictures. You should put a bid in because she'll be giving it to charity."'

I had been to see Geoff Crawford, who handles Diana's public relations at the Palace, wanting to know what lay behind her AIDS work, why she dedicated so much time to it. I'd heard there was opposition, initially at least, from within the court, a mild form of disapproval and suspicion. Huffing outrage was left to the likes of John Junor who, in his *Mail on Sunday* column, pondered whether she could 'really want to go down in history as the patron saint of sodomy?' Crawford was delighted to talk, but could tell me little, even off the record. He put a few things in the post: a list of her official AIDS engagements and some speeches she'd delivered at these events. There had been 26 engagements since mid-1990, not including tonight: some big gigs (national women's conferences and management forums), some gala showbiz (the première of *Prince of Tides*, the upcoming Concert of Hope with George Michael and kd lang) and some cool little stuff (St Mungo's Community Trust's Patrick House in Hammersmith and Bethany, a home for people living with HIV/AIDS in Bodmin, Cornwall).

The speeches were calls to arms, plaintive warnings of a dire future. She had seen the future in New York and Zimbabwe. 'In New York two years ago I visited a ward in Harlem for babies with AIDS whose short lives were already drawing to an end,' she told a conference on children and HIV/AIDS at the Queen Elizabeth II Conference centre in 1991:

Many of them are now dead, their places taken by new children. In our own cities, I have met young men and young women whose lives have been forever changed and probably shortened by the virus. In New York I was told that HIV was like an invading army, already inflicting terrible casualties. In other parts of the world, especially Africa, the picture is even bleaker. In this country the main invasion has not yet arrived. I hope we will not be deceived. It is waiting – just too far away to be seen clearly, but not nearly distant enough to be safely ignored.

As for motivation, there were few clues. But in February 1993, addressing an audience of researchers and health-care professionals at the Langham Hilton in central London, she spoke publicly for the first time of the personal impact of AIDS. One of the first patients she met was incontinent. Her body

was being eaten away by fungal disease, weight loss and a chronic chest infection. Her wasted hand reached out for help and support. She had been abandoned by her family, seen as an unbearable embarrassment and disgrace. And still I am meeting patients like her ... It is hard to find words to express the aching loneliness and rejection I have found them experiencing as they approach the end of their lives.

Heavy on the melodrama, but a heartfelt sentiment; unroyal, perhaps, and rather un-British. That was another thing, she said; she felt out of place with such a display. 'It is doubly difficult to deal with AIDS in a country like Britain, where there is still an understandable reluctance to have frank and open discussions on emotional issues.' Why understandable? She didn't explain.

Several of her friends had been affected by AIDS and she had seen the epidemic devastate the art worlds which she loved – ballet and music. Her interest in AIDS began before the illness of her close friend Adrian Ward-Jackson, the fine-art dealer and former chairman of the Contemporary Art Society, who died in 1991. But it was with Ward-Jackson that she tracked the course of the virus up close, and his demise almost certainly strengthened her resolve to learn and do whatever she could. When his health deteriorated, Diana visited him frequently at home and in hospital. These were not fleeting visits borne out of a sense of duty; occasionally she would take her children to see him; her eyes were red and wet as she left him each time. At the end she drove through the night from Balmoral to be with him at St Mary's (supposedly 'without the Queen's permission'), and stayed at the hospital for three days.

'I wish to help her,' wrote former judge James Pickles in the *Sun* after Adrian Ward-Jackson's death, but it was not the sort of help Diana wished to receive. 'I believe her constant, high-profile, all-embracing support for AIDS victims is both wrong and highly damaging to her.' Pickles believed caring for 'blameless' victims was all right, but it was dangerous to express the same concern for men who became infected 'by indulging in sleazy, unnatural sex with other so-called "gays"'.

'I've talked to her about how she feels about the [negative] reaction,' says her friend Angela Serota,

> and I think she finds it very hurtful. It's very undermining for her and it's usually out of ignorance. People doubt her motivation. I've heard so many strange things – people say she's doing it for the publicity. The point is that she does all this in the face of knowing that people are misjudging her, but she's got the sense to follow her own inner beliefs. If she moved in a different time, she'd be acclaimed as a most remarkable healer.

Angela Serota nursed Ward-Jackson for many months before he died and observed that Diana is 'driven by this sense of wanting to make life change for people. She's got great loyalty as well, so she's able to sustain that drive. She feels the same about anyone who is suffering or in trouble. That sounds terribly naff, but it's genuine.'

Shortly after their friend died, Diana wrote of her experience to Serota: 'I reached a depth inside which I never imagined was possible. My outlook on life has changed its course and become more positive and balanced.'

Ten minutes or so, and we've each had a tenner's worth of champagne. Mr Malcolm looks at a photograph of a sculptor's hand in the catalogue and asks, 'Henry Moore – was he a boxer?' 'And a damn fine one,' I say. He explains that Continu-Fix is a photo-chemical company, but that he used to have another life back in Edmonton, where he owned a newspaper. And that was where he had his only other brush with royalty: 'It was the Queen Mother. She raises Aberdeen Angus cattle, and I met her through that.' Do we, as a group, think he should mention this when Di comes round?

John Russell Taylor has also met royalty, Fergie, whom he compares unfavourably with the work being done tonight by Diana. 'She arrived about half an hour late for an opening, made some bumbling comments, said, "Hello everyone, I'm happy to say this place is now open. Thanks. Bye!"'

The conversation then turns to the Queen Mother and that old cracker, what the BBC will broadcast when she dies and how they've been planning it for years and how Radio 3 will play blah-de-blah and yackety-schmackety. Then back to Diana: is she more popular than all of them put together?

Here she comes, quite ungloved. I've never understood the dress frenzy, but this one looks all right, a black velvet number with a red motif down one side like the holes in a roll of film. Up the steps with her frequent companions Captain Edward Musto and Anne Beckwith-Smith, great smiles, taller than on the television. You shouldn't gawp of course, but it's hard not to, especially as she's down that end with Group 1. Still no sight of Prince Hannibal Reitano. Another crass thought on motivation: maybe she does all this because she sees herself as a victim too.

Group 4 now, with people from the Photographers' Gallery. Diana asks them: 'What do you think of the prices here tonight? Are they fair?' Someone answers. Then she says, 'Where actually is the Photographers' Gallery?' Someone else explains, saying it recently held a show called Positive Lives, a large photodocumentary of personal responses to HIV, which was seen by 100,000. 'That sounds like a great success,' she says, as she moves on.

And now it's our turn. She's introduced to John Russell Taylor by a member of the Art Works For London Lighthouse Committee. 'John is also a member of the Committee and is art critic of *The Times*.'

'Oh yes,' Diana says, 'that's cheaper now, 30p, isn't it? I don't suppose the *Independent* is very pleased about that.'

'No, not too thrilled,' I say. She looks at me, smiles. I think: she's tall, she flashes her eyelashes a lot. She looks around for another hand to shake. 'This is Mr Chris Malcolm, Ms Kathy Tallman and Ms Kristy Tallman,' our host says.

'We're the Canadian contingent here tonight,' Mr Malcolm beams.

Diana says, 'How nice to see you.'

'Mr Simon Garfield.' I want to give her the Arnie handshake, something a little meaningful, but she just won't let you in that close; so she gets the old three-fingered wet fish. This is it: my line. I suck up. I say, 'Your AIDS work is very valuable – what motivates you to do it?' Pathetic, but there you are.

She smiles and blushes and flaps the lids. 'You have to, really, don't you?'

'And this is ...' Our eyes have parted. Still no Prince Hannibal. And then she's off, smiling with Group 10. In a few minutes she'll be up on the podium, getting a free book from Christopher Spence, the Lighthouse director. He'll make a speech, noting Diana's show of strength. Then he'll say:

> Even in this relatively rich country, where we have probably spent more per capita on this issue than any other country in the world, there is a substantial shortfall between the revenue we raise from statutory sources and what we actually need to maintain our services for people living with HIV and AIDS. As the epidemic moves into its second decade, there are worrying signs that the political consensus on AIDS policy and funding is beginning to fray round the edges.

Spence then takes a seat in the front row of the auction room. Hockney by Snowdon went for £1,000; the Canadian woman got her Marilyn for half that. Every time a photograph fetches more than a grand, the room draws a little more breath. But Diana has already gone, motoring off with her friends to a dinner maybe, or to ready herself for tomorrow's visit from John Major. The evening is just beginning; the evening is over.

24 November 1993

Baroness Julia Cumberlege, Parliamentary Under-Secretary of State for Health, with a special responsibility for AIDS, is sitting in the basement of the Royal Society of Arts near Charing Cross at the launch of World AIDS Day. WAD is, as ever, on 1 December, but so much is happening in the run up that we now have an unofficial World AIDS Week to get through. For Britain this means all manner of things: the launch of a payslip leaflet produced by the Brook Advisory Centres called 'Play Safe at Office Parties'; the play *Love Bites* performed in schools and young offenders' institutions in Darlington and Teesdale; a silent vigil and prayers at Hereford Cathedral.

Lady Cumberlege has a crib sheet in front of her, a three-page document that tells it from the Conservative point of view. During question time she will refer to it often. It begins:

When the HIV/AIDS epidemic emerged in the early to mid-80s, the Government responded quickly to the serious threat. Little was then known about the virus and its effects; but it soon became clear that it could be transmitted through heterosexual as well as homosexual sex though, as now, the majority of cases in the UK occurred among the gay community ... Early action was taken to:

• protect the UK blood supply;

• run a series of high profile campaigns to inform the public about the risk of HIV infection and how they could be reduced;

• ensure that young people received both formal and informal education about HIV, more recently through the National Curriculum;

• establish harm reduction policies, such as needle exchange schemes, to counter the threat of HIV transmission associated with drug misuse.

And on for quite a while, an impressive array, although some of it was already out of date (all references to HIV/AIDS were removed from the national curriculum after an amendment in the Lords at the beginning of July). The latest predictions indicated that the epidemic had plateaued among gays, Cumberlege said, and was declining among drug users. The heterosexual figures would continue to increase steadily. The UK now had one of the lowest estimated HIV prevalence rates in Western Europe; the rates were about three times as high in Italy, four times as high in Spain, six times as high in France. Overall, she was led to the conclusion that 'the government's policies have been vindicated'.

It depends on how you define vindication. In June 1993, a Working Group chaired by Professor Nick Day of the MRC Biostatistics Unit at Cambridge produced a new set of predictions for the Public Health Laboratory Service. These could be used by anyone to show all manner of things. Lady Cumberlege claimed that the epidemic had plateaued among gays; the Day report predicted a levelling off of AIDS cases, but warned that new HIV cases might in fact be increasing among gay men.

He also emphasized that the risk to heterosexuals was not as negligible as some had begun to claim. 'The number [of heterosexual infections] is several thousand,' he announced:

It's something like three times the number who are infected by drug use. It's growing. The more heterosexuals we have infected, the more the risk is that at a chance encounter your partner will be infected. It would be a disaster if the Government decided that a heterosexual epidemic was not a realistic prospect for the future. If they did that, and acted accordingly, I think it will greatly increase the risk that in fact just such an epidemic would occur.

Using data available at the end of June 1992, the group projected that there will be between 2,015 and 2,720 new AIDS cases in England and Wales in 1995 and between 1,945 and 3,215 new AIDS cases in 1997. For planning purposes a figure of 2,375 was projected for 1995 and 2,440 for 1997. The corresponding planning projections for new AIDS cases among the main exposure categories were: gay men 1,490 and 1,350; injecting drug users 145 and 165; and heterosexual transmissions 605 and 770.

The Working Group suggested that levels of HIV infection had been heavily under-reported, giving an estimate of 23,400 HIV infected people (living) at the end of 1991 compared with the reported figure of 11,140. Thus almost 48 per cent of people living with HIV had not been identified.

There was one other big stat at the World AIDS Day: the concept of life-years lost. A lot of people shared the views expressed in a lot of newspaper columns that all this AIDS stuff had gone quite far enough, and what about cancer and heart disease and liver disease and road accidents and all those things that weren't being written about as much? Well yes: if you worked in the AIDS field there was no answer to this. You argued that HIV was entirely preventable and so you needed all the education money, but still: still fewer than 9,000 AIDS cases by 1 December 1993, still fewer than 6,000 AIDS-related deaths … In 1992 many more men died on the roads and in other accidents than died of AIDS – 9,330. Of all male deaths in 1992, 73,713 (29 per cent) died of heart disease, 71,391 (28 per cent) died of cancer, 27,777 (11 per cent) died from respiratory diseases and 23,393 (9 per cent) died from strokes. Amongst women, 65,301 (24 per cent) died from cancer, 62,405 (23 per cent) from heart disease, 38,733 (14 per cent) from strokes and 28,988 (11 per cent) from respiratory diseases.

In the past the most used counterattack had been that the amount the government actually spent on AIDS care was quite proportionate with spending on other diseases. In 1993, AIDS accounted for 0.7 per cent of total health spending in Britain, compared, for example, with 14 per cent for mental illness.

But now there is a new angle. Life-years lost reflect the young age of those who died from AIDS-related illnesses and, as it relates only to people under the age of 65, a measure of loss of economic productivity. At the end of December 1992, 79 per cent of people with AIDS and 87 per cent of women with HIV were aged between 20 and 44. In the same year, an estimated 43,594 life-years were lost as a result of AIDS. This placed AIDS tenth in a table drawn up by the Department of Health in 1990, behind heart disease (178,708 life-years lost), car traffic accidents (117,175), suicide (75,845), lung cancer (58,000), breast cancer (56,025) and others. The trend for all these figures is downwards, except suicide and AIDS. The important point was that projections estimated that by 1997 AIDS would account for 76,421 life-years lost, placing it third in the table.

Did these figures make much difference to anything? No. The argument didn't change: the government had spent about £880 million since 1986 on prevention, treatment, care and research, and for some this would be too much, while for others it would not be enough (8 per cent of this figure was spent on prevention campaigns, 12 per cent on training, testing and surveillance services, while 70 per cent was spent on treatment and care; the cost to the NHS of each person with HIV was estimated at £75,000). Apologists would say, 'If only all health issues could have this much spent on them ...'

We were now at a key moment. Policies were being reviewed and spending was being redirected and in some cases reduced. The Section 64 funding, only available to voluntary organizations providing a national service, was cut back earlier in the year, ostensibly to free more money for other areas of health care. The grant to the Terrence Higgins Trust was cut, over three years beginning in 1994–5, from £450,000 per annum to £150,000; London Lighthouse's was cut from £300,000 to £150,000 over three years. Another charity, AIDS Ahead, which provides information and advice for the hearing impaired, had its total allocation of £40,000 (about 25 per cent of its total budget) cut in one go.

This didn't seem to make much sense, not after the Health Secretary Virginia Bottomley had said the government would from now on be targeting the specific at-risk groups. But for Bottomley there was a logic to everything. 'What we can now do is fashion our policy according to fact, not fantasy,' she said at the time of the cuts. 'For a voluntary organisation £150,000 is still a great deal of money. I think we're past the time when money was needed for pump priming ... I think that there have sometimes been people who can't see the wood for the trees, and that HIV/AIDS has to be seen in the context of other very serious diseases, and there has to be a spirit of practical realism.'

Baroness Cumberlege takes the same line, of course. For today's launch, she is on a panel with people from London Lighthouse, the Terrence Higgins Trust, the National AIDS Trust and the Health Education Authority. This year's theme is 'It's Time To Act', a statement which many regard as a stab in the heart: what the hell have they been doing over the last decade?

'I like Julia a great deal,' David Mellor had told me, 'but I think it says something about changing priorities that once AIDS was the responsibility of the highest minister of state and now it's the work of a junior minister in the Lords.'

Cumberlege says it has not been de-prioritized; it has, however, been mainstreamed.

'I'm very keen that HIV and AIDS is seen as important, but not seen as totally special,' she says after the launch. In practice this means more care in the community, the inclusion of HIV/AIDS in the Health of the Nation programme and the end of ring-fenced money for treatment and research. 'When it's a new epidemic, clearly you have to treat it differently. Now AIDS should be more people's business than before.' By making AIDS less special you destigmatize it; but you can also create administrative hell. Ring-fencing for treatment and care was due to disappear on 1 April 1994, after which even the smallest voluntary organizations would be obliged to muscle in to the bureaucratic maelstrom of fund-holding and purchasing and service provision. In effect, the autonomy of the voluntary sector has been shot to pieces.

This is not necessarily a terrible thing: it may make voluntary sector services more accountable; in this new jargonized world of 'performance indicators' they must produce only what a purchaser requires (the purchaser is increasingly a district rather than a regional health authority). But extreme rationalization has a downside too: a small organization, perhaps one for deaf people with HIV, must convince an authority that its services are worth supporting, even though they are used by few people. If it cannot, it must either seek funds elsewhere, which means more time-consuming paperwork, or it may go to the wall. And with no statutory requirement to fund certain HIV/AIDS organizations and prejudice still rife in many non-metropolitan districts (and political sensitivities ever present) local authorities may find it increasingly easy to ignore requests for funding.

Lady Cumberlege believes things will shake out all right in the end:

I do understand that the voluntary organizations are finding it much more complicated, but I think they can't be totally detached from the rest of the world. It's up to them to ensure that their services are of the quality that people want to purchase and they are relevant and I'm not sure that the government is best placed to make those decisions, it's better left to people on the ground.

But she does foresee problems:

We've got a tremendously long way to go. We had a case about nine months ago of an infected health-care worker, and a helpline was set up in the hospital and health workers were ringing up the helpline asking the general manager to fumigate the hospital. This was Bromley [east London]. I mean, to think that health-care workers still think you can catch it as an airborne disease ...

Cumberlege has seen the effects of AIDS more closely than most ministers, first as chair of Brighton Health Authority (Brighton has a large proportion of positive gay men), and from visiting her sons while they worked in Kenya. She reiterates the life-years lost factor:

I think that really what I find most distressing is the age of the people affected. Some of those in the gay community have suffered the loss of so many young friends; I think it's a terrible toll for any individual to come to terms with. But in all these tragedies something good somehow comes out of it and the thing that's impressed me enormously is the way that AIDS patients have begun to alter some of the attitudes of health professionals. Health professionals say that it has to be a partnership, that they recognize the knowledge that is now around in lay people in this field. The whole thrust of the thing is empowering the people who are suffering, and I hope that will spread into the rest of medicine.

What has the UK achieved in terms of scientific progress? Cumberlege looks at her notes. Not much there. 'I don't think they're very great yet,' she says. 'It's interesting when you discuss HIV and AIDS with scientists and researchers, because it's an area that you're very conscious that there isn't a lot of evidence, unlike cancer or heart disease or tuberculosis where you ask questions and you get very quick answers.'

26 November 1993

At the National Museum of Photography, Film and Television in Pictureville, Bradford, a local man of 20 has paused at the section on the AIDS wards at the Middlesex. He looks at a series of photographs about a 29-year-old called John; he likes the fact that John's parents were there, 'and obviously cared for him – it must be hard for parents'.

John has died since these pictures were taken. He was in and out of the Middlesex for years; towards the end it became a home and his mother and partner would sleep over. The exhibition visitor, Peter Wells, is surprised at the informality of these pictures, two men close on a bed, clothes all over, fruit and cards and mugs and bad light, just like any crowded ward, 'but this is AIDS and I know you can't just catch it, but it is still different'.

'Positive Lives', a joint project between the Terrence Higgins Trust and Network Photographers, began life in 1990. The plan was to roam Europe in search of images that would portray it all – medical research, medical practice, sexuality, even the role of transport, illustrating, an early mission statement says, 'the failure of society/the state to provide for the needs of people'. There were many objectives: 'to promote the perceived relevance of HIV to all ... to emphasise the responsibilities internationally of governments, commercial and business sectors, to reinforce the standing of the THT internationally (amongst peer organisations, in the public eye, as a diverse and effective organisation) ... to create immediate possibilities for fund raising'. This was some ambitious project, and when it finally opened three years later it had limited its subject matter to Britain. Levi Strauss & Co picked up the sponsorship tab of about £100,000.

It was a terrific and popular show, starting in London and then touring the country before heading for Europe and the United States. In Bradford it was accompanied by a series of talks and discussions, some of them of interest to professional photographers, others community-based events looking at parental responsibility and HIV infection in pre-school children. The pictures covered all the bases in all styles, tough grain for the Edinburgh druggies, saturated colour for the drag queens, some mantelpiece portraits, some religious melodrama, some Utopian landscapes. There was an impressionist set on Rupert Haselden's life, and some doctored, half-glimpsed Polaroids of mothers and children. 'It is difficult to photograph illness in any meaningful way,' said Steve Mayes, the co-curator of the project, but his show is probably the closest art has come to defining its impact.

All photography is about death, as Roland Barthes observed, because every captured moment is also lost for ever. 'Each of the photographs ... is a *memento mori*,' Edmund White noted in a foreword to the accompanying book, 'even as they are also reminders of all those unexpectedly joyful instants afforded by AIDS: the permission to be as different from the others as one has always longed to be; the courage to comfort the ill even in the cold heart of institutions; the inspiration to devise new ways of expressing either faith or grief ...'

Michael Scott was on the ward with John when a member of staff said a photographer was coming in later and would it be all right if he hung about a bit? 'They were looking for someone who wasn't a typical AIDS patient, who didn't conform to that image that most people may have of someone pathetically wasting away,' Scott says. 'John was always so cheerful and always looked so good, and he said he didn't mind. He always loved publicity.'

Scott is 32, a Welshman, a computer worker. He'd only known John six months before he died. They met in a bar in December 1992, by which time John had been ill for two years. He was the first person he knew who was infected. 'I was chatting with him, trying to pick him up basically, but he was quite withdrawn, didn't want to get too involved. He was very careful about what he said, but eventually he did say, "Look, I'm HIV positive." I think he was surprised I didn't walk away.'

John had spent most of his time in the East End, where he worked as a decorator. He had broken up with his boyfriend after seven or eight years; his boyfriend was ill also. He was out of hospital for a short while, but went back two weeks after he met Michael and never left. He had had PCP. In March they found brain lesions.

The photographer came in so many times and took thousands. He'd always show us the contact prints and John's main concern on some of them was that he had the scruffiest clothes on or that his hair wasn't combed. John signed a consent form for all the photographs, but after he died his parents had doubts about the photographs being used at all; in the end they didn't show the ones that his parents didn't want used. They went along to the opening and that was all fine.

When I saw them on the opening night I was pleased the pictures were there; there was no sadness. There were only six photographs, only six moments, and you can't see the real pain, the real tears. They show the positive side of things, that was the idea, but people might not realize that there was also this awful side. Nothing prepares you for the immense variations in someone's condition – the way one day he would be perfectly well and the next desperately ill. He got tired so easily, even walking down the stairs. First time I met him I didn't realize how much he felt the cold, and he was wrapped up so much.

28 November 1993

Officially it's the annual Gay Lifestyles exhibition at Olympia, but most people call it the Ideal Homo. Last year seven thousand people visited, this year they're expecting twice that. A lesbian and gay superstore for a couple of days: videos, bookstalls, motorbikes, plants, paintings, candles, leatherware and T-shirts that say 'I Can't Even Think Straight' and 'From Queer to Eternity'. On the main stage, drag act Regina Fong talks about Coronation St ('Corrie') and does that song about a little mouse with clogs on. And in an upstairs room there's a sparsely attended debate on sexual behaviour entitled 'Are gay men who cruise their own worst enemy?'

There are six on the panel: Ford Hickson and Peter Keogh from Project SIGMA, the extensive Socio-sexual Investigation of Gay Men and AIDS based at the University of Essex, Julian Hows from London Lesbian and Gay Switchboard and Gay Men Fighting AIDS, Matt French, gay men's health education officer at the THT, Paul Sigel from the gay London policing group GALOP and John Campbell of the UK Coalition of People with AIDS.

We may learn a lot. Since 1987, Project SIGMA has interviewed over a thousand gay men, many of them more than once, and Peter

Keogh also talked to other men for a St Mary's Hospital survey on cruising and cottaging (gay sex in public lavatories). The SIGMA research indicated that 60 per cent of gay and bisexual men in Britain had a casual partner in the last year. Twenty-six per cent of respondents met a partner in a cruising area (usually heath or common), and 27 per cent met a partner in a cottage in the past year.

The St Mary's research suggested that the most common sexual activity when cruising or cottaging was masturbation; sucking was next, with only a tiny percentage of participants coming in each other's mouths. A third of subjects usually kissed, but half reported that they would like to do so. About 25 per cent fucked after making contact when cottaging or cruising, but often this would be at someone's home. About 5 per cent said they had fucked without a condom in the last year, and this in a context where there was a very high degree of knowledge of the risks of unprotected anal sex.

Why do men go cottaging or cruising? In many cases it is not a last resort. The majority of respondents mentioned the excitement involved, including the physical danger and danger of arrest or discovery (fantasy played a large part in this: most respondents had experienced unwelcome physical or verbal abuse or harsh treatment by the police). Anonymous sex was rated high, far higher than the potential for meeting new partners for long-term relationships; indeed, many men who cruised or cottaged were already in such relationships. Others just enjoyed having sex *en plein air*. Few in the survey only cruised when they were drunk or stoned and few did not have sex in other situations; cottaging and cruising were simply seen as enjoyable elements in a wider repertoire of sexual experience.

Julian Hows lost a lot of sleep between August and October 1993, as GMFA and Switchboard established a basecamp in the corner of Jack Straw's Castle car park on Hampstead Heath – a table, a lamp, tea and coffee, lots of condoms and literature, on Thursdays, Fridays and Saturdays between 11 p.m. and 3 a.m. 'We got rid of two thousand condom packs,' he said,

and we were only giving them to people who asked. A lot of men brought their own. We were only giving them out to about one-third of all the people who passed us, and we thought we were only accessing about 40 per cent of the people using the Heath at any one time. So there was an awful lot of sex going on. We reached the conclusion that it was possible to materially change the environment in which we cruise, to make it safer.

Matt French opened with a confessional. Cruising is not just about going to the Heath or Clapham Common or the underside of Clifton Suspension Bridge:

We cruise in the street, in the bars, I cruise in Tesco and Sainsbury. I may not end up having sex with those people, but I cruise them constantly. In a lot of ways I often equate cruising with shopping: you know what you want, you know where to go and get it. You might on the way find another shop that takes your attention and you wander off down there. You usually get something and you're usually fairly happy about it.

French had learnt one thing above all during his time as an HIV educator for gay men: the best campaigns are the ones which demand the minimum change necessary:

It's no good asking them to fundamentally change their behaviour, to stop cruising, stop going to the Heath, or as we heard earlier on in the epidemic, stop fucking. These are never going to work. What we must do is continue to make our cruising and other activities safer. We have experience of that, but what we need is more support and acceptance from the wider community. So of course gay men who cruise aren't their own worse enemy. Almost all the difficulties seem to stem from the outside, from those who won't accept cruising as part of our sexual identity.

From the side of the room, Steve Coote, the organizer of this debate for the National AIDS Trust, amplified the dilemma:

I've been out at work for about twenty years. When I first started talking about my activities, perhaps saying I'd met someone in a supermarket that lunchtime, I could tell my colleagues and there wouldn't be a real problem. Since AIDS that became less possible. They would all talk about their families and what they get up to, but I felt more constrained in being honest about what I got up to.

29 November 1993

From the towering pulpit of St Martin in the Fields, close by Trafalgar Square, an Australian judge called Michael Kirby, a middle-aged man with thin ginger hair, delivers this year's Doughty Street Lecture. Doughty Street law chambers are home to Helena Kennedy, Geoffrey Robertson and other liberal barristers, and if you were looking for a leading figure of the law to talk about AIDS in the same liberal spirit, Kirby would always be your first choice. He is president of the New South Wales Court of Appeal, chairman of the executive committee of the International Commission of Jurists and a former member of the World Health Organization Global Commission on AIDS. He wears a red ribbon, too.

Given its size, AIDS is a relatively minor problem in Australia, at least if you just play the numbers: 4,258 cases of AIDS reported up to the end of 1993 and about 25,000 cases of HIV. This is partly due to the dissemination of preventative information, which is in turn made more effective by the right signals from the lawmakers. This was Kirby's main message: the law has an important role in containing HIV, and a punitive legal system will only make matters worse. He echoed Jonathan Mann's view that there was a close inter-relationship between limiting the epidemic and protecting the human rights of those infected or at risk. As in Britain, gay men account for the bulk of AIDS cases in Australia, but the incidence of heterosexually transmitted cases of HIV is growing. The key point was: given its size, the potential for HIV infection in Australia is immense.

Overall, Australia does not present a bad legislative model for dealing with an epidemic and English and Scottish law could still benefit from heeding its enlightenment and its errors. While each state passes its own legislation, all states still look to London for their legal moorings. Kirby explained that some over-anxious and prejudicial laws had been passed in recent years, but these had been outnumbered by good ones. In the former category there is a law in Western Australia obliging any person with HIV to inform the driver of any public bus of his or her condition. As Kirby put it, 'One can only imagine the robust response of a bus driver in Perth.' In the State of Victoria the Crimes (HIV) Act 1993 stipulates that a person who, without lawful excuse, recklessly engages in conduct that may place another person in danger of death (i.e. infecting another person with HIV) is guilty of a new offence punishable, upon conviction, with a ten-year jail term, a throwback to the earliest strategies for dealing with HIV by punishment. Kirby concluded that

> the notion of imprisoning for such very long periods a person already infected with HIV is self-evidently farcical. The only explanation I can offer for the legislation is that it was enacted by a government out of office for most of the 1980s which saved up this legislative gem and enacted it for political rather than for public health purposes.

On the good side, and in contrast with England, there exists the Disability Discrimination Act 1992, which applies throughout Australia and makes it unlawful to discriminate or harass on the grounds of disability – the definition of disability extending to the presence in the body of organisms capable of causing serious illness. A week before Kirby flew over from Sydney, he read of a man receiving an award of $60,000 for discrimination on the grounds of his HIV status. In New South Wales an act also prohibits discrimination on the grounds of homosexuality or assumed homosexuality, or HIV infection or assumed infection. This came about partly to protect gay men in Sydney from the increase in queer bashing. In Britain, no such protection is enshrined in law: indeed, at 18 the age of consent for gay men is deliberately discriminatory.

Kirby emphasized that the above legislation was extremely hard won; the battles showed that the Australian response was far from uniformly idealistic or courageous. None the less, he felt that most of the new laws regarding gay men in the wake of AIDS had been 'supportive of self-respect and aimed at the reduction of alienation and low self-esteem', attitudes which provide a barrier to the effective protection of people at risk. 'By protecting them,' he attests, 'we protect the whole of society.'

He closed by talking a bit about the history of St Martin in the Fields, then read some Spender and sat down. Shortly before thanking him and presenting him with one of her own books, Helena Kennedy asked what he thought of AIDS charters, declarations of human rights and the like; we had all been given the 'UK Declaration of the Rights of People with HIV and AIDS' on our arrival. Very limited value, Kirby thought. 'A charter is not a law; it won't enforce anything. The law of the land is the way to lay down your principles.'

Someone then asked him about HIV in Australian jails. The judge quoted Churchill: we judge a civilization by the way it treats its prisoners. Some jails had made some progress in issuing condoms and bleach tablets, he said, and he hoped others would follow. He was also asked about the coverage of AIDS in the *Sunday Times*, and whether, since Galileo, we should all be sceptical of everything, and whether the AIDS issue had 'been hijacked by liberals for liberal political ends'. Kirby said he read yesterday's *Sunday Times*, an edition which quoted new Nobel laureate Dr Kary Mullis, the inventor of the Polymerase Chain Reaction (the DNA amplification system much used by AIDS researchers); Mullis now had many problems with the belief that HIV caused AIDS. The *Sunday Times* had many doubts about this too, as well as about 'the myth of heterosexual AIDS', and it had run a tireless campaign attacking what it called 'the AIDS establishment'.

Kirby said he was appalled by the paper's coverage. 'You should look at good figures,' he said:

The WHO's figures show that globally 71 per cent of all reported cases are heterosexual and it's not an excuse to say, 'Oh yes, anal sex is a form of contraception in the developing world,' because it's not in Thailand or India. What really offended me about yesterday's paper was the passage at the end which said something like 'remember, we were right about Thalidomide'. There's a world of difference between them. Thalidomide was an alert, a moral thing to do. What they're doing now is an irresponsible immoral act, willing people into false security. The *Sunday Times*, a high-standing newspaper, is ignoring, blindly, the great mass of evidence.

1 December 1993

'We know quite a lot,' said Jane. 'It's not shocking. I think we know more than boys now.' Jane is on a bench with six others, having packed lunch at Southwell House Youth Project, a Jesuit enterprise near Swiss Cottage, north London. The girls are 14 and 15, from local schools, and have come for an all-day World AIDS Day seminar; topics include Sex and Sexuality, HIV/AIDS and Special Needs, and AIDS and Religious Perspectives. 'People open up here far more than at school,' says the project's deputy director. The conversation continues through the lunch hour.

Jane: I saw about it first on TV. My parents hadn't told me anything.

Catherine: I was getting quite worried. I thought that if so many people are going to get this, our generation are going to be wiped out.

Another Girl: Now they're saying it's nothing, like it was all a joke, whereas in fact it's all quite serious.

Catherine: What it's meant is that people talk about sex now, and about being gay. I'm not homophobic, I'm not scared of people who have AIDS. On the other hand I don't pity them. I don't feel they need our pity.

Jane: Now we have an AIDS night at our school to keep the parents up to date. We've got our school's policy on AIDS here. Mr Power wrote it.

Me: If I was to ask you what the main modes of transmission were, would you know?

All: Yeah.

Me: What are the first things that come into your mind when you think of AIDS?

Jane: Needles.

Catherine: Newspaper headlines. It will always be around. Even if they find a cure today it won't go away that quickly.

Another Girl: Older people don't understand it.

Jane: Because of celebrities people accept people being gay. There's talk about sex on the TV all the time now, whereas before they wouldn't talk about it.

Me: Do boys understand as much as you?

Jane: I think boys accept that if they don't use condoms they could go on to get HIV and die.

Another Girl: I know boys who carry condoms around in their wallets to show off. I saw this programme on TV about these lads going on holiday to this beach, basically just to hit on girls. One of them said, 'Well, I only use a condom because I want to keep my willy clean.'

Jane: I saw that.

Catherine: When we had sex education at school everyone was laughing.

Another Girl: That's only because you had Tatiana and Tara in your class.

Jane: It wasn't just girls laughing. Mr Dean was going 'Hur Hur.' He's not actually trained to do it; he's an English teacher and he has to teach us PSE [Personal and Social Education].

Another Girl: We had Mr deSouza. He's a science teacher.

Another Girl: Yeah, but Mr deSouza … come *on*.

3 December 1993

'I was in negotiation with Diana's office for her to come and do something locally,' said Christopher Spence in his office at the London Lighthouse. 'And they rang up and said, "The answer's going to be no ... there's going to be an announcement."' The announcement came at London's Hilton Hotel, at a gathering for another good cause; she'd done enough public healing for a while. 'She's been to the Lighthouse many times,' Spence continued, 'and I've never met anybody who's got her extraordinary capacity to make a really good and appropriate human connection with one person after another, after another, after another, never misses a beat. She came here once on a private visit and a service user who's now dead came in absolutely blind drunk and screamed at her, "Diana is that you?" She was completely unfazed, but didn't just ignore him like others would do. She said something that took the sting right out of it. My sense is that she'll come back, because although it must be very hard dealing with all the intrusion, she *does* love working the crowd.'

14 December 1993

At the Edinburgh New Town home of Joy Barlow, manager of Brenda House Project, a residential and day-care centre for women with HIV and AIDS and their children. Since it opened here in 1989, it has been witness to the changing face of the epidemic in Scotland, drawing people not only from the local area, but also from Dundee and Glasgow. The number of women infected is not as large as first feared and only about 20 per cent of their children are positive (not the 80 per cent talked of in 1985), but the dynamics of the problem have changed.

Almost all the women seen at Brenda House have a link with drug use, but increasingly these are not first-generation transmissions; more and more, women believe they have become infected through sleeping with a drug user rather than by using drugs themselves.

Sleeping with a drug-user is still a high-risk activity, of course, although it is dismissed by those wishing to play down the limited extent of the heterosexual crossover. But Barlow says we deceive ourselves if we think the numbers of people infected are our only concern. This is a family issue, she says, and she talks of one extended family that her staff work with regularly which includes an infected woman, her three children, her current partner, her former partners, their families and her mother. It sounds like a bad joke.

'But they're all part of the picture of her illness. They will all be part of her dying. There'll be a big custody battle if she doesn't make her own plans before she dies.'

She continues:

I cannot imagine a situation before in modern human history, where we go to a funeral and sit by the side of people who are dying of the same illness as the man or woman in the coffin and whose families will be coming back again and again and again. A young woman stood up at the World AIDS Day on 1 December and said, 'I just want you to remember my three brothers', and gave their names and sat down. At a recent funeral I attended the mother was burying her second son and will be back to bury her daughter and back even maybe to bury another son.

That's when it hits me. Just the huge impact. And the numbers may not be enormous, but thank God they're not. Goodness knows how we would have managed, if there had been the numbers that were projected. I'm glad, of course I am, but I don't think we should run away with the belief that everything is wonderful either, that we've got it taped, that all the services are marvellous.

10 January 1994

At Wells Street Magistrates the Benetton Nine are charged with offences under the Public Order Act, and two men are also charged with assault. The case is brought not by the clothing company, but by the Crown Prosecution Service, and 12 police give evidence. Benetton staffers appear as witnesses.

After a four-day trial, the protesters are acquitted of all charges. Outside, supporters lay down their posters of Luciano Benetton with his mouth stuffed full of money, and embrace.

18 January 1994

Professor Michael Adler's office in James Pringle House, Middlesex Hospital's genito-urinary clinic. The last time I saw him he was sitting next to Diana, clapping along to George Michael on World AIDS Day. Just to think: 12 years before it was all genital warts and non-specific urethritis, and now it's also glamorous fundraisers and pop stars and royalty. An energizing decade:

> Quite right, one is in this contrary position that this is a human tragedy, but at a personal level it's been very exciting, incredibly exciting to be part of medical history, part of a new disease unfolding, to actually have been given the chance that one normally wouldn't have of developing services on the run that were new and imaginative, and to actually get involved with the media and to get involved with politicians.
>
> On a personal level extremely interesting and very fulfilling.

And will it continue to be?

'No, I don't think so, I think that whole initial excitement of the first few years is not there any more. AIDS has become much more mainstream, and pedestrian.'

24 January 1994

Some seven years since it was first planned and six years after it was canned by Margaret Thatcher and colleagues, the survey of sexual behaviour in Britain is published by Penguin and Blackwell Scientific Publications, with the financial support of the Wellcome Trust. It is the biggest such survey ever conducted: 19,000 people aged between 16 and 59 in 1990–91 took part both in face-to-face interviews and in less threatening questionnaires. The main aim of the survey was to understand the risks people take with their sexual health, and thus help us map out the future shape of the HIV/AIDS epidemic. The resultant report is massive and intricately detailed, and contains some controversial findings. Principal among these are:

1 24.9 per cent of men and 17.7 per cent of women who had more than two heterosexual partners in the last year never used a condom. 9.7 per cent of men aged between 16 and 25 fell into this group. Two-thirds of men and women who had slept with more than ten partners of the opposite sex believed they were taking some risks; one third thought they were taking no risk at all.

2 Serial monogamy was in vogue: there was a strong commitment to fidelity and less than a fifth of both men and women considered sex the most important part of a relationship; over two-thirds

303

regarded companionship and affection more highly. A small group of people across the age range did have many partners. 9.1 per cent of men who had homosexual sex reported 10 or more male partners in the previous five years, compared with 5.2 per cent of those who only had heterosexual sex. 3.9 per cent of gay men had had 100 or more partners. Among heterosexual men, only 0.8 per cent reported more than 100. Of some significance for the potential spread of HIV was the finding that men who had had ten or more women partners were twice as likely as men who had had sex with only one woman to have also had a homosexual partner.

3   Frequency ranged from absolute celibacy to 4.8 times a day and the range of lifetime partners went from none to 4,500.

4   The survey suggested that homosexuality was not as common as most believed – at least not the 'one in ten' of common lore. 90.2 per cent of men and 92.4 per cent of women claimed exclusive heterosexual attraction and experience. One man in 100 said he had sex exclusively or mostly with other men. Fewer than three in 1000 women said they had been exclusively or mostly lesbian. 2.2 per cent of men and 2.6 per cent of women said they were attracted to their own sex but had not had a homosexual experience. In the written questionnaires, the experience was higher: 3.6 per cent of men and 1.7 per cent of women wrote that they had had homosexual sex involving genital contact, about the same result found in surveys in the United States and France.

Homosexuality may, after all, be 'just a phase'. Of the 3.6 per cent of men who had had a male partner at some point in their lives, only 1.4 per cent had had one in the previous five years. More than 90 per cent of men and 95 per cent of women who had had a homosexual experience had also had a partner of the opposite sex.

5   Less than half of the men who reported having a homosexual partner in the past five years had taken an HIV test. The same was true of male injecting drug users.

1 February 1994

Visiting the Terrence Higgins Trust in Gray's Inn Road is never an entirely pleasant experience. You sign in, peel yourself a visitor's sticker, and when you call on any of its 50-plus staff you appreciate at once that this sector of the AIDS world at least is not overrun with money. The lift rarely works, which isn't much fun if you're sick and want to consult the medical journals in the fourth-floor library. All the offices are crammed with people, and there is insufficient space even for the basics, for decent desks or a good filing system. All the trust's services are run from here – buddying, fundraising, housing, education, counselling, legal – and it is no wonder people complain of inadequate facilities and look enviously towards the conditions at the London Lighthouse. The atmosphere warms up in late morning and early afternoon. Gossip spills over into intrigue and occasionally paranoia; for reasons that have nothing to do with clients, staff members have been known to spend inconsolable minutes bawling outside the building.

The office of the chief executive barely has room for one visitor. A few shelves hold videos and some directories from the Berlin AIDS conference; on one wall is a poster signed by Keith Haring, a familiar Silence = Death image.

On this particular day, Nick Partridge, 38, looks out at a clear view of rush-hour traffic. For him this is a good view, because it means Gays Against Genocide haven't gathered to protest this afternoon. Partridge has been on staff longer than anyone, joining as one of the earliest paid staff in 1985 and becoming chief executive in 1991.

Before he took the helm, the trust had lost three chief executives in quick succession, owing to a series of financial miscalculations, managerial shortsightedness and what some have called downright ineptitude. Oh, and there was another reason: some of the staff hated their guts.

Partridge, a gay man, followed a woman and a heterosexual married man into the post and appears to be more than holding his own; certainly he has much support from the board. But like his predecessors he has seen his organization lurch from crisis to crisis and has presided over painful job and service cuts in order to keep it solvent. A year after he heard that the trust's statutory funding would be cut by two-thirds, by £300,000 over three years, he is still coming to terms with its consequences.

A hint of bad news had leaked out several weeks before Partridge and the trust's chairman Martyn Taylor visited Julia Cumberlege at the Department of Health, but he was surprised by the extent of the cut and its delivery. 'It was a classic good cop/bad cop routine,' he says. 'Cumberlege sat us down with a number of other officials from the department, and really very apologetically announced that our grant was going to be cut and talked about how it was going to be tapered, so that we can have time to plan the impact.' And then, without knocking, in came the Secretary of State. 'Nick, you can blame me,' Virginia Bottomley said. She went on, 'When I saw that man jump into the lion's den, I thought, "Well, he won't be leaving any money to mental health charities in his will." Nick, you must really look on this as our confidence in you that the trust is a mature organization, and you're so successful at fundraising. You're so good at it.' And then, according to Partridge, she swept out again.

Partridge feels the trust is misunderstood, and not only by the Secretary of State. Not all gay men are rich because they're single; not all gay men are bound to leave money in their wills to AIDS organizations. The chief executive believes that Bottomley and her officials have begun to fall into the familiar traps, thinking that the trust's high profile attracts the high rollers.

Well, sometimes it does, albeit posthumously. When Freddie Mercury died, the royalties donated from the re-release of the *Bohemian Rhapsody* single netted almost £1 million. A great windfall, but not enough, because the million pounds from Queen went straight into the reserves that had been depleted by the huge deficit the trust had accrued from its over-expansion by 1991. And Partridge says it enabled Virginia Bottomley to send out all the wrong messages: by cutting funding to the trust, it would make many believe that the epidemic was over, or that the work it did for gay men was not important. Certainly it was another sign of shifting priorities:

I think that she was getting very conflicting messages. On one level she was being applauded internationally for what the UK had done; in parts, quite rightly so. But at another level, she was being hit both by commentators on the right, and one assumes fellow MPs, fellow cabinet members, who were presumably being asked 'Why are you spending money on queers and junkies?' and by Act-Up chaining themselves to the railings of Richmond House or lying down in the traffic, saying that she was not doing enough. I think that there was just a growing level of frustration and when she could see a way out, which was provided by what she perceived as being an everlasting fund of money coming from the music industry, she took that way out.

One line of thinking holds that a charity dedicated to care and welfare and education should repeatedly overspend and draw on its reserves; its services would appear to be expanding and in increasing demand. This line suited the trust well, although in a period when some other AIDS organizations had failed some wondered how it had survived at all. In June 1991, Frontliners, the trust offshoot organization established in 1986 as a self-help group run for people with AIDS by people with AIDS, was forced to cease trading. A subsequent report, commissioned by the Department of Health, cited lack of managerial and financial experience as the main reason for closure, but it also mentioned a lack of direction and purposeful development, features that have also afflicted the trust.

'A problem I never got to grips with, but which I think is a much bigger problem now, is what exactly were we all for?' So says Naomi Wayne, chief executive at the trust between 1990 and 1991. 'When the trust had started it was the only thing. I think it never worked out what to do when it stopped being the only thing. An industry got created. There'd be a massive increase in unemployment if there was a cure for AIDS tomorrow. What the trust never worked out was, if there is this industry around the country, what did it specifically have to contribute?'

Partridge confronted this dilemma anew in the spring of 1994, when forced to make budget savings of over £400,000. In the past, cuts had been met by a reduction in staff, but all services had been maintained. This time the prison work and the education roadshow were stopped, the spending on printed material was reduced and eight posts were lost. A comprehensive independent review of all its services was commissioned at the same time.

Despite the fact that the number of AIDS cases continues to rise each year, Partridge believes that too many politicians, journalists and members of the public believe that AIDS is almost over as an issue, a crisis contained. The proceeds from bucket rattling and other fundraising events on World AIDS Day (1 December) was down last year, and partly he blames the *Sunday Times* and Virginia Bottomley for both sending out wrong, although different signals:

We thought that the general public wouldn't buy it. They hadn't bought it the first time round, we managed to create a consensus about AIDS and we didn't think they'd buy it this time round, but they have. It's all come together – the cuts, Concorde, the *Sunday Times*, the fact that there are no new drugs, the fact that the figures are not as huge as some thought. You can lose sight of the very thin ice that you're skating on and the fragility of that support.

Things will probably get worse, he thinks. The introduction of a national lottery traditionally has the effect of directly diverting funds away from charities, as people feel that they have already donated by buying tickets. 'The organizations that will benefit will be the very large national charities, the RSPCAs, the NSPCCs and so on because they will be able to have contacts in Whitehall in general to be able to make the bids to get money when it's distributed from the lottery. The people it will harm will be those who rely far more on charity premières and small-scale local collections.'

As an organization providing a national service, the trust will also be adversely hit by the ending of ring-fenced funds and the gradual reduction in the number of regional health authorities; its future in London and large cities will be secure, but the new contracting culture will be less supportive of a diverse provision of services to a less identifiable and fewer number of people in rural areas and small towns.

'I think we're bound to see voluntary organizations closing over the next few years,' Partridge says. 'My greatest fear is that those who are most vulnerable and find it most difficult to access services will be the ones who will be hurt first.'

7 February 1994

An hour alone with Tom Hanks, movie star, who is at the Regent Hotel, London, to talk about *Philadelphia*, Hollywood's first $30 million AIDS movie. This is a plaintive tale of prejudice, discrimination and justice, for which he has been nominated for an Academy Award. He plays Andrew Beckett, a gay lawyer who is dismissed from his firm when a senior partner notices a lesion on his forehead.

Hanks is smart box office. The real issue of the movie, he believes, is fear and loathing – why so many people fear and loathe gays. 'It makes great sense to have someone who is not particularly fear inducing or loathsome in the role and I'm not. Very few people fear me. There might be some people out there that loathe me, but I'm pretty much the absolute apex of a charming, disarming, likable kind of personage.'

Hanks did much research for his role. He talked to doctors and to people with AIDS. He even talked to his hairdresser:

I asked the man who did my hair what the bathhouses were like. He said, 'Oh, the baths, it was this amazing place where you could walk in and have anonymous sex.' The techniques are fascinating stuff. I can hardly believe that it exists and I want to read every detail. And I did in fact and some of it was shocking and I thought they must be embellishing ... I mean *rimming* ... that stuff's *amazing*.

Before Hollywood became serious about him in the mid-1980s, Hanks used to live in Times Square, the crotch of the world's sex industry. 'I visited the belly of the beast any number of times in my early days,' he says, but he never experienced the gay scene. He thinks he was a little envious of it, and that there probably wasn't a young heterosexual man in the world who wouldn't want to live the same kind of hedonistic life for a while, 'especially when there's no information as to how dangerous that can be. I just thought it was wild. I wondered how often in the history of the world does this come along. Is this Berlin in the thirties? Is this Rome in the first century?'

Hanks grew up mainly in San Francisco. His mother left when he was young, his father remarried many times, but he says he remained sheltered and naïve until his late teens. He was shocked when he learnt that his high school drama teacher and several of his college classmates were gay.

These days he knows lots of gay men and many with HIV. A good school friend died of AIDS, as did a cousin. He says he feels a little uneasy about cashing in on the disease. He is sympathetic towards the criticisms levelled at Philadelphia, of which there have been many. He recites them almost as penance:

The gay community says that the film is not a real accurate reflection of their lives, that my character is not your average gay man. They say he's not political enough, not taking a bold enough stance. They say he's in the closet. They say that his family is too supportive of him. We're damned if we do and damned if we don't. These are all valid criticisms, but they don't come from the people whose lives are really like that. They said there wasn't any close love scene, but if there had been, they would have said, 'Are we supposed to accept that Tom Hanks and Antonio Banderas are *believable* as they lather each other in the shower?' There's no sleep to be lost by reading bad reviews. I've read great reviews that I thought really got the movie and I've read horrible reviews that I thought also really got the movie.

Hanks has never played gay before, and he's no activist. 'I have no political ... [he searches for the right word] ... *bent*.' *Wrong* word. But surely this will change now and he will take up AIDS as a great cause and rattle tins?

No. I'm very sceptical about anyone using their Hollywood celebrity in order to sway anything. I remember being thirteen and seeing Sonny Bono at the Republican National Convention and thinking, 'What is that guy doing there?' People's minds are already made up. I don't think it does any good. There are a lot of organizations that keep coming at you all the time, wanting you to do this for them or that for them, but if you do ...

Uh-oh, the slippery slope; too far in to rescue himself now: 'If I was to go out and try and truly believe in something and crusade for it, then I wouldn't be an actor.'

But Hanks does do some stuff – he turns up for an American Foundation for AIDS Research (AmFar) benefit alongside Barbra Streisand and he 'tithes' anonymously. It's just that he doesn't believe in those red ribbons:

It just becomes a trifle after a while, a nothing. It becomes an issue of who *didn't* wear it. Anything that happens on TV now, they have a red ribbon. So do you *have* to wear it? Is it still an option? Is it just a publicity thing? I don't know any more. It's like Kafka after a while! My God, I mean how much do you have to do? I didn't wear one at the Golden Globes and someone called up my publicist. I mean for crying out loud. It ends up being comical, but tragically comical.

We meet during the period Hanks calls his 'six week window of specialness', that hype time between nomination and Oscar night where 'the tension and the nerves can just screw your head right off'.

Has he thought about what he will say if he wins? 'The important thing is to get on and get off without doing or saying something that will embarrass you for the rest of your life.'

But will he say something about AIDS?

'Of course, but I don't know what yet.'
Maybe he'll ask his hairdresser.

10 February 1994

Professor Ian Weller is working in his cramped office in Charlotte Street, London. It is still several weeks before the official publication of the full-length Concorde report, the report that will tell us whether AZT has any effect in slowing the onset from HIV to AIDS. As a co-ordinating British investigator he has helped write more than a dozen drafts of the report, every word pored over at the Medical Research Council trial centre at the Royal Brompton Hospital in London and at Villejuif, the headquarters of the French side of the study. Back and forth every week, countless officials flying around with all this confidential information in their cases, and yet Weller says we all already really know the results and there are no surprises.

Indeed. There was a letter in the *Lancet* ten months earlier that set it out pretty clearly. AZT was next to useless in symptom-free HIV infected adults. These were only preliminary results, but they made front pages worldwide.

Concorde was the biggest clinical trial of AZT ever conducted: 1,749 patients over three years. It did not examine how effective AZT was in treating people who were seriously ill with AIDS but, just as important, it looked at how effective the drug was in treating those with HIV, before they became unwell and showed symptoms of AIDS. The preliminary results suggested that it made no difference to either mortality rates or disease progression if one took AZT early.

In this double-blind study, AZT was given to 877 people and 872 were given a placebo. As soon as a patient developed any AIDS symptoms, he or she (15 per cent were women) would be offered 'open-label' AZT. The mortality rates appeared to be shocking: over the three years of the trial, there were 79 AIDS-related deaths in the AZT group, but only 67 in the placebo group. The researchers explained that among so many patients this figure was not statistically significant, but if you were HIV positive and read of this in the newspapers, you were bound to question all the great hope that had once been invested in AZT. More people got AIDS and died on Concorde than on any previous trial.

There were other causes for concern. Those on AZT developed more side effects than those on the placebo. The results of the tests also cast doubt on one of the fundamental ways we measure a person's immunity to disease. Those given AZT early increased their CD4 or T-cell count; but the fact that, even with this higher count, patients did not live longer or develop the disease more slowly, appeared to strike at one of the basic tenets of AIDS research.

Most people with AIDS and many with asymptomatic HIV take or have taken AZT. Other drugs have emerged in the past few years that work in a similar way – ddC (produced by the Swiss company Hoffmann-La Roche) and ddI (made by the American company Bristol-Myers Squibb), but AZT is still the market leader. It is hard to think of another product that is so dominant in its field. You read the showbiz autobiographies and those three little letters snap out of the page.

Earvin 'Magic' Johnson, the basketball star who tested HIV positive in October 1991, was advised to take AZT immediately. He agreed. 'There was a lot of public interest in the fact that I was taking AZT, which was originally used only in the later stages of the illness,' he explained in *My Life*, his autobiography. 'These days it's used as a preventative, but not everybody knew that. That may be why some people, including a few reporters, concluded that I was sicker than I actually was.' People wrote to Johnson telling him that AZT was not the answer. Somebody advised him to drink all his blood and replace it with new blood. 'Even now I can't go anywhere without somebody coming up and saying, "I know this friend who knows this doctor who has a cure."'

'To my relief, I tolerated AZT fairly easily,' Arthur Ashe said shortly before he died in February 1993. 'In 1988, no one was sure of the optimum dose. I started out taking ten capsules a day (1,000 mg) … By the fall of 1992 I was down to a daily dose of three. I refuse to dwell on how much damage I may have done to myself taking the higher dosage.'

As would be expected, Wellcome plays up the good news. When, in 1989, two double-blind placebo trials of the effects of AZT on asymptomatic and less seriously ill patients showed that it could delay the progression of the disease, much was made of the results and the share price rose by 30p. But when, four months later, the company admitted that AZT had caused cancer in rodents, it explained that the rats and mice were given ten times the dose prescribed to humans and that several other drugs in use by humans had also produced tumours in animals when administered over long periods. Wellcome's share price went down one penny.

After the release of the preliminary Concorde results, Wellcome had another damage limitation exercise on its hands. The company's share price was hammered by the results, falling 10 per cent to 670p, before rallying to 692p; about £500 million was wiped off the value of the company in a single day. (When the full report was published a year later, the share value had slumped to 557p. Although not all of this was blamed on AZT, Wellcome did announce that sales of AZT fell by 16 per cent over the last financial half-year.)

Five days after the preliminary results appeared, Professor Trevor Jones, Wellcome's director of research and development, told a press conference that he was unhappy with the way the results were released, without peer review or advice to patients, and said it had caused panic among those with HIV. He hoped that a more beneficial picture of early intervention with AZT would emerge at the ninth International AIDS Conference in Berlin in June. He also outlined that the protocol of the study had changed from that agreed in 1988. When an American study reported in 1989 that AZT did have beneficial effects on people with asymptomatic HIV, the Concorde officials decided that people on its trial could switch to AZT if they wanted to; this may have led to a diluting of the results.

'When Wellcome saw the preliminary results,' Professor Weller says,

> it was the first time they raised objections to the trial. The company had two representatives on the co-ordinating committee [of the trial], and for five years they hadn't said a dickybird. They suddenly had statistical concerns, for which we had strong counter-arguments. They wanted to analyse it in a way that many many senior statisticians would think would be uninterpretable, in a way that would give a bias to the AZT group. We refused then and we refuse now to do that, because it would be completely misleading.

As for peer review, Weller states that Wellcome didn't argue for peer review when they released the more favourable results of O20, a much smaller European/Australian study conducted in people with high CD4 counts. 'Basically,' he says, 'the results came as a shock to a lot of people. What else could Wellcome do? If you want to defend your compound, you have to attack the study, there's no other way round it.'

I told Weller that a month after the *Lancet* letter, Professor Jones had invited me to lunch at Wellcome and told me why AZT might still be beneficial and why doctors should continue to prescribe the drug early:

We have gathered together ten studies on asymptomatic patients. Five of these are control studies with placebos and five are cohort studies, in which we simply give the drug and observe what happens. These studies involved more than 6,500 patients and ranged from one to four years in duration. We believe we have accrued sufficient data to show that taking the drug when you're asymptomatic does delay the onset of further symptoms.

Weller had heard this one many times before:

The thing about company studies is that they ask a specific question, and they often know the answer to it before they pose it. They are product orientated, and as soon as there's the earliest sign of efficacy they will stop. Whereas the government-sponsored trials look at bigger questions – in the mid to long term, does this early treatment do any good? In my view Concorde stopped too early, and everyone else said it was a long trial.

Weller reaches for a chart that he hopes will appear in the forthcoming full-length *Lancet* report. Look, he says, pointing to figures that Wellcome insisted be removed from the final analysis. This was a record of those people who died unexpectedly while on Concorde, but not through AIDS-related illness (often they were just found dead at home, an unexpected death, including suicide, with no apparent clinical link to HIV). This accounted for 16 people overall: 13 of them were taking AZT, three were not.

Wellcome has a presence at all the chief AIDS conferences, and will occasionally organize gatherings of its own. In June 1992 it launched Positive Action, 'an international initiative in support of those with HIV and AIDS'. For the launch conference in London, journalists flew in from all over Europe to hear Wellcome executives describe how £1 million was being distributed to many educational organizations. An emotional climax of sorts was provided by Jerry Breitman, the company's US director of professional relations. He was there to present the 'workplace initiative' and his speech contained a little surprise at the end. Like the wig salesman whose *coup de grâce* is to rip off his own toupee, Breitman declared himself HIV positive. 'I thought long and hard before deciding to tell my management,' he revealed. 'But ... when you are part of an enlightened organization such as Wellcome, I am absolutely convinced that communicating your HIV infection is a positive action ... It is, truly, one of the best decisions I have made in a very long time.' A few journalists felt distinctly queasy at the theatricality of it all.

One of the initiatives raised was Wellcome's involvement with the Terrence Higgins Trust. This first surfaced in 1991, with the publication of four information leaflets. In March 1993, staff at the trust and volunteers read in their newsletter that the link had been strengthened. The newsletter explained that

> THT, along with the Wellcome Foundation, is about to begin producing an important new medical information series. THT are providing a series of medical updates for all staff and volunteers. We will be providing them on a regular basis every two months in the evening. Costs will be met by the Wellcome Foundation, which also funds our series of general booklets.

The preliminary Concorde results were a disaster for some staff at the THT, but in a way that they could never have dreamt possible. Shortly after learning of the results, a small group of men began gathering outside the trust's London offices in Gray's Inn Road, near King's Cross, and demanded immediate resignations of management and staff. Soon this group had a name: Gays Against Genocide. Its leaders were Michael Cottrell, a former volunteer at the trust, and his partner Karl Burge. As their picket continued they were intermittently joined by several others who had themselves had bad experiences with AZT, including members of the alternative self-help group Positively Healthy.

So what had the trust done wrong? It had taken money from Wellcome plc and included positive information about AZT in several leaflets and documents (several other organizations, including the National AIDS Trust and the National AIDS Manual, had also accepted Wellcome funding). Cottrell and his friends felt they were being betrayed by the very organization that they had believed existed to act in their best interests; they felt that what was once an invaluable institution was acting as a mouthpiece for a multinational pharmaceuticals company. This was some ironic turnaround: people with HIV picketing the trust and shouting 'Murderer!' at those entering the building each morning.

One placard dubbed Nick Partridge, chief executive of the trust, 'Nick the Sick'; another claimed 'Nick sold our lives to the drug companies'. In reply, Partridge called them 'New Age flat-earthers who have a naïve hope that Holland and Barrett will produce a herbal tea that will be effective against HIV.' Partridge said that the trust actively pursued funding from a wide range of companies and government agencies, and that it was 'quite clear that none of that funding involves an ability by those companies to influence the information we produce. We would be neglecting our duty if we were not in regular contact with Wellcome, Bristol-Myers Squibb and Roche, arguing for greater investment in HIV research and fair and balanced information. The leaflets [we produce] are not about treatment issues.'

But once they were. In 1991 the trust produced a 24-page booklet on HIV and its treatment; nine pages were devoted to AZT, but only half a page was given to other therapies. The copyright on the leaflet was held by the Wellcome Foundation, which also paid for its printing. 'It was only available for eight months,' Partridge says. 'Information changes quite rapidly. The main fault of that leaflet is that it is too hopeful. By 1991 the hopes around early intervention had probably gone further than we realize, in retrospect, was wise.'

Wellcome's involvement with the leaflets stemmed from a financial crisis at the trust. 'Wherever we could get money from and wherever we could be seen to be tackling our deficit, then that is what we should do,' Partridge remembers saying at the time:

> The theme of World AIDS Day that year was 'Sharing the Challenge' and one of those was sharing the challenge with Wellcome. Bluntly it was the only way we were going to be able to pay for a new set of leaflets. So it's management based on hope and inexperience, rather than mismanagement ... For all its faults, our leaflet was still a lot more realistic than the material that Wellcome was putting out on its own.

By the summer it had all turned rather sour for the protesters Cottrell and Burge. After they began abusing and physically impeding trust staff and clients (some unwell with AIDS), the trust gained a High Court injunction to prevent them continuing. After repeated breaches, they were sentenced to four weeks in Pentonville.

Shortly after their release they were outside the trust again, but now their horizons had expanded and they had joined those dissidents who supported Professor Peter Duesberg, the Californian scientist who believed that HIV was not the cause of AIDS. They spoke tearfully and movingly at some anti-AZT/anti-Wellcome conferences, and Michael Cottrell talked of suing Wellcome for hastening the death of his former partner Kevin Bills (one woman from Birmingham had already been granted legal aid to pursue a similar case, claiming that her husband, an infected haemophiliac, was symptom-free when he began taking AZT).

But it wasn't long before the increasingly extreme nature of their tactics alienated all the Duesberg supporters and anti-AZT campaigners who had originally supported – some might say used – them. At one stage Cottrell claimed he had bought a nuclear warhead in Amsterdam and threatened to use it against his enemies; several doctors received physical threats for continuing to prescribe AZT. At the trust, Nick Partridge says that his confrontations with GAG were one of the worst periods of his life, but he maintains some concern for their well-being. 'You can see how people might get like that, how they might despair,' he says. 'Basically they need a lot of help.'

In his office, Professor Weller is reading a new document that has just arrived from Wellcome, a draft of a leaflet intended to guide patients through the controversy, ahead of the release of the full Concorde results. He consults it in disbelief: the only reference to Concorde is that AZT is non-toxic in asymptomatics. 'But they could have been a lot more open. The point remains that if you have AIDS, AZT can be of definite benefit.' Doctors who administer AZT for symptom-free patients (and the licence only extends to those with a CD4 count below 500 and rapidly falling) do so on the optimistic assumption that some other drug will be available when symptoms appear; others prefer simply to hold AZT back, knowing they at least have something in their armoury when AIDS takes hold.

Despite the disappointments of Concorde, Weller remains very optimistic about the future of HIV/AIDS treatments and care. No magic bullets, he says, but some valuable new drugs on the horizon. He runs through the current state of play with some enthusiasm. Of the nucleosides, which work in the same way as AZT by providing compounds that block the enzyme that stimulates HIV to multiply, ddI is probably of similar efficacy to AZT, but it hasn't had a chance. If there were placebo-control trials of ddI in symptomatic disease (which there aren't, for ethical reasons), there would most likely be marked, if transient, benefits. However ddI is unpleasant to take and has the rare but potentially life-threatening side effect of pancreatitis.

The nucleoside ddC is regarded as inferior; a recent study, a head-on trial between AZT and ddC in symptomatics, was halted when it was detected that the mortality was higher in the ddC group. There is some hope that these nucleosides may prove beneficial when used in combination, but the first large-scale trial, Delta, is unlikely to report until 1996 (tellingly, the drop-out rate for the trial increased as a result of general disillusionment with nucleosides post-Concorde). But until Delta reports, doctors employing combinations could be doing as much harm as good. By mid 1994, AZT remained the only anti-HIV drug to be granted a UK licence.

Of the non-nucleosides in development by Upjohn and Janssen and several other companies, the first reports were exciting: they have very specific efficacy against the virus and seem to be of low toxicity apart from rash. Wonderful news. The sad news emerged swiftly: resistance to the drug developed very rapidly. In people with AIDS, it takes between six months and a year for resistance to develop against AZT, but with these drugs it's there within four to eight weeks. Then there are the HIV-protease inhibitors, a very precise designer drug which works in a far more direct way than the others, but requires almost 20 stages of manufacture. Toxicity is unknown because of the shortage of the drug for trials.

'But everyone talks about the anti-virals,' Weller says. 'Sometimes I think we don't focus on things that we're doing best. We've had too high an expectancy of how fast we would develop the really important drugs. Remember that hepatitis B virus was discovered in 1970. By 1994 we still do not have an effective anti-viral therapy.'

Weller emphasizes the advances made in PCP prophylaxis:

In the days when we only had high-dose Septrin and intravenous Pentamidine, the mortality from Pneumocystis was 50 per cent. Now it's probably less than 10 per cent. Now, when you get your dreadful rash from Septrin, you switch to Pentamidine, and when you have your severe hypertension, then there's this and that, all these other second-line agents. Nobody talks about how we've prolonged so many lives.

Other new drugs are effective against other opportunistic infections, against CMV and fungal growths. There are even trials of the anti-HIV effects of thalidomide. Then there are all the advances in patient care, in hospice care, in community care and the increased amount of money that goes into looking after AIDS patients. And not all of this care focuses on conventional medicine; many HIV positive patients hold great store by acupuncture, by traditional herbal remedies, by holistic therapy in general. 'People came back from Berlin [the 1993 International AIDS conference] with their heads down,' Weller says, 'but I think there may always have been too much optimism.'

11 February 1994

Eight weeks ago I had visited Esmee Seargent, the newly appointed director of the Black HIV/AIDS Network (BHAN), an organization for African, African-Caribbean and other ethnic minority communities. She told me the charity exists principally because 'You may be able to hide your sexuality, but you can't hide the colour of your skin.' There was a double jeopardy to being HIV and black – twice the discrimination, twice the homophobia, additional problems of telling your community and, if you were African, the compounded obstacles of being blamed for starting the pandemic.

BHAN saw 131 clients, about 20 of them children aged between three and 12. It received funding from more than a dozen sources, including the South West Thames Regional Health Authority, the Department of Health, district and local authorities, all of whom appeared supportive of its many counselling, prevention and consultancy services.

But this morning came some bad news. The Metropolitan Police had been called in to investigate the disappearance of over £500,000 from the organization's funds. Seargent had uncovered the fraud when she attempted to reorganize the accounts and commissioned an audit that found that tens of thousands of pounds were untraceable and that about £250,000 in cheques had been made payable to Bijon Sinha, BHAN's former treasurer, who had since disappeared. Mr Sinha had been with BHAN since its inception in 1989 and was believed to have been involved with the company that had previously audited BHAN's accounts. Detective Inspector Simon Goddard, heading the inquiry at Shepherds Bush CID, west London, said he was treating the case as 'systematic theft' and was urgently trying to track down Mr Sinha.

Esmee Seargent declined to comment on the investigation, but assured her clients that services were being maintained. The organization appeared to have the continued support of its principal funders, though there was much talk of tightening the financial checks on the voluntary sector as a whole.

19 February 1994

On the beach at Dungeness, it's those nuns again. The Sisters of Perpetual Indulgence are saying their 'Hail Saint Derek's and Derek Jarman is 'lying in state' in his wooden Prospect Cottage. In his coffin he wears a golden robe, the robe of Edward II in his film, the robe in which he was canonized by those nuns. His hands hold a plastic frog. On his head, a cap marked 'controversialist'.

In the afternoon, the coffin is driven a few miles to the Norman spire and cool stone of St Nicholas Church in New Romney, Kent. It is a traditional service, a George Herbert psalm and 'Abide With Me', a bit subdued for Derek. The action comes with the speeches. First Nicholas Ward-Jackson, then Norman Rosenthal of the Royal Academy:

> Derek ... Instantly after meeting you in 1970, I was able to help you organize an exhibition of your work and that of two of your friends. I felt myself at that time little more than a hanger on, but you enthusiastically gave me the opportunity. To others you gave their first canvas or camera and they became real and good photographers. Students of literature became your scriptwriters, young musicians made music for you and dancers danced, and boys and girls who chanced into your life found parts in your movies – all of us refugees from institutional constrictions imposed on us by the fake values of the moral majority. Together, and much inspired by you, we found ways to be creative ourselves ...

Then Sarah Graham, who had demonstrated with Jarman for Out-Rage. And Nicholas de Jongh, the theatre critic:

> All down the exciting road of his life, as the first and greatest gay English icon, he blazed a trail. And he dared to show in our unkind

and unfeeling times what it was and is to be outcast, reviled and persecuted for a sexuality in which he rejoiced and in which he could see no shred of natural evil ... He lit so many gay candles in a hard world. No one else lit more. None shone more clearly.

We emerge into shards of sunshine. We hang around outside, four hundred or so, a few pop and film people, plenty of media, some in pale blue ribbons to mark his last work. He is buried privately at the church of St Clement, Old Romney, beneath a yew tree.

That morning, Tony Pinching, his principal doctor at Bart's, was giving students the HIV basics in an informal session called an academic half-day: this is what we know, this is what we're doing. Lots of questions from the floor and two student papers going round: 'The Pathology of AIDS' and 'Epidemiology of AIDS'.

These students knew much more than their counterparts a decade ago. The biology of HIV-I infection (to distinguish it from the less virulent HIV-II present mainly in West Africa) was relayed in language quite opaque to the casual visitor; all lipid envelopes and gp41 glycoproteins and altered monocyte functions resulting in decreased chemotaxis.

The natural history is a little more penetrable. After contact with the virus, seroconversion (the formation of antibodies) occurs within three to 17 weeks. After a variable latent period, the following are observed: an acute viral-like illness in 30–50 per cent of patients; persistent generalized lymphadenopathy; AIDS-related complex (ARC) characterized by persistent fever, weight loss and diarrhoea. There is a reduction in CD4 (T-helper) cells, as well as anaemia, and thrombocytopenia (a reduction of platelets leading to bruising and bleeding).

Current estimates suggest that 25 to 30 per cent of infected patients develop full-blown AIDS in five to seven years. This is marked by a wide variety of opportunistic infections; Pneumocystis *carinii pneumonia* occurs in 50 per cent of cases; aggressive Kaposi's sarcoma occurs in 25 per cent of patients; diseases of the nervous system, including meningitis and encephalitis (inflammation of the brain) occur in 75 to 90 per cent of cases. With AIDS, 85 per cent of patients die within five years.

At the end of one of the papers there was a paragraph on euthanasia. 'A BMA working group set up to investigate the legalisation of euthanasia, wrote in its report that they rejected the need for legalisation, and felt instead we should be "reaffirming the supreme value of the individual, no matter how worthless and hopeless that individual may feel".'

When Bart's was threatened with closure in May 1993, Jarman wrote an eloquent letter to the *Independent*, so eloquent and lucid that it appeared on the front page:

I have been here for two weeks, first in the casualty ward, and now in Colston, which cares mainly for the dying. My 'own' ward, Andrewes, is full; and the construction of the new purpose-built AIDS ward has been postponed. Over the road is Rambling Rose, who was sedated out of kindness after two days clucking like a chicken and screaming abuse. I escape to the 18th-century court-yard and read in the pavilion to the sound of the fountain, before retiring to the hospital church of Saint Bartholomew, which itself is cool and filled with the peace of time.

Jarman quoted Virginia Bottomley's comment that she was 'not in the heritage business'. He asked, 'Aren't we all in the heritage busi-ness? Without our past our future cannot be reflected, the past is our mirror. Every profession has a history, and the medical profession's starts here.' Founded in the eleventh century, Bart's is the world's oldest hospital. It is still not 'one of the new Habitat hospitals; its rooms are high and cool, but the voracious cashflow snake is out to strangle it'. He closed with the comment that 'Bart's is my second home and my life here is cherished.'

In his office, Tony Pinching says:

I still owe a duty of confidentiality to my patients. But I will say that as a person he was an extraordinary man by any standards. He combined a matter-of-factness about things with an extraordinary vision. He didn't hang about intellectually. He was always several steps ahead; whatever we were talking about, he always had some-thing interesting and different to say. In many ways the way he dealt with his disease publicly was a reflection of this. Things that other people agonized about he just did and moved on.

Most people are able to make something positive in their lives of HIV and AIDS and the insights that it brings. Disease in general does and AIDS does it with a particular brightness. Derek was just doing that, but on a bigger scale. He had at least two different visu-al problems as part of his illness, and as somebody who is such a

THAT THE LAW PROTECTED

visual person, that's a really raw deal. But Derek's approach was always, 'How interesting!' You never exchanged a trivial word with Derek. There was no question that this was a guy of real genius. One sensed that he had maintained the childlike enthusiasm for colour and shape; he retained that sense that it was always fresh and exciting and meaningful and he never took anything for granted. He was a stunning person to look after. He did a great deal for all of us at all sorts of levels. I just hope we were able to do something for him.

21 February 1994

A late-night vote at the House of Commons. For the past month, anal sex has been on the agenda like never before, as MPs, health officials, charity workers and evangelicals debate the age of consent. Edwina Currie had proposed to reduce the age for gay men from 21 to 16 and thus make it equal with that for heterosexuals.

Apart from the ethical/ideological/religious debate that might have characterized the issue a decade ago, AIDS now presented a health dimension, which was being used by all sides. Those who wished to maintain inequality at 21 claimed that the law protected society from the virus and that a reduction to 16 or 18 would spread the virus faster. Some Bible thumpers even used the old 'divine retribution' line again. Those who favoured equality at 16 argued that the present law and Section 28 meant that many sexually active young men were likely to be practising unsafe sex because they were cut off from the education they needed in order to protect their health.

Those who supported this line of reasoning included the Health Education Authority, the British Medical Association, MIND, the National Children's Bureau, the Family Planning Association, the Family Welfare Association, the Save the Children Fund, the National Association of Probation Officers and Barnardos. 'The present laws prevent us from giving practical support and information,' said Carol Lindsay Smith, development officer for HIV services at Barnardos. 'We find ourselves in a ludicrous situation of handing out condoms to girls who are 16 and to heterosexual boys who are 16, but not to gay 16-year-olds.'

After a three-hour Commons debate, the vote to equalize at 16 failed by 307 to 280. The amendment to adopt 18 was passed by 427 to 162. Thirty-five Labour MPs, including health spokesman David Blunkett, voted for 18. There was a mini-riot after the result, as some of the five thousand people who had gathered outside tried to gain entry. Sir Ian McKellen, who had campaigned tirelessly for equality (an act which Bernard Ingham, Mrs Thatcher's former press secretary, had likened to a 'party political broadcast for the Buggers' Party'), claimed that they had won the arguments, if not the votes, and they would be back soon to win.

28 February 1994

Paul Muldownie began with a knife, raiding a garage in Sittingbourne, Kent, and stealing £80. Then it was a London hairdresser's, with the knife covered with some of his own blood. Then two clothes stores and a hotel giftshop, where he threatened staff with a syringe. The syringe also had blood on it, infected blood, he said, as Muldownie told his victims that he had AIDS. Speaking in his defence, Nicholas Doherty told Southwark Crown Court that his client learnt only yesterday that he had less than four years to live (though he did not explain how this figure had been reached). Doherty said Muldownie had committed the crimes to raise money for the Terrence Higgins Trust: 'He feels a cure has to be found to this disease'. Charles Davidson, the recorder, acknowledged that these were 'exceptional and personal circumstances' as he sent him to jail for two and a half years.

1 March 1994

'We have actually done extremely well on a small amount of money.' So says Professor Alan Stone, the head of the AIDS secretariat at the MRC. This small amount of money, a figure which has reached over £60 million since the MRC became serious about AIDS research in 1987, has yielded a lot of scientific advance, little of it appreciated by the patient. Researchers believe they understand more about HIV than any other virus, and yet the more they learn, the less certain they become.

On his desk at the MRC headquarters near Regent's Park, Professor Stone has a list of advances (he loathes the word 'breakthrough') achieved with MRC money; an impressive list, especially when he explains the terminology. But he knows that what he's got isn't enough. 'We have not yet managed to deliver to the patient drugs which will prolong their life substantially,' he admits. 'You can prolong the life of someone with AIDS by two or three years with treatments, but what everybody would like to be able to do is say, "This poor chap's discovered he's infected – what can we give him which will ensure he lives for another thirty or forty years?" We haven't been able to do that.'

Stone attended the international Keystone meeting in January 1994, another annual gathering of the leading people in the field. Researchers weren't depressed when they returned, he says, but there was a renewed feeling of realism: only by stepping back from the mountain could they see the true scale of their problem. It had been an indifferent year on several counts. The vaccines they were all set to try didn't neutralize the field isolates of the virus; the new drugs that people had read about (and there were more than 60 of them) were mostly still unavailable for Phase 1 trials; and then there was Concorde.

I tell him what Baroness Cumberlege had told me: that she believed that scientific advances had been slight. What about the advances in terms of genetics, Stone asked, or the progress made in the molecular biology of HIV (what keeps it dormant, what activates it), or the increased knowledge about the immunological changes in the body when one becomes infected? He reached for his document and began to read. There had been key advances in:

1 Studies on the molecular organization of HIV and on the structure of the molecules known to be important in the infection and replication processes.
2 The work on reverse transcriptase, viral protease, p24 core protein and the T-cell CD4 receptor, which has provided valuable information of potential importance for the rational design of anti-viral agents.
3 Studies on the immune response to immunodeficiency viruses which have thrown light on the various components of the immune response to HIV and SIV, including mucosal immunity.
4 The effects of HIV infection on antigen presenting dendritic cells (cells involved in the early stage of infection).
5 The role of the human T-cell components in experimental vaccines based on chemically inactivated SIV (although the MRC had also been criticized for wasting much money on monkey vaccine experiments that had already been conducted in the United States).

There were many more. One of the most important was the work conducted on mother-to-child transmission of HIV. The MRC co-ordinated a European study in 1991 which found that out of a study of 721 children of infected mothers, 104 were presumed infected (14 per cent). It was found that vertical transmission from the mother was not associated with intravenous drug use (80 per cent of mothers had a history of such use), but the more important factors were the current clinical health of the mother, early birth and breast feeding.

This dovetailed with more particular studies. In February 1994, a study conducted at 59 medical centres in the United States concluded that AZT might be useful in helping to prevent a pregnant HIV positive woman infecting her baby. Such transmission normally occurs about 15 per cent of the time. This study involved 477 positive women, half of whom were given AZT, the other half placebos. In the placebo group 26 per cent of newborn babies had HIV, while in the AZT group the figure was only 8 per cent. Dr James Curran, one of the chief co-ordinators of the American effort against AIDS at the Center for Disease Control in Atlanta, called this result 'a real breakthrough with worldwide implications'. He called for an immediate rethink of the recommendations for treatment of HIV during pregnancy. But many questions remain. Only an extended follow-up will show whether HIV will develop in the uninfected children when they grow older and comparative tests still have to be done looking at the optimum time to administer AZT. The predictable debate ensued, cheered on, no doubt, by Wellcome: should all pregnant women test for the virus and should AZT be administered to infected mothers who are only contemplating childbirth?

Potentially there was more good news for women – a new MRC programme to develop vaginal virucides. This is a relatively simple thing, a form of disinfectant that kills the HIV, and the trick is to find something a woman can insert before sex that will be safe and undetectable. The spermicide nonoxynol-9 can inactivate HIV in laboratory studies, but there was also evidence that it could inflame the vaginal mucosa and therefore increase the risk. The challenge is to find a substance that causes no inflammation; this could have enormous impact in countries where condoms aren't available.

In May 1994 it was announced that the MRC's entire AIDS programme would be re-evaluated and overhauled. At the same time it was announced that its ring-fenced AIDS budget would disappear from the autumn, thus bringing it into line with the end of ring-fencing for treatment and care. Henceforward, HIV/AIDS research will have to compete for finance as it did in the days before the Directed Programme, against all the other scientific projects demanding funds. This will not necessarily mean less money will be available (though this is thought likely), but it will almost certainly mean that the speed of grant allocation will slow down.

This was not greeted with an expected outcry from within the AIDS community. 'To go on demanding more and more for AIDS research and care, in isolation from all the other specialist services – care for the elderly, the mentally ill – is very difficult,' Ian Weller says. 'Money should be concentrated on high-level research; now fairly inferior projects could easily be funded.' In terms of hospital provision, Weller says that when he visits non-AIDS wards he sees a much inferior standard of care. 'People might say that it's all got to be brought up, but I'm afraid we haven't got the money to do that. So the resources we've got have got to be spread around a bit more equitably.'

There is another factor at work here too, a familiar one. Because AIDS in Britain is not on a scale that some had feared and appears not be growing as fast as it did when the serious money began coming through in the late 1980s, there is a slender but visible financial retreat. As the political priority of AIDS declines, so its effect is felt in terms of research and care. The principal of mainstreaming is widely welcomed; after many years of protection it is right that AIDS should be regarded as an important and general societal problem and treated as such in all areas of the community. What is less certain, because it is still much too early to say, is the extent to which the worst aspects of stigmatization and callousness may return to impede scientific and medical progress, progress that will also have a crucial impact on the wider global epidemic.

16 March 1994

After the Terrence Higgins Trust, Naomi Wayne found a new job with older people, but AIDS remained on the agenda. Not long after she began work at Age Concern Lewisham, Tara Kaufman, who was writing a report on AIDS and the over-fifties, arrived. According to the official PHLS figures, about 11 per cent of people with AIDS are 50 and older.

Kaufman gave a talk to the Libertines, the local gay group for men who no longer find an evening at Bang in Tottenham Court Road an enticing prospect. About 20 Libertines meet each week; their average

age is about 60. Kaufman found that although many of them were still sexually active, they knew almost nothing about HIV or AIDS and less about safer sex.

'The assumption was that it wasn't for them,' Wayne says. 'You know that excuse that gay men use: "If I only sleep with young men I won't get it"? Well, this was: "If I only sleep with old men I won't get it."'

With a local grant, Wayne put together two leaflets, one of which was specifically aimed at older gay men. She had some help from Kingsley, one of the Libertines, who told her, 'You must say put the condom on first and then the lubricant. It's not that they're stupid, they just haven't a clue.'

'They were very clear they don't like stuff from the trust,' Wayne says:

They don't like the street language, they don't like the explicitness, they're not interested in pictures of pretty young men. And I was totally taken aback, because it had never crossed my mind. The last thing I thought of when I got here was that I was going to be doing HIV work. What touched me about AIDS was young men dying before their time. Others had thought this way too and what had happened was that there had been very little thought about HIV-related service provision for older people.

Age Concern Lewisham also produced a leaflet for heterosexuals, and people seemed pleased that there was some acknowledgement that sex doesn't stop at 50. During the writing, Wayne asked her insurance worker, who's in her late sixties, what terms she should use for different bits of the genitalia. She said, 'People don't have terms if they're my age, they say, "down there".' Wayne said she thought 'down there' wasn't on. 'But when I was picking up literature in Bromley, I got a leaflet from Beckenham Hospital which somebody else had written and the front cover is "Taking Care of Down There".'

Wayne claims the leaflets have been a great success and continue to be in demand nationwide. She says 'people are having sex in the oddest places'. And what of safer sex in her greying gay community? 'Kingsley says the Libertines is a changed group.'

21 March 1994

Tom Hanks wins his Oscar. The studded jewellery on his tux lapel forms the shape of a ribbon. In the hottest speech of the evening, he recalls his gay drama teacher and cousin. He talks about angels in heaven mopping feverish brows. He thanks God and he says God Bless America. Oddly, no mention of rimming.

25 March 1994

The latest figures from the European Centre for the Epidemiological Monitoring of AIDS are dispatched from Saint-Maurice, France. There have been a total 109,858 AIDS cases reported in the countries of the WHO European region up to 31 December 1993; the centre, like all other past sources, regards the actual number of cases to be considerably greater. There are, for instance, no cases reported from Albania, Azerbaijan, Kazakhstan or Tajikistan and only 22 in the Ukraine, 47 in the Czech Republic and 132 in the Russian Federation.

Taking countries with more than 300 cases, the comparative table looks like this:

Austria	1,100
Belgium	1,555
Denmark	1,356
France	28,497
Germany	10,858
Greece	891
Ireland	378
Italy	20,336
Netherlands	2,912
Norway	368
Portugal	1,641
Romania	2,635
Spain	22,655
Sweden	948
Switzerland	3,561
United Kingdom	8,529

France, Italy and Spain account for 65 per cent of all cases reported in Europe. The highest cumulative rates per million population are reported in Spain (579), Switzerland (509), France (481) and Italy (352). The UK's rate is 147 cases per million. Between 1992 and 1993, the increase in AIDS cases is 11.6 per cent. Just over half the reported cases are known to have died.

There is a continuing increase in the number of female cases. Of cases diagnosed in 1991, 17.4 per cent were female; by the end of 1993 this had risen to 19 per cent. The number of reported cases due to heterosexual contact continued its steady rise, from 11.9 per cent in 1991, to 13.4 per cent in 1992, to 15.3 per cent in 1993.

The average age of adult cases increased. Between 1991 and 1993 the proportion of AIDS cases in men aged 25 to 29 decreased from 23.2 per cent to 17.7 per cent; in women it went from 31 per cent to 28.2 per cent. By contrast, in the 30 to 34 age group, the proportion increased from 25.9 to 28.8 (men) and from 23.1 to 30 per cent (women). The number of paediatric cases (children under 13) increased to a total of 4,505, almost half of these reported in Romania.

30 March 1994

'I don't think Virginia Bottomley listens any more, and she used to.' Increasingly, Professor Tony Pinching can see it all slipping away, very slowly. Perhaps not all: the treatment and care have improved beyond recognition and he's proud of the reputation Bart's now has in the AIDS field (once it was the last place you'd go). But he reads about how it's all been overblown, how AIDS isn't this great plague after all – 9,000 cases, 20,000 infections, is that *all*? – and he's seldom consoled, because his own caseload just seems to get bigger.

If the figures are not cataclysmic, we should learn from our success; we should have learnt that this is a preventable epidemic; we should learn from France, where comprehensive public education came far later. Pinching says he told Virginia Bottomley some time ago that what we needed was some consistency, just to keep things ticking over. 'All they needed to do was to smile,' he says, 'and not lose their nerve. But now there's this meddle and interference and change, as if this was a problem you could just deal with by a quick political fix. If the problem's gone, why are we seeing a rising rate of HIV amongst young gay men?'

When Pinching moved from St Mary's, west London, to Bart's, he encountered not only a different ethnic population, but another group of gay men quite separate from the recognized peer group. Last year he says he saw an active gay man who presented with PCP but had never heard of AIDS. These men don't self-identify as gay, but they have sex with other men. Educationally, they are very difficult to access. He sees substantial numbers of people from parts of the world where the heterosexual epidemic is more advanced, particularly Uganda. And

> there are other populations who are still there waiting to be zapped. There's a very large Turkish population for example. Ask them about AIDS, where are the Turkish leaflets? They didn't have them, and they don't hear anything from their peer group. There are all sorts of problems about how to get new messages across to certain cultures that are not used to health messages, and certainly not messages about sexual health.
>
> There's an enormous epidemic there waiting to happen. So suddenly you look eastwards and you find a whole range of communities which aren't part of this general sort of feeling of 'Oh, we've fixed AIDS'. These are people who are just the other side of London. They haven't heard that we've fixed this epidemic. In some cases, people don't even know it's started.

9 April 1994

On the day the full report of Concorde appears in the *Lancet*, I remember something Ray Brettle said up at the City Hospital in Edinburgh. He talked about the huge disappointment his patients felt about the lack of progress. 'When people first came in they had this feeling that in three years' time things would be a lot better. Some things have improved, but it's been slow and gradual and learnt through experience. The optimism that was there – they'll find a cure, a cure just around the corner, and I'll be OK – that's all gone.'

Brettle said he couldn't continue to do his job if he thought there was no hope. 'We still feel we can make a difference, make people's lives better, but we still can't save their lives. We still can't crack it. But the man who trained me said, "Because there's no magic treatment, you've just got to be a better doctor."'

Brettle is 45. I ask what he'll be doing in five years' time. 'I'm not sure whether I can keep doing this,' he says:

> It does get to you. It's changed: early on it was all drug use and few people were actually dying. Now a lot of people are dying. I used to be able to cope OK, but now it's one a week. Your whole cohort of people being wiped out.

What happens a lot in America is that people who have been doing it for years now see far fewer patients. They're not really in the wards nearly so much. But it's quite addictive, that's the trouble.

We lose about thirty or forty people a year now, and we gain about fifty new patients a year, so we're still ahead slightly.'

12 April 1994

Nine o'clock on a Tuesday morning at the Royal Free Hospital, north London, finds Dr Margaret Johnson contemplating her increasing caseload. In 1989 Dr Johnson became the first designated HIV/AIDS consultant in the country, a job that entails overseeing all aspects of a patient's treatment, from her hospital's pioneering same-day test through to terminal care.

This year her caseload has gone up by 30 per cent. She looks after about 1,100 with HIV and about 280 with AIDS. About 20 per cent of her patients are women, of whom one third are from African countries with a high prevalence of HIV, and another third are injecting drug users (mostly from abroad, particularly Spain, France and Italy). The final third, about 60 women, are white Caucasians who have caught the virus heterosexually,

who you wouldn't in any way feel had any risk factors. The figures are small for the heterosexual cases, but women *have* been infected that way and epidemics start in small ways. The women I look after on average have half the amount of sexual partners compared to those who come in to test at our clinic. So they're not a particularly promiscuous group of women, they've just been unlucky. Most of them really do say, 'Look, I knew about it, but I really didn't think it would happen to me' – the classic line.

The Royal Free's same-day testing clinic operates three days a week, during which it sees about 80 new people. If you're there at 10 a.m. you'll know your results by 4 p.m., and a positive finding is checked twice. The traditional two- or three-day wait is just 'too painful, too stressful', Johnson says.

The incidence of infection hasn't changed over the years. The sero-prevalence of gays who test is only 6 per cent, much lower than general London figures, especially from the genito-urinary clinics which often report a 20 per cent rate (Johnson believes her hospital's figures reflect a more accurate picture of spread amongst all London gay men, rather than those who may be more promiscuous and report to GUM clinics for other STDs).

The future is not a merry prospect. 'I think the type of care and treatment we are going to be able to deliver will be less good. Because it's no longer ring-fenced, my director of public health is looking and thinking, "If I can save some money on the AIDS budget, I can use that for cataracts."'

With the opening in 1992 of the Ian Charleson Centre (a former patient at the hospital), the Royal Free pre-dated the Department of Health's push towards fewer beds and reduced overnight stays by offering day-care for such things as chemotherapy and blood trans-fusion. Since it opened, HIV-related hospital admissions have dropped by 50 per cent, a trend hugely welcomed by the patients. But there are clearly limits to outpatient and community care, and Dr Johnson believes the trend may be getting out of hand:

I actually think that AIDS is the most complicated medical problem around and it's complete nonsense that it should be community based. People are confusing very much what is appropriate in the community and what is appropriate in hospital. Certainly looking after Pneumocystis or CMV retinitis is not appropriate in the com-munity and is incredibly complicated. You're using very toxic drugs, combinations of different drugs for different things that may all interreact with each other – it really is very inappropriate general practice medicine, but it's a bandwagon that is gaining huge momentum. Certainly my director of public health, our purchaser, has written in the *BMJ* to say that treatment doesn't work for HIV and we should spend it all on prevention. He quotes one reference – Concorde. To me that's complete lunacy. Are we really going to have 24-year-olds with CMV retinitis who we're going to let go blind?

The 1994–5 funding, though no longer ring-fenced, will remain much as it did in the previous year, but next year things will probably be different. 'The survival of my patients is as good as anywhere in the world, and I want to ensure that that continues,' Dr Johnson says. 'But next year I may not be able to prescribe ganciclovir for CMV retinitis; I may have a budget that tells me that it's just too expensive. There is this view now that we're not getting value for money in AIDS care and it's not true.'

There *has* been some loony spending, she says, citing community centres that give patients free lunches and great gyms:

I think that's wonderful, but if at the end it jeopardizes their basic medical care, I think it will be a tragedy. Mainstreaming is right, but it is important that definite protections are in place to make sure the important treatments are available. At the end of the day there *are* prejudices and HIV care is very expensive hospital and trusts are into things that will make money. If HIV isn't going to make money you'll quickly find that your colleagues won't be so keen on treating it, and they'll start saying, 'Well it might be dangerous' and all those old things might come back again.

12 April 1994

Lunch with Lindsay Neil at the Health Education Authority. She has some perplexing news. She has recently heard that forces 'on high' (her board members) have agreed to suspend temporarily all future HIV/AIDS and sexual health promotion work. The exact reason for this isn't clear (or at least she won't divulge it), but it comes after a period of sustained criticism of the HEA's work. First the condom campaigns banned by Lady Cumberlege, then last month the withdrawal of *Your Pocket Guide to Sex*, an HEA publication written by Nick Fisher, agony uncle at *Just Seventeen*. Dr Brian Mawhinney, Minister of State for Health, found the book 'smutty' and agreed with the objections to it first raised by the HEA's own board members, the Bishop of Peterborough and Esther Rantzen. Lindsay Neil has heard that the book may soon be bought from the HEA and published by Penguin.

Five months after the Lee Report was due to survey the HEA's role and relationship with the government, there is still no sign of it. It is now expected in late summer. Many in the AIDS world predict the HEA will come in for a hammering. Neil believes at least a name change is imminent, to the Health Education Commission. She is unmistakably disturbed by the way things are going: with HIV/AIDS removed from the national curriculum (by an amendment from Labour peer Jock Stallard) and parents able to remove their children from sex education classes, many young people may leave school with little or no awareness of sexual health issues, be they matters of HIV transmission, other STDs or contraception.

19 April 1994

London International Group, makers of Durex, announced some bad news. Condoms were moving out of Chingford, Essex, and would in future be made in Italy, Spain and, alongside the company's rubber gloves, in the Pacific Rim.

The company talked of losses and the need for refinancing, and said it was to lay off about a thousand British workers. This was some contrast to 1987, when the company announced a pre-tax profit increase of 13 per cent. Worldwide sales of condoms were up 20 per cent, due mainly to the government's recent advertising campaigns. But sales had since fallen and Durex was no longer as dominant as it was: In 1987 it claimed 96 per cent of the UK market, but by 1994 this had fallen to 75 per cent. Mates and the other brands had clearly done all right out of AIDS.

On the same day, an important meeting was taking place in the offices of the British Standards Institution. The technical committee on mechanical contraceptives had gathered to address the big condom questions – falling standards, rising standards, new standards. The committee had a guest speaker this morning, Dr S. J. Tovey from Guy's Hospital. Dr Tovey had recently become a minor celebrity on the condom circuit for publishing a report in the *BMJ* which said that 20 per cent of men attending his clinic had found standard condoms to be too tight. Of these men, 73 per cent complained of condoms coming off during use and 68 per cent had reported condoms splitting.

This morning Dr Tovey illuminated his findings, presenting a graph from the World Health Organization showing the distribution of penis circumferences in three ethnic groups – white American men, black American men and men from Thailand. Amongst other things, this showed that most men from Thailand had a circumference between 101 mm and 112 mm and that most white and black Americans had a circumference of 113 mm to 127 mm.

He also presented a video, in which the bigger man, the man with a circumference in the range 138 mm to 150 mm, was shown having trouble fitting the condom designed for the regular man. As the minutes of the meeting record, 'the subject experienced difficulty in rolling the bead [the base of the condom] over the glans penis and down the shaft, the bead tending to become stuck in the sulcus'. Dr Tovey said that these difficulties disenfranchised a large proportion of people from condom use and from the protection condoms conferred against HIV transmission.

The meeting then went on to discuss particulars of the bead, and how it became stiffer the longer the shaft of the condom that was rolled around it. Dr Tovey suggested that there was a need to study other means by which a condom could be held securely in place. A certain Dr W. D. Potter, chairing the meeting, thanked Dr Tovey and said that hitherto his committee had concentrated on the width of the condom during use, as well as comfort, sensitivity and strength. The difficulty of putting one on was a relatively new dimension to the debate, but one that would be considered with vigour at future meetings.

Nine months earlier, *Which? Way To Health*, a magazine of the Consumer's Association, had been blowing up 17,000 condoms until they burst and the results were a little worrying. Nine out of 34 brands showed weaknesses and failed new draft EC standards. The 'airburst' test proved just too much for some samples of Gold Night Extra Shield, Aegis Ribbed and Aegis Rugged, Durex Gold, Mates Natural, Red Stripe, flavoured Rubbers, Skinless Skin and coloured and flavoured Streetwise. Three of these carried the BSI Kitemark. The magazine urged the government to ensure regular inspections of all condom manufacturers and frequent testing of all brands against the EC standard.

But there were already stringent standards. The BSI revises its guidelines on condoms – BS 3704 – every few years. The first edition of BS 3704 was made in 1964 after a proposal by the Family Planning Association. A new edition with more stringent tests was published in 1972. In 1979 a third edition took account of the growing demand for coloured condoms and for condoms with a textured surface. The fourth edition of 1989, the first to be published after the advent of AIDS, introduced requirements of uniformity of wall thickness, the provision of more explicit instructions for use and provisions for different sizes of condoms. The latest standards, appearing in 1992, introduced requirements and new test methods for bursting volume and pressure. There were no standards concerning condoms to be used for anal sex; indeed there were no condoms available in the UK that could be recommended or marketed for such use.

16 May 1994

Sir Donald Acheson has had several jobs since he retired as Chief Medical Officer in 1991. He has worked with the World Health Organization in Bosnia and he became chairman of the Prison Service Health Advisory Committee. It was in this last role that today he presented a report to Home Secretary Michael Howard, recommending, 'despite the inherent difficulties', that condoms be made available for use by prisoners in England and Wales.

The official figures also published today showed there had been 377 reported HIV cases in prisons in England and Wales since 1985, with 51 reported in 1992–3. Still a small number, but more were being reported every year and this probably represented rather fewer cases than actually existed. For the first time, the Home Office reported a case of a prisoner becoming infected while in custody; again, there were almost certainly many more. The latest figures also showed a 63 per cent increase in the number of drug-dependent prisoners on admission. Sir Donald again regarded this with great concern. But he had been down this path many times before; he needed little reminder of how politically unacceptable the provision of condoms or clean needles in jails continued to be to Home Office ministers.

17 May 1994

A drink with Simon Watney, the critic and art historian. Watney is in his mid-forties. He says this is the worst time in the epidemic; the cycle of death is ceaseless:

> To say 'A friend of mine just died' doesn't mean anything any more, but that friend could be someone you lived with for two years in the seventies and whom you saw through all his subsequent relationships as he's seen you through all yours. That network is qualitatively and quantitively specific to how gay men live. Deaths in those networks mean deaths of whole areas of memory and association. Death for most heterosexuals means family deaths most of the time, up to the age of about sixty, and then it begins to mean friends. It's so different for gay men in the epidemic.
>
> And you know there's more to come and it's going to get worse before it gets better, because you know so many people who are positive. Anyone living in metropolitan London is living that life

around the clock. That means you fight fiercely for pleasure too, for holidays, for Saturday nights, for getting off your face totally at least once a fortnight.

I'm very moved by the numbers of people I see on the streets of London wearing red ribbons. You see many more people wearing them here than in Paris or New York and yet we have this disproportionately small epidemic. But that tells us something I think about the people who are dying. They are people who are fun and sociable, who have opposed bigotry, who have come to London from all over the country, a particular range of people with a lot of friends. They are a vital part of a city, not just London, but Manchester and Newcastle and others too, and they are greatly missed. Most of them are kids, boys who are getting infected in their early twenties, become diagnosed with HIV in their late twenties, and dying in their early thirties. That's an appalling process; a whole quarter of an entire subculture is dying. I think a lot of people in London are aware of that and are in grief. You know, 'The gay boys are dying.' One could never have begun to imagine, in one's wildest nightmares, how absurdly wrong things have gone in lots of ways.

22 May 1994

As you enter Trafalgar Square you get a pack with a programme, a candle, a candle shield and a book of matches.

There are thousands of people here, looking towards the column and down towards Whitehall and Big Ben. At 8.15 p.m., the broadcaster Paul Gambaccini takes the microphone. 'You may notice camera crews from the BBC and Channel 4. You may also see representatives of the press. As the effects of AIDS increase in this country, so the attention from the press increases. Some day in this country we'll have a government that pays attention.' Mild applause. This is an annual event organized by the Terrence Higgins Trust to remember those who have died with AIDS in the last year.

'1994 is the International Year of the Family,' Gambaccini continues:

Through your response to HIV and AIDS, you have shown what family is all about. You have proved that there is such a thing as society and there are such things as brotherhood and sisterhood.

When people who knew me as a boy in the sixties ask me why I got involved with popular music, I simply and honestly say, 'It is what there was in my time.' Now, even though we haven't asked for it, AIDS is what there is in our time and it is in response to this duty that we are measured.

In an hour there will be a service at St Martin in the Fields, at which a choir will sing a requiem and Helen Mirren will read from Christina Rossetti. We need at least an hour for all the names: the names of people who died last year, recited by representatives from various AIDS organizations. The names go on and on, a devastating list, numbing in their number. William, Frank, Jed, Paul, Jerry, Jack, Terry, Glenn, Mary, Little Pete, Joanne, Paul, Alice ... then the next person reads and then twenty more, and on until it gets dark. When it was dark, candles were lit. There was a minute's silence and people held their candles aloft and called out the names of their lost loves.

27 May 1994

Roy Cornes, 26, the Birmingham haemophiliac accused of deliberately infecting four women, died today. Cornes was the 'AIDS Romeo' (*Today*), the 'Sex Bomb' (*Daily Mirror*), the 'AIDS Maniac On Killer Sex Spree' (*Sun*), the man who two years ago made clear that heterosexual transmission was a relatively easy thing to achieve.

Cornes was the youngest of six brothers and one sister. He contracted the virus from contaminated Factor VIII and was diagnosed HIV positive in 1985, along with two of his brothers. Garry Cornes was also 26 when he died in 1992, but Gordon Cornes, 39, has survived.

By the spring of 1992, Birmingham health officials had already known for some time that a man whom they knew to be HIV positive was behaving irresponsibly by sleeping with several women. One of these women, Gina Allen, 20, died of AIDS-related causes in May. 'There were concerns about a particular individual,' the district's director of public health confirmed at the time, and a case conference was called to discuss him. What could they do? They could not stop him having sex or force him to wear condoms. They could confine him only if there was proof of his intention to endanger the health of others, which there was not. But before the conference was called, the story was broken by the *Birmingham Post*, and for a week later the tabloids were interested in little else. Gwen Gray, Roy Cornes' mother in law, sold the video of Roy and Linda's wedding to a local news agency for £2,000.

Cornes was accused of deliberately spreading the virus, something he always denied; but he did admit to hiding his condition from at least one woman and not always using a condom. In interviews, for which he demanded payment, he claimed to be misunderstood and exploited. Before the media descended on him and he went into hiding, he claimed he had never been made fully aware of what the virus was or what it could do. 'I knew it was an illness, but at that time I didn't know the full extent of the disease and never fully understood the consequences.'

His wife Linda defended him after death. 'People made him out to be a monster,' she said,

> but Roy was a kind, caring and lovely man ... If it hadn't been for all the lies and gossip, I am convinced Roy would still be alive today. Those girls who pointed the finger are as much to blame as Roy. They knew about his condition, they knew about condoms, but they still insisted on sleeping with him ... People tried to tear us apart, but they couldn't manage it.

On one level, the story of Roy Cornes was the best health education campaign money couldn't buy: his case 'proved' the risks that many had dismissed. But there was an explanation within days. The *News of the World* and the *Sunday Times* both reported that in at least two cases, the virus had been transmitted by 'unnatural' acts, i.e. anal intercourse. The *Daily Mail* gave it another spin, blaming promiscuity and moral impoverishment. 'For most ordinary heterosexual people, AIDS does still remain a remote, million-to-one possibility.' The *Daily Express* noted that it was 'downright wrong to continue using the Birmingham case to terrify normal heterosexuals that they are as much in jeopardy as homosexual men – who are infinitely more at risk'. This was a convincing argument of course, albeit one that had evolved little from the beginning of the epidemic (the difference now was that some more reliable figures backed it up). But did those who were not considered 'normal' not deserve to be continually educated? Apparently not. 'The gay community has already been warned of the dangers.'

Back in Birmingham, Rose Allen had just returned from visiting her granddaughter Gina's grave when she was told of Roy Cornes' death. 'She made one mistake and paid dearly for it,' she said. 'I am satisfied Cornes knew what he was doing when he slept with Gina and those other girls.' And then a fearful phrase from a vanishing world: 'God pays debts without money.'

29 May 1994

The latest statistics show that the rates of HIV infection and of AIDS cases, reported quarterly, are still increasing. A total of 9,025 AIDS cases had been reported in the UK since 1982, 8,298 male and 727 female; 6,031 had died. Five hundred and one of these cases were reported in the first three months of 1994.

The number of AIDS cases reported in the twelve-month period to the end of March 1994 was 1,704, a rise of 9 per cent on the preceding year's total of 1,561. In these two periods the number of cases reported in women increased by 44 per cent (from 149 to 214). The numbers of men and women probably infected through heterosexual intercourse increased by 33 per cent (226 to 300). AIDS cases of people infected through injecting drug use increased by 61 per cent (from 83 to 134).

A total of 21,718 HIV infections had been reported to the Public Health Laboratory Service by the end of March 1984. Sexual intercourse between men accounted for 60 per cent of this total and 57 per cent of the 2,507 cases logged in the last twelve months; though still by far the largest single group, it was gradually declining, while the proportion of infected women showed a steady increase.

Sixteen per cent of all HIV infections (3,374) were contracted through sexual intercourse between men and women; this proportion was 28 per cent of the reports received in the last year (696 of 2,507). Just under 73 per cent of all heterosexual cases (2,454 of 3,374) were believed to have been the result of exposure abroad, notably in African countries.

Of the other cases, 456 (14 per cent) had a sexual partner considered to be at high risk, 258 (8 per cent) were not known to have had sexual intercourse with a high-risk partner or intercourse abroad. The remaining 206 (6 per cent) were still under investigation at the end of April 1994.

A footnote accompanying these figures from the Public Health Laboratory Service still strikes an ominous note after all these years: 'Due to the length and variability of the period between infection with

HIV and development of AIDS (estimated to be between 8–10 years on average), reports of AIDS cases do not give a picture of the current spread of HIV infection.'

4 and 5 June 1994

The first day was a wash-out, but the second was glorious. Quilts of Love, a display of the international AIDS memorial quilt in Hyde Park, had taken seven months of preparation, and on Saturday it rained so hard that people huddled in marquees all day and saw almost nothing.

The plan was to lay out 300 of the quilt panels made to commemorate those who had died of AIDS. These panels were often 'grief projects', *memento mori* made by loved ones as the fancy took, using any combination of materials and personal artefacts. Each panel was a unique testament and, when stitched together with others into huge blocks, provided a moving visual commentary of the impact of the epidemic.

The Quilt began in San Francisco in 1987; the NAMES Project (UK) started 18 months later. There were more than 60 similar initiatives throughout the world and an estimated four million people had visited displays. There had been many small-scale displays in Britain over the years, particularly at schools and community projects, but Hyde Park was the big one and here we were, crowded in a tent, looking at the sky as steam rose from our clothes. There was a little consolation: the Terrence Higgins Trust had organized a 'Wall of Love', a collage of five-inch-square cards on which supporters had written or drawn or pasted a dedication to a dead friend. Some just stuck a photo to a name, some wrote poetry, others inscribed private thoughts in crayon. It was an instant, spontaneous memory store, making tearful reading. There were a lot about Freddie Mercury.

There was grief of another sort, too, as some protested against the reappearance of the Benetton 'branding' advertisement in some promotional literature. Benetton had spent £26,000 on the printing costs of the official programme, into which they had hoped to insert a 'resource pack' containing the offending advert. OutRage made a noise again and drew support from the THT. For some the row wrecked the weekend.

On Sunday the sun shone, the panels were rolled out and thousands came to sigh and weep. Many hundreds of these had just completed the annual 'Walk for Life', a ten-kilometre sponsored stroll that raised about £160,000 for the hardship fund of the charity Crusaid.

During the display, people read the names of those on the panel. It was the same pattern as the candlelight memorial: reps from the major organizations and the odd celebrity reading about ten names each, adding their own friends at the bottom. More than one told of how a friend had died earlier in the week.

There were names from all over the world, names I knew, names I didn't. Tom, Chris the Lad, Gerald 'Dog', Paul, Mark Ashton, Roderick Macneill, Peter von Werfelli, Ian Charleson, Kevin Bills, Simon, John Macintyre, Alisdair, Jim M, Jamie Fraser, Peter Turnbull, Scott Lago, Jack Babuscio, Philip Core, Douglas McCusker, Howard Sasportas, Keith Haring, Amanda Blake, Diva Dan Danny, Gareth Allinson, Manic Mary, Rev Virgil Hall, Andre, Michelle Cross, Wilton, Anthony Brahame, Elaine, Starlight Express, Farouk, Wendy, Paul, Mark, William, Mal, Paul, Sue, Rock Hudson, Amanda Hegg, Ulla Guldborg, Herman Meeske, Raymond Clarke, Oggie La Farga, Richard Fuller, Victor Richardson, Robyne Gibson, Scott Engel, Tom Woolison, Jay O Freeman, Luiz of Boston, Akello, Harriet, Janne, Kasirye, Kisarale, Nabasaala, Shelly, Waldo Suarez, Valeriano Suarez, Carol Belove, Larry Witlock, Michael Torrey, La Fabulous Miss Thing, Bobby Quercio, Eric Lawson, Antony Gallucci, John Philip, Larry Foster, Robert, Jim L, Tracy Brown, Claudia Sharon Washington, Jocelyn Theriault, Gregg Dagg, Tony Martin, Myles Yates, Steven Hill, David Lewis, Christel, Hans Faasse, Danja, Piet Stuvoet, Willem Boode, Martin Golding, Karin, Marco, Maria, Claudine, George, Baby Jessica ...

The names ring in my ears all night.

14 June 1994

He's not a monster, this Neville Hodgkinson, despite what the casual reader might think from a glancing acquaintance with his work. A few days before the science correspondent of the *Sunday Times* left the paper to write a book about his life as a vilified journalist, he sits in what appears to be a makeshift newsroom at Wapping, all bespectacled refinement and cautious intent. It is Tuesday, the slowest news day on a Sunday paper, and Hodgkinson, 50, is happy to talk about how his work has angered 95 per cent of those involved with AIDS in Britain.

Back in the mid to late 1980s, when he was medical correspondent,

Hodgkinson churned out the same sort of stuff all the other newspapers were printing – the biggest health threat of our generation, numbers as big as pools wins – most of it spoon-fed by the Department of Health or the HEA. He wrote a story which suggested that the pattern of our AIDS cases was mirroring exactly what had happened in the United States. This suggested that in time all sexually active people might be at risk. Even as late as August 1989, Hodgkinson wrote that although the British epidemic showed signs of slowing down, the potential for its heterosexual growth was only too visible elsewhere in the world. 'A striking illustration of the virus's ability to sweep suddenly forward has been provided recently in Thailand, where at the start of 1988, only 198 people were identified as infected. By the end of February this year the number had reached more than 4,000, and it is expected to be several times higher again before long.' In Africa, he wrote, 'its spread is almost exclusively associated with heterosexual promiscuity and prostitutes. In countries like Malawi, Tanzania and Zaire, at least half the prostitutes are infected. Widespread venereal disease facilitates the spread.'

Earlier stories had inspired a memo from the editor, Andrew Neil. In 1987, Neil had devoted a whole issue of the *Sunday Times Magazine* to just this sort of thing, but two years later had grown more sceptical. 'Where is this threatened heterosexual spread?' one of his memos to Hodgkinson read. 'Is it really happening?' His reporter sent back a memo saying you can't actually see it at the moment and the numbers are very tiny, but the whole point is that there is this long time-lag between infection and developing the disease. 'He accepted that,' Hodgkinson says. 'If you give him a reasoned case on something he doesn't impose his prejudices. But he had these doubts.'

Shortly afterwards, and for the best part of two years, Hodgkinson left the paper to join the *Sunday Express* as health editor. During this time, a *Dispatches* programme for Channel 4, made by the independent company Meditel, offered the hypothesis that AIDS was not an infectious disease; three years earlier, in the same slot, Meditel had argued that HIV might not be the cause of AIDS, a programme for which it won an award from the Royal Television Society. Hodgkinson thought these hypotheses were mostly rubbish and he was distrustful of Professor Peter Duesberg, the Californian virologist whose work had inspired them.

Duesberg was nicknamed Snoozeberg by his many detractors, and his theories were widely trashed as the obsessive workings of a crank.

344

For his part, Duesberg liked to quote Lewis Carroll in *Through the Looking Glass*: "'It's too late to correct," said the Red Queen. "When you've once said a thing, that fixes it, and you must take the consequences.'" In a paper published in 1992 he also expressed a fondness for Sherlock Holmes, whom many have convinced themselves is not a fictional character: 'Circumstantial evidence is a very tricky thing,' Duesberg quotes Conan Doyle's hero as saying in the late 1920s. 'It may seem to point very straight to one thing, but if you shift your point of view a little, you may find it pointing in an equally uncompromising manner to something entirely different.' Running against the great body of scientific expert opinion, Duesberg claimed that HIV was a harmless retrovirus that infected less than one in ten thousand T-cells. AIDS, he said, was not transmitted sexually. So what did cause AIDS? Drugs, especially poppers (amyl nitrites), and the lowering of natural immunity (which he said explained both gay and haemophiliac infection). And what about Africa? In Africa, the professor said, AIDS is probably a myriad of other diseases that have existed for hundreds of years but are now dressed up as an epidemic.

Hodgkinson himself accused the Duesberg line of being irrational when he received an MRC report about a haemophiliac cohort in Scotland. This showed that for a number of years two groups of haemophiliacs had been tracked. All of them had been exposed to contaminated Factor VIII at about the same time. Some had become HIV positive and that group was declining; the ones who hadn't were fine and stable. This seemed to answer one of Duesberg's objections, that there hadn't been a controlled trial to demonstrate HIV's ability to cause disease. Hodgkinson wrote an item saying that this trial showed HIV to be a key factor in the causation of AIDS.

Meanwhile, the Meditel television programme, directed and produced by Joan Shenton, was widely criticized for being unrepresentative of the mass of international medical opinion and was subsequently criticized by the Broadcasting Complaints Commission after protests from Wellcome and others.

When Hodgkinson returned to the *Sunday Times* as science correspondent in 1991, the paper had already serialized *The Myth of Heterosexual AIDS* by Michael Fumento. This had largely been Andrew Neil's decision, and it provoked outrage. In America bookstores had boycotted it; at the *Sunday Times* the letters editor was inundated. This was the beginning of the newspaper's challenge to the AIDS orthodoxy. Henceforth it would run along two crisscrossing tracks: the theory that heterosexual AIDS was a serious threat to the population was merely an attempt to make us feel bad about sex, and HIV was not the cause of AIDS. Interviewed in *Continuum*, a magazine for long-term survivors of HIV and AIDS, Andrew Neil spoke of how, at the end of the 1980s, he began to feel 'that there was a kind of conspiracy beginning to develop – almost an unholy alliance among the Government, the militant gay lobby and a sort of Christian moral majority Right'.

A few weeks after he had returned to the newspaper from the *Sunday Express*, Hodgkinson spoke to Joan Shenton at Meditel. She told him that she still had great faith in Duesberg's theories and that she was suspicious of the MRC haemophiliac survey. She claimed it didn't compare like with like, because those who became HIV positive were different from the ones who didn't: they had been on Factor VIII for longer, and had a number of different genetic dispositions; loaded with more foreign antigens, they were already sicker. 'I was really bugged to hear this,' Hodgkinson says:

> It meant that I had done something that was wrong, which I didn't like to accept, and it meant that the whole mindset that I had with a lot of stories I'd written might also be wrong. I got the paper that Joan said demonstrated these haemophiliacs were different and it was true. So I thought I ought to look again at what Duesberg was saying.

With the forthcoming general election filling up most of the paper, Hodgkinson found he had a lot of time on his hands. He says he spent about a month studying Duesberg's papers and poring over his references. 'I checked out what people had written in response to what Duesberg had done and found that it was abusive, but it usually didn't answer his arguments.' He concluded this was 'poor science'.

At first he couldn't get any interest from his news desk. 'Challenging the HIV causation was too mind-boggling. They didn't see how we could do it as a news story.' He then composed a 5,000 word memo to an assistant editor, setting out what he had discovered during his research. It was passed on to Neil, who said it should run almost in its entirety. This was in April 1992, a double-page spread. 'Neil said he wasn't persuaded by it,' Hodgkinson remembers, 'but he felt there was enough logic to it that it ought to be put out.'

According to Roy Greenslade, who worked with both men as an editor at the *Sunday Times*, 'It only needed one man to gradually do something that was broadly appealing to [Andrew Neil's] prejudice. This was no conspiracy, it just happened to be a conjunction of two separate individuals, one who was ready to receive, and one who was ready to give.' The classic active–passive roles, in fact.

After the article appeared, the paper again received a huge number of vituperative attacks, from doctors, the HEA and the Chief Medical Officer. One virologist wrote to Hodgkinson, inviting him to see the work they were doing with this 'harmless' virus. 'When I got there I got two hours of earbanging from him. He was really angry. He didn't tell me anything that answered the criticisms. The fact the general response was so emotional, not reasoned, made me feel that, even though I didn't know where the truth lay, I really wanted to do more.'

In the next few months, Hodgkinson tried to place other doubting articles in the paper, with little success. Many of his colleagues were suspicious of their content and possibly of his motives.

The turnaround came in the spring of 1993. The preliminary Concorde results appeared. If AIDS was not a viral disease, then the value of AZT was clearly also brought into question and Hodgkinson spared no opportunity in subsequent articles to stress its negative side. He also got hold of a leaked early copy of another nationwide anonymized screening survey which, when extrapolated, suggested that the epidemic was on a far smaller scale than had been predicted previously (i.e. on a smaller scale than had been predicted previously in the *Sunday Times*). It estimated that there were 23,000 HIV positive people nationwide, a figure similar to the one thought likely five years before. The *Sunday Times* seldom suggested that this might be a good thing, a sign that Britain had done something right.

The campaign then took off, with articles appearing every few weeks. In headlines, AIDS became 'The Emperor's Clothes' and 'The Plague that Never Was'; the paper soon demonstrated 'Why We Won't Be Silenced'. Hodgkinson didn't see it as a campaign: 'I just felt that we were putting out various pieces of information that came up and were judged on their news merits. It wasn't like we were looking to write about this week by week, although there was an acceleration towards the end, in the wake of the *Nature* attack.' At the beginning of December 1993, the leading science journal had run a blistering attack by its editor John Maddox on the *Sunday Times*' AIDS coverage. Maddox accused it, among other things, of being wholly irresponsible: 'Impetuously, the newspaper seems not to have considered how much damage it will have done by recruiting young and adult people to the ranks of those who consider the discomforts of "safe sex" to be tiresome encumbrances.' Maddox promised to keep his readers up to date with further *Sunday Times* aberrations by summarizing them in future issues and thus saving people the cost of buying it themselves.

The gloves came off after this, as the *Sunday Times* not only repeated its arguments, but launched an offensive on Maddox for failing to print the dissidents' letters. The newspaper occasionally appeared to veer from its course. Sometimes it would use the 'world ain't flat' argument and claim that it was doing the world a great service by being bold enough to challenge accepted but inconclusive science (who could argue with that?) At times it even distanced itself from some of Duesberg's more extreme theories, such as one which suggested that anal sex posed no additional risk to infection. And sometimes it came out all guns firing, reinforcing Andrew Neil's view that 'we are not just dealing with something that the medical profession got wrong; I think we are now dealing with one of the greatest peace-time scandals of the 20th century'. Neil believed that 'the AIDS establishment has killed thousands and thousands of people, particularly in Africa. Young African kids who are diagnosed as HIV positive are regarded as untouchable. They are not looked after and then they die – not of HIV but of neglect. Much of what is going on really discredits science.'

Hodgkinson says he doesn't know when he and Neil and his paper will be proved right – a few months, a few years, perhaps 20 years. But it will happen, he says, though it will take great courage for so many doctors and scientists to admit they were wrong. He derives some sustenance from the fact that both Luc Montagnier and Robert Gallo, the co-discoverers of the virus, have already accepted that HIV may not be the sole cause of AIDS and that there may be co-factors which determine the rate to which those infected progress to disease (though they both maintain that HIV is paramount).

Andrew Neil left the *Sunday Times* (at least temporarily) for Fox Television in May 1994, and Hodgkinson has also decided to throw in the towel, at least temporarily, to write about his experiences. He says he has become fascinated by the concept of paradigm shifts. Any regrets?

The stories I feel least happy with are the ones where we reverted to the conventional viewpoint, believing that HIV still has some role.

I felt that I was betraying the way I really see things by going back into that mode of reporting. Maybe also there should have been a bit more detachment and we should have just continued gently to put forward the facts. Maybe people would have come to terms with those facts a bit earlier if we hadn't been quite so strident. But it's the *Sunday Times*'s style to put things out in force.

Neville Hodgkinson says that there is still 'ostensibly' very little support for the dissident view in this country, but that when he has given talks to younger scientists, they have no difficulty seeing that the conventional theories are in great difficulties. He claims that GPs tell him, privately, that they're very glad that the *Sunday Times* has been so courageous. Those I talked to – people Hodgkinson would call the establishment – remain horrified.

'I'm very concerned,' says Alan Stone, who has helped compile the MRC's official response to the *Sunday Times*:

I meet intelligent people at dinner parties and school parents' committees, and they say, 'Oh, I understand that HIV may not actually be a dangerous thing.' These are lawyers, bankers, people who should know better. It's wishful thinking: wouldn't it be nice if there was no risk and if this was a harmless little virus. It's doing an awful lot of damage. If people believe they can have sex without any great risk, or they can inject themselves with drugs without any risk, it would be wonderful.

Stone believes that the evidence for HIV causing AIDS is overwhelming, and points to a recent MRC study of 15 villages in southwest Uganda. This study, published in the *Lancet*, examined 9,389 people, and suggested that those who were HIV positive and aged between 25 and 34 were 60 times more likely to die within two years than if they were HIV negative. These people, mostly subsistence farmers and their families, had blood samples taken in 1990 and were then monitored for two years. The general mortality rate in those who were HIV positive was 115.9 per 1,000, but only 7.7. per 1,000 in those who were negative.

I think the *Sunday Times*' definition of a balanced debate is invalid. They think that by giving the left-hand page to the Duesberg idea and the right-hand page to the majority view is balanced, even

349

though very few people can quote very little evidence in favour of one and an enormous number of people, fully trained, can quote evidence for the other. What they're looking for is a hundred per cent watertight proof and you don't get that in anything. Look at the number of people who smoke who don't get lung cancer, yet nobody is going to argue that smoking can't cause lung cancer. The same with polio – a lot of people are infected with the virus that don't get it. If it weren't so serious it would be a very bad joke.

Many doctors and scientists accept that Duesberg needed to have his airing and that he had plenty of opportunity to speak at scientific forums. They say that he raised some valid points and some inconsistencies early on, but stress that these have all been systematically addressed and refuted. Many of these doctors and researchers have complained of difficulties in getting these refutations published as letters in the *Sunday Times* (Andrew Neil has insisted that this is because many have been 'abusive'). But they have had more luck with the *Independent* and *Independent on Sunday*, whose science correspondent, Steve Connor, has been a forceful opponent of Duesberg and his supporters. In one letter, three Nobel prize-winners working at Cambridge University asserted that support for this 'fringe hypothesis' was misleading and dangerous. Laureates Sir Aaron Klug, Cesar Milstein and Max Perutz, along with Abraham Karpas, the assistant director of research at the university's department of haematology, wrote: 'There is no question in our minds – as in the great majority of scientists who have acquainted themselves with the facts – that HIV is the cause of AIDS.'

In January 1994, Connor tracked down a doctor working in Nairobi who felt he had been unfairly treated by the *Sunday Times*, which he claimed had distorted his views. Angelo d'Agostino ran a hospice in Nairobi for orphans infected with HIV and was an important witness in a recent *Sunday Times* story about the 'myth' of African AIDS; the article claimed that because only one out of 45 HIV positive children in Dr d'Agostino's care had died, the doctor was beginning to question 'whether HIV is really the killer disease it has been made out to be'. D'Agostino was said to suspect that those who test HIV positive are not the victims of a new and inevitably lethal disease. The doctor told the *Independent on Sunday* that 'I want to categorically distance myself from the gross distortions and quite incorrect implication made as a result of his [Hodgkinson] interviewing me.' He believed that

Hodgkinson had a hidden agenda, and said that he had faxed the *Sunday Times* details of his objections after it appeared, but received no acknowledgement or promise of correction. 'One cannot help but wonder at the motivation for such irresponsible journalism,' he wrote, 'and, more so, decry the terrible effects on the unsuspecting public who are given a false sense of security and run the very real risk of contracting an incurable disease as a consequence.'

Less qualified critics had their own theories as to the motivation behind the *Sunday Times*' coverage. Edwina Currie, for instance: 'Andrew Neil has a non-monogamous heterosexual lifestyle,' she observes,

> and it suits him fine that there should be no risk attached to that, and that's the argument that he's making. I've had heated debates with him on TV about it. I've actually had him on my own TV programme last summer, and I was disgusted with him and I said, 'You're just having this campaign against gays and saying that it's just a gay disease and that there's no risk for heterosexuals because you wish that to be so. You are misleading people and you will encourage people back into taking risky, taking on board risky behaviour. You deserve to catch something.'

And how did he react to this? 'He got a bit shirty, because it was true.' (Neil has insisted that his newspaper has never consciously run anti-gay articles and that its AIDS policy is not motivated by homophobia.)

James Fenton, the poet and journalist, is a former *Sunday Times* writer and believes he has seen something like this before. 'The people conducting the *Sunday Times* campaign on AIDS like to compare their fight with the thalidomide battle of the Seventies,' he wrote in the *Independent*. 'I should say that a closer comparison would be with the Hitler diaries.'

There is no doubt that the *Sunday Times*' line has had a direct and detrimental effect on the voluntary sector. The Terrence Higgins Trust has reported far more scepticism and reluctance to donate during casual collections, and Action Aid, an organization that supports several projects in the developing world, cancelled a Christmas campaign in the belief that its supporters would be discouraged by the newspaper's reporting.

'I find the whole thing deeply troubling,' says Professor Tony

Pinching at Bart's. 'I know that people will die as a result, but what am I to do? I'm one of the 'AIDS establishment', anything I say is of course because I have some 'vested interest'. What this vested interest is, other than caring about patients, I'd love to know.'

Pinching took part in a Channel 4 *Right To Reply* programme following the first Meditel AIDS documentary. 'I probably looked pretty cross on the programme,' he says, 'although I was very cautious to avoid getting angry. But it's very difficult when Joan Shenton tells you that she's an expert and you don't know anything more than she does. If anything got me uptight I guess it would be the extent to which people deny the reality of an epidemic that's been such a reality to me for so many years.'

Professor Pinching fears that the paper's coverage, widely disseminated and internationally influential, may have a detrimental effect on policy making where the virus is most prevalent – sub-Saharan Africa and South and South-East Asia. He believes much of the coverage has been purposely 'anti-science', and that the dissidents have totally reversed the hierarchy of data and hypotheses that science depends upon. Logically, if the data do not fit the hypothesis, you throw the hypothesis out, not the data. Pinching suggests that Duesberg and his supporters have done the reverse:

What is really troubling is that the level of scientific literacy amongst journalists is such as to allow people to get away with it, in a sort of seductive, journalistic reasoning that conceals this complete reversal of scientific thought. I know it will end in tears for some people. And of course the people who sell those stories won't be there to pick up the pieces, it will be us.

17 June 1994

Michael Cottrell and Karl Burge, the two men behind Gays Against Genocide, the AZT protest campaign, are arrested and charged with 11 joint offences, including criminal damage and threats to kill.

1 July 1994

Do you have many different hobbies? Do you stop to think things over before doing anything? Does your mood often go up and down? Have you ever taken the praise for something you knew someone else had really done? Are you a talkative person? Would being in debt worry you?

If you are a healthy long-term survivor with HIV, these are the questions you have to answer these days. In the last two years, AIDS researchers have increasingly turned their attentions to 'non-progressors'. This entails studying those who have been infected for between five and 14 years, have shown no sign of an AIDS-related illness and without the aid of anti-viral drugs have maintained a high CD4 count (usually above 500). One such study is actively recruiting at the Kobler Centre at Chelsea and Westminster Hospital.

When you join, you get a couple of hours with the eight-part MRC questionnaire. Question 90: Would you feel very sorry for an animal caught in a trap? Then some questions on health: Have you been getting a feeling of tightness or pressure in your head? Have you lost much sleep over worry? Have you thought of the possibility that you might kill yourself?

Later there are questions on religion, nutrition, complementary therapies and a lot of intricate stuff on your sex life.

Dr Philippa Easterbrook, who runs this study, presents me with an editorial she has just completed for the international publication *AIDS*. The piece discusses all the factors that might determine why one person infected in 1983 might still be not only alive but fighting fit, while most infected in that year are dead (the average period between infection and AIDS is 9–10 years). The gist of the article is: we don't really know.

There are two distinct lines of thought: one subscribes to the view that non-progressors are nothing unique, that they merely represent one end of the continuum; in any disease cycle there will always be a small proportion of people who live longer than others. Others think there may be something particularly noteworthy about them and suggest they should be studied. What is it about their natural immunity that makes them different? If this could be found out, the vaccine development strategy would benefit greatly.

Easterbrook has recruited 56 people to her study, about 95 per cent of them gay men. One of her patients is a 14-year-old haemophiliac boy infected in 1981. Her team had to construct a special questionnaire for him, removing all the sex questions.

At this early stage in her work, there are a few speculations that tie in with similar studies in the United States and Europe, but nothing conclusive. It appears that non-progressors have a very vigorous cellular immune response right from the start. It also looks as though they may have picked up a far less virulent strain of the virus.

That's what the researchers believe. Intriguingly, the non-progressors themselves have a rather different view. 'We asked them what did they think was the reason for their good health,' Dr Easterbrook says, 'and almost unanimously they said, "It's my attitude, my lifestyle, the control I've taken of my life."'

This is not to say that lifestyle or mental attitude is never important, but it does look as though such factors may only affect a proportion of non-progressors. Easterbrook posits the existence of three distinct groups. The first have 'received an unlucky roll of the dice', they have been infected with a virulent strain and have a poor immune response. Then there are those with a robust immune response infected with a mild viral strain. Finally there's the in-between group, and it is here that there is the greatest potential for lifestyle changes and psychological factors to influence disease progression. However, as she explains in her paper, all the studies that have specifically examined lifestyle factors found that past history of certain sexually transmitted diseases, the number of sexual partners, frequency of specific sexual activities, or recreational drug use had little bearing on the rate of progression. One study suggests that some micronutrients, including higher levels of vitamins C, B1 and niacin, may decrease the rate of progression. 'But it's still early days on this sort of work,' Easterbrook says. 'In five years' time we may have an entirely different picture.'

7 July 1994

I think the phrase is demob happy. In two weeks Sir Norman Fowler will be relieved of his duty as Conservative Party Chairman in order to spend more time with his business interests and yet more time with his family. Up at Conservative Central Office it is a champagne day: Shirley Oxenbury, who runs the chairman's office, is celebrating her birthday. The only cloud in Sir Norman's sky is that he must race to the Commons every 30 minutes to vote in another clause of the Criminal Justice Bill.

On his desk is a large axe, a prop from a comedy show, inscribed with the words 'British jobs cut'. The walls are crowded with signed photographs of past cabinets and maps of parliamentary constituencies. His bookshelves contain one volume called *All You Need to Know*

About Exchange Rates and a video from Saatchi & Saatchi entitled *PPB on Europe, June 1994.*

With all this behind him, Sir Norman talks about AIDS. Many regard his period dealing with the issue in 1986 and 1987 as his finest hour. Others, driving the backlash, see the force of his campaigns as rather overheated, a trifle melodramatic. The two views are not wholly mutually exclusive.

'I feel very unrepentant,' he says:

On the information we had at the time ... we would have been criticized far more now for underreacting rather than overreacting. Had we underreacted, had we continued with our full-page boring advertisements in the broadsheet press, I think our results in this country in terms of AIDS would be measurably worse, and more people would have died. Every day you delay giving the message more people can contract the virus. So I think it was the right thing to do and I think the general public felt it was right too, even the public who even had not the slightest prospect of ever getting into the [risk] category of catching AIDS.

But the Prime Minister felt that it was not the right thing to do?

There were obviously a number of people close to Margaret who thought that we were doing the wrong thing and emphasizing it too much. They didn't particularly like the television pictures that came back from the United States, because here was a government minister who was shaking hands with AIDS victims, and was this really how the government and the party wished to be portrayed? But to be fair to Margaret, that was certainly never a view she expressed openly to me. I think she perhaps felt that we did too much, that we overdid it. Her initial instinct was that this was not a big problem, and at any rate the people who get AIDS, it's entirely their fault, their responsibility and we shouldn't spend a lot of time upon it. But I think as she became more aware of the size of the problem, I think she acquiesced in our policies and certainly never sought, as far as I was concerned, to undermine them. With the benefit of hindsight I think she would concede that her instincts would have led her to have underdone it in a fairly dramatic way.

18 July 1994

Thirty-five years after David Carr checked into the Manchester Royal Infirmary with what is believed to be the first recorded case of AIDS, the press officer at the Health Education Authority sends out another copy of a popular video: *HIV and AIDS Information for Seafarers*. The video, which lasts 15 minutes, features a mixture of stock footage of docking ships and new animation by Aardman Animations, the company that won Oscars for the films *Creature Comforts* and *The Wrong Trousers*.

A captain explains to his helmsman about the virus and safer sex: how you can catch it, how best to avoid it. The captain metamorphoses into a woman, a syringe, a penis. He talks about shore leave, about prostitutes, about first aid, about oral sex, about gay sex. We get condom demonstrations. 'When I was young,' the captain says, 'the worst I could get was gonorrhoea.' It's a good package. We have travelled far.

APPENDIX, NOTES AND REFERENCES AND INDEX

TABLE 1 AIDS cases and deaths by exposure category and date of report: United Kingdom to 30 June 1994

How persons probably acquired the virus	Jul 92 – June 93		Jul 93 – Jun 94		Jan 82 – June 94			
	Male	Female	Male	Female	Male	(Deaths)	Female	(Deaths)
Sexual Intercourse								
between men	1102	–	1149	–	6917	4805	–	–
between men and women								
"high risk" partner[1]	2	23	8	28	30	16	92	51
other partner abroad[2]	95	78	141	97	527	298	334	165
other partner UK	13	6	12	11	53	32	43	29
under investigation	2	–	9	4	15	6	4	1
Injecting drug use (IDU)	64	30	101	42	365	229	153	91
IDU or sexual intercourse between men	30	–	22	–	149	100	–	–
Blood								
blood factor (e.g. for haemophilia)	55	2	51	–	412	358	6	4
blood/tissue transfer (e.g. transfusion)								
abroad	3	6	3	9	14	8	40	23
UK	2	2	5	5	24	18	26	22
Mother to infant	18	12	17	21	60	29	67	32
Other/undetermined	13	2	18	3	92	64	13	7
Total	1399	161	1536	220	8658	5963	778	425

1. Men and women who had sex with injecting drug users, or with those infected through blood factor treatment or blood transfusion, and women who had sex with bisexual men.

2. Includes persons without identified risks from, or who have lived in, countries where the major route of HIV-1 transmission is through sexual intercourse between men and women.

TABLE 2 UK AIDS cases by quarter of report and death[1]

Quarter		Reported AIDS Cases	Known deaths[5]
1982 or earlier[2]		3	3
1983	1 & 2	8	8
	3 & 4	18	16
1984	1 & 2	21	21
	3 & 4	56	54
1985	1	33	32
	2	33	31
	3	45	41
	4	47	45
1986	1	48	45
	2	59	59
	3	96	88
	4	95	89
1987	1	147	140
	2	143	137
	3	197	174
	4	154	146
1988	1	202	189
	2	167	157
	3	194	176
	4	193	178
1989	1	207	192
	2	178	161
	3	272	223
	4	185	156
1990	1	321	276
	2	277	241
	3	366	304
	4	304	242
1991	1	350	283
	2	303	229
	3	317	230
	4	389	264
1992	1	335	220
	2	360	227
	3	412	229
	4	378	204

Continued

TABLE 2 *Continued*

Quarter		Reported AIDS Cases	Known deaths[5]
1993	1	415	205
	2	360	135
	3	427	175
	4	414	140
1994	1	500	126
	2	417	87
Quarter unknown[3,4]		–	–
Total		9436	6388

1. Reporting of recent diagnosis and deaths is incomplete.

2. One AIDS case was diagnosed in 1979, 4 in 1981, and 13 in 1982. Three reports were received in 1982. One death occurred in 1981 and 7 in 1982.

3. Two AIDS cases were diagnosed sometime in 1984, 2 in 1985, 5 in 1986, 3 in 1987, 5 in 1988, 5 in 1989, 4 in 1990, 4 in 1991, 1 in 1992 and 1 in 1993. Both the year and quarter of diagnosis for another 14 were also unknown.

4. Two deaths occurred sometime in 1985, 1 in 1988, 3 in 1989, 1 in 1990 and 2 in 1991. Both the year and quarter of death for another 28 were also unknown.

5. Of the cases reported in each particular quarter, these are the numbers known to have died by end June 1994.

Tables 1 and 3 to 6 were prepared from voluntary confidential reports by clinicians and microbiologists sent directly to the PHLS AIDS Centre at the Communicable Disease Surveillance Centre and to the Scottish Centre for Infection and Environmental Health, returns by haemophilia centre directors to the Oxford Haemophilia Centre, and returns to the British Paediatric Surveillance Unit. Paediatric data in these tables is compiled at the Institute of Child Health, London, in collaboration with CDSC and SCIEH.

Data included in tables 7 to 9 was compiled at the Institute of Child Health, London, in collaboration with CDSC and SCIEH. Data sources include returns by obstetricians to the National Study of HIV in Pregnancy, returns by paediatricians to the British Paediatric Surveillance Unit, reports by haemophilia centre directors to the Oxford Haemophilia Centre, and reports by clinicians and microbiologists to the PHLS AIDS Centre and SCIEH. All reporting is voluntary and confidential.

TABLE 3 HIV–1 infected persons by category and date of report: United Kingdom to 30 June 1994

How persons probably acquired the virus	Jul 92 – Jun 93			Jul 93 – Jun 93			Oct 84 – Jun 94		
	Male	Female	NS[4]	Male	Female	NS[4]	Male	Female	NS[4]
Sexual Intercourse									
between men	1547	–	–	1432	–	–	13381	–	–
between men and women									
"high risk" partner[1]	14	69	–	10	37	–	84	387	–
other partner abroad	262	263	–	260	259	–	1373	1216	5
other partner UK[2]	21	41	–	25	24	–	105	176	–
under investigation	12	12	–	30	38	–	80	98	–
Injecting drug use (IDU)	157	58	–	135	60	1	1775	809	4
IDU or sexual intercourse between men	28	–	–	28	–	–	298	–	–
Blood									
blood factor (e.g. for haemophilia)	8	1	–	3	–	–	1216	11	–
blood/tissue transfer (e.g. transfusion) abroad/UK	11	5	–	7	8	–	78	77	1
Mother to infant[3]	27	36	1	15	17	–	121	122	1
Other/undetermined	31	7	–	89	15	2	553	99	31
Total	2118	492	1	2034	458	3	19064	2995	42

1 and 2. As for Table 1.
3. By date of report that established infected status.
4. Sex not stated on report.

362

TABLE 4 Geographical distribution of AIDS cases and deaths by date of report: to 30 June 1994

Country or region of first report	Jul 92 – Jun 93		Jul 93 – Jun 94		Jan 82 – Jun 94	
	Cases	(Deaths[1])	Cases	(Deaths[1])	Cases	(Deaths[1])
England:						
Northern	19	8	26	4	149	104
Yorkshire	36	23	34	15	227	169
Trent	32	21	59	19	219	153
E Anglia	23	15	31	11	138	89
NW Thames	560	255	541	123	3371	2234
NE Thames	285	112	406	91	1880	1146
SE Thames	203	122	205	70	1083	763
SW Thames	57	27	90	31	371	248
Wessex	40	22	43	15	231	162
Oxford	35	17	60	28	229	159
S Western	24	11	35	20	192	146
W Midlands	37	18	42	17	224	163
Mersey	14	12	30	18	116	93
N Western	64	37	20	7	313	249
Wales	20	12	24	15	130	108
Northern Ireland	9	6	7	2	45	35
Scotland	102	54	103	42	518	367
United Kingdom Total	1560	773	1756	528	9436	6388
Ch. Islands/Isle of Man	1	–	–	–	6	4

1. These deaths are of patients referred to in the previous column and known to have occurred at any time up to 30 June 1994.

TABLE 5 Sexual orientation of adult (15 years or over) AIDS cases: United Kingdom to 30 June 1994

Sexual orientation (regardless of exposure category)	Jul 92 – Jun 93		Jul 93 – Jun 94[1]		Jan 82 – Jun 94[1]	
	Cases	(%)	Cases	(%)	Cases	(%)
Homosexual men	970	65	994	59	5982	66
Bisexual men	160	11	176	10	1086	12
Heterosexual men and women[2]	359	24	507	30	2044	22
Total[3]	1489	100	1677	100	9112	100

1. Period during which reports were received.
2. Includes those exposed through injecting drug use or infected through blood factor treatment or blood transfusion.
3. Excludes other/undetermined cases.

Table 6 Sexual orientation of adult (15 years or over) HIV-1 infected persons: United Kingdom to 30 June 1994

Sexual orientation (regardless of exposure category)	Jul 92 – Jun 93		Jul 93 – Jun 94		Oct 84 – Jun 94	
	Number	(%)	Number	(%)	Number	(%)
Homosexual men/bisexual men	1575	63	1460	62	13682	66
Heterosexual men and women[2]	931	37	896	38	7194	34
Total[3]	2506	100	2356	100	20876	100

1. Period during which reports were received.
2. Includes those exposed through injecting drug use or infected through blood factor treatment or blood transfusion.
3. Excludes other/undetermined cases.

Table 7 AIDS cases and deaths in children[1] by exposure category: to 30 April 1994

How children probably acquired the virus	May 92 – Apr 93		May 93 – Apr 94		Jan 82 – Apr 94	
	Diagnosis[2]	Report[2]	Diagnosis[2]	Report[2]	Total[3]	(Deaths)
Mother to infant	36	27	22	43	126	61
Blood						
blood factor (e.g. for haemophilia)	–	2	–	–	24	20
blood/tissue transfer (e.g. transfusion)	1	1	1	3	13	6
Other/undetermined	–	–	–	–	–	–
Total	37	30	23	46	163	87

1. Aged 14 years or under when AIDS was first diagnosed.
2. In any given period the number of cases reported does not equal the number diagnosed due to reporting delay.
3. Includes 1 child infected through mother to infant transmission, 11 haemophilia patients (7 died), and 1 blood recipient who were aged 15 years or over at 30 April 1994 or at death.

TABLE 8 HIV-1 infection[1] and deaths[2] in children[3] by sex and exposure category: cumulative to 30 April 1994

How Children probably acquired the virus	England, Wales and N. Ireland			Scotland			Total[4]	(Deaths[2])
	Male	Female	NS	Male	Female	NS		
Mother to infant	111	109	1	10	13	–	244	64
Blood								
blood factor (e.g. for haemophilia)	245	–	–	21	–	–	266	45
blood/tissue transfer (e.g. transfusion)	14	14	1	2	1	–	32	8
Other/undetermined	1	–	–	1	–	–	2	–
Total	371	123	2	34	14	–	544	117

1. Includes all children with AIDS, or with virus detected, or with HIV-1 antibody at age 18 months or over.
2. Deaths in HIV-1 infected children without AIDS are included.
3. Aged 14 years or under when infection was first diagnosed.
4. Includes 1 child infected through mother to infant transmission, 220 haemophilia patients (30 died). 9 blood recipients (1 died) and 2 in undetermined category, who were aged 15 years or over at 30 April 1994 or at death.

TABLE 9 HIV–1 infection status and deaths[1] by year of birth of children born to HIV–1 infected mothers[2]: to 30 April 1994

Year of birth	Infected[3] England, Wales and N. Ireland AIDS	Infected[3] England, Wales and N. Ireland not AIDS	Infected[3] Scotland AIDS	Infected[3] Scotland not AIDS	Indeterminate[4] England, Wales and N. Ireland	Indeterminate[4] Scotland	Not infected England, Wales and N. Ireland	Not infected Scotland	Total	(Deaths[1])
1979–83	5	7	1	–	–	–	–	–	13	3
1984–85	10	8	3	6	4	5	3	9	48	9
1986–87	15	19	3	2	11	7	15	31	103	8
1988–89	21	25	2	1	9	5	26	25	114	11
1990–91	34	31	1	2	36	4	41	21	170	22
1992–93	30	15	1	1	88	9	21	6	171	18
1994–95	–	1	–	–	9	5	–	–	15	–
Total	115	106	11	12	157	35	106	92	634	71

1. Deaths in children known not to be infected are excluded.
2. Due to ascertainment bias the rate of vertical transmission cannot be estimated from surveillance data.
3. See footnote 1, table 8.
4. Aged less than 18 months when last tested positive for HIV–1 antibody and without other evidence of HIV–1 infection. Includes 33 children who were lost to follow-up.

367

Notes and References

Personal interviews have been by far the most important source for this book. Between April 1993 and July 1994 I talked to over 120 people, the vast majority tape-recorded sessions on the record and for attribution (a list appears in the Author's Note). Others provided background material off the record, particularly for Chapters 6 and 10. In order to avoid repeating every sourced quote in the text again in the notes, I have indicated the key interviews used for each chapter.

I have also relied on a large selection of minutes and other documentation from several committees and advisory groups. These are identified in these notes except in those instances where a reference would reveal the source of confidential material.

Unless otherwise stated, all UK statistics quoted derive from the Public Health Laboratory Service Communicable Disease Surveillance Centre and the Communicable Diseases & Environmental Health (Scotland) Unit. European and worldwide figures come from the World Health Organization.

In addition to the articles cited, I have also drawn useful general information from the *British Medical Journal*, the *Lancet*, *New Scientist*, *Nature*, *National AIDS Manual*, *AIDS Matters* (produced by the National AIDS Trust), the *Digest of Organisational Responses to AIDS and HIV*, *AIDS*, The Falmer Press series on the Social Aspects of AIDS, *Parliamentary AIDS Digest*, *WorldAIDS*, *Campaign*, the *Pink Paper*, *Capital Gay*, *Gay Times*, *Phase*, *Attitude* and the publications of Project SIGMA.

PART I
Chapter 1: Thirty-Five Years
Principal interviews: Dr John Leonard, Dr Trevor Stretton, Dr George Williams, Dr David Ho, Rupert Haselden.

4.	They wrote the case up: G. Williams et al., 'Cytomegalic inclusion disease and Pneumocystis carinii infection in an adult', *Lancet*, 1960, ii, pp. 951–5.
5.	'Could [our patient] have had AIDS?': G Williams et al., 'AIDS in 1959?', *Lancet*, 1983, ii, p. 1136.
6.	HIV infection before 1970: for a good general discussion on the origin of AIDS and some early cases see 'Case Shakes theory of AIDS origin', *Chicago Tribune*, 25 October 1987; M. Essex, P. Kanki, 'The origins of the AIDS virus', *Scientific American*, 1988, 259, pp. 64–71; Mirko D Grmek, *History of AIDS* (Princeton University Press, 1990), Chapter 12; Walter S Kyle, 'Simian retroviruses, poliovaccine, and origin of AIDS', *Lancet*, 1992, 339, pp. 600–601; 'The Birth of AIDS', *Out* magazine, April 1994.
8.	There was much interest: G Corbitt et al., Letters to the editor: 'HIV infection in Manchester', 1959. *Lancet*, 1990, 336, p. 51. See also 'How the first AIDS case was unravelled', *Independent on Sunday*, 8 July 1990.
23.	an article for the *Guardian*: 'Gay Abandon', Weekend section, 7 September 1991. See also 'Forum: Glad to be gay... honestly', *Guardian*, 14 September 1991.

Chapter 2: Subway
Principal interviews: Peter Scott, Tim Clark, Linda Semple, Rupert Whittaker, Alastair Hume, Tony Whitehead, Roy Greenslade.

27.	Taken to Subway: Holly Johnson, *A Bone in my Flute*, Century (London, 1994), pp. 143–4.
28.	'Who needs his lover's pick-up germs?': 'They say there isn't a plague', *Gay News*, 235, March 1982.
30.	'The moral was clear': 'Gay cancer or mass media scare?', *Gay News*, 228, November 1991.
	'The alleged connection': 'Cancer, poppers and gay men', *Gay News*, 245, July 1982.
	two French Kaposi's patients: Isabelle Gorin et al., 'Kaposi's sarcoma without the US or "popper" connection', *Lancet*, 1982, i, p. 908.
34.	'I was not next of kin': transcript of interview with Rupert Whittaker conducted in February 1993 in San Francisco for *The Plague*, made by Barraclough Carey for Channel 4.
	'There were people in there': ibid.
	'US Disease Hits London': *Capital Gay*, 26 November 1982.

35. 'I'm amazed at the ignorance about it': 'Crossing the pond', *Gay News*, 262, March 1983.
    A man called Floyd: 'US Disease Hits London', op. cit.
    The *Horizon* programme: 'Killer in the Village', BBC2, 25 April 1983.
    He listed the 'eerie invitation to diseases': *Observer*, 1 May 1983.
36. 'newly fashionable': 'AIDS: The price of promiscuity?', *Daily Telegraph*, 26 April 1983.
    'hundreds of patients with anxiety': 'AIDS scare is making people ill, say doctors', *Capital Gay*, 19 August 1983.
37. 'We would like to see the great public concern': reported in *Capital Gay*, 27 May 1983.
    'I don't think it will be very long': ibid.
    'I hope you get very scared': ibid.
40. 'Although the risk': 'Surveillance of the Acquired immune deficiency syndrome in the United Kingdom, January 1982–July 1983', Editorial prepared by the Public Health Laboratory Service, *BMJ*, 1983, 287, pp. 407–8.
41. 'Mystery disease kills gays': *Guardian*, 10 December 1981.
    'Cancer one of the "gay syndrome" illnesses': *Times*, 11 December 1981.
    'A deadly new illness': 'Mystery new killer disease', *Sunday Times*, 5 September 1982.
42. '"Gay Plague" may lead to blood ban on homosexuals': *Daily Telegraph*, 2 May 1983.
    'Indiscriminate promiscuous homosexuality': ibid.
    full-page specials: 'AIDS is here', *Times*, 27 July 1983; 'The lurking killer without a cure', *Guardian*, 2 November 1983.
    'Killer Love Bug Danger': *Sunday People*, 16 January 1983.
    'What the gay plague did to handsome Kenny': *Sunday People*, 24 July 1983.
43. 'special on the disease doctors can't cure': *Sun*, 11 November 1983.
    'My doomed son's gay plague agony': *News of the World*, 30 December 1984.
    'Fleet Street does not like homosexuality': Derek Jameson, *Open Space*, BBC2, quoted in *Panic* by Robin McKie, Thorsons (Wellingborough, 1986).
    'Scared firemen ban the kiss of life': *Daily Express*, 18 February 1985.
    'AIDS: Now ambulance men ban kiss of life': *Daily Mirror*, 19 February 1985.
    'Policeman flees AIDS victim': *Daily Express*, 24 August 1983.
44. 'I did not want to expose': *Daily Express*, 2 November 1983.
    'AIDS is far from being a well-studied disease': *World at One*, BBC Radio 4, 2 November 1983; quoted in *Times*, 3 November 1983.
    'Expert refuses "AIDS death" probe': *Daily Express*, 2 November 1983.

44. 'Top doctor shuns "sex death" victim': *Daily Mirror*, 2 November 1983.
'Body blacked in AIDS scare': *Waltham Forest Guardian*, 4 November 1983.
'Torture of Innocents': *Sunday Mirror*, 4 December 1983.
45. 'Shock finding by doctors': *Private Eye*, June 1983.
46. 'I suppose you know what GAY stands for': *Private Eye*, 4 November 1983.
a detailed critique: letter from Julian Meldrum to the director, the Press Council, 30 June 1983.
European Conference on AIDS: 'AIDS and the Press', paper by Julian Meldrum, written 3 January 1984.
Unwittingly, early hysteria: I. V. D. Weller et al., 'Gonorrhoea in homosexual men and media coverage of the acquired immune deficiency syndrome in London 1982–3', *BMJ*, 1984, 289, p. 1041.

Chapter 3: False Negative
Principal interviews: Professor Anthony Pinching, Professor Ian Weller, Professor Michael Adler.

50. 'Acquired Immunodeficiency Syndrome: No UK Epidemic': Editorial, *Lancet*, 1983, 1, p. 487.
51. applied to the MRC: An Investigation into the immunology and aetiology of AIDS, MRC Application for a project grant submitted 8 July 1983.
were awarded £160,000: minutes of meeting of MRC Working Party on AIDS, 25 October 1984.
Working Party on AIDS: minutes of first meeting held 10 October 1983.
52. what those doctors knew: a very basic summary of some points expressed in meeting above.
53. doctors gathered again: minutes of meeting, 20 December 1983.
54. the announcement in April 1984: in Washington, 23 April 1984. Robert Gallo et al.'s paper, 'Frequent detection and isolation of cytopathic retroviruses (HTLV-III) from patients with AIDS and at risk for AIDS', appeared in *Science*, 4 May 1984, 500.
55. 'Virology have not been able to cope': minutes of meeting of the AIDS Collaborative Group held 6 February 1985. This group, which included Professor Adler, Dr Weller and a dozen others working at or connected with the Middlesex met monthly from 1984 to 1988 to discuss new advances and issues such as funding, safety and testing.
the considerable number of 'false positives': minutes of Aids Collaborative Group, 5 June 1985.
study of the prevalence of HTLV-III: R. A. Weiss et al., 'Prevalence of antibody to human T-lymphotropic virus type III in AIDS and AIDS-risk patients in Britain', *Lancet*, 1984, 2, pp. 477–80.

59. a terrible accident: Editorial, 'Needlestick transmission of HTLV–III from a patient infected in Africa', *Lancet*, 1984, 2, pp. 1376–7.
What no one knew then: interview with Dr Peter Jones. See Chapter 4.

Chapter 4: The Fridge That Day
Principal interviews: Simon Taylor, Dr Peter Jones, Professor Anthony Pinching, Sir Norman Fowler, Caroline Guinness, Tim Clark.

61. The worst you could get: C. R. Rizza, R. J. D. Spooner, 'Treatment of haemophilia and related disorders in Britain and Northern Ireland during 1976–80: report on behalf of the directors of haemophilia centres in the United Kingdom', *BMJ*, 1983, 286, pp. 929–33.
62. only two British haemophiliacs: G. C. White et al., 'Chronic hepatitis in patients with hemophilia A: histologic studies in patients with intermittently abnormal liver function tests', *Blood*, 1982, 60, pp. 1259–62.
60 per cent of all Factor VIII: Rizza, Spooner, op. cit.
haemophiliacs representing one per cent: C. Marwick, 'Contaminated plasma – no automatic recall', *Journal of the American Medical Association* (*JAMA*), 1983, 250, pp. 1126–7.
a question from Edwina Currie: Edwina Currie, *Life Lines*, Sidgwick & Jackson (London, 1989), Chapter 4.
In the same month the *British Medical Journal*: Peter Jones, 'Acquired immunodeficiency syndrome, hepatitis, and haemophilia', *BMJ*, 1983, 287, pp. 1737–8. This is also the reference for the first four chapter sources cited above.
63. Ninety-nine patients with severe haemophilia A: Peter Jones et al., 'AIDS and haemophilia: morbidity and mortality in a well defined population', *BMJ*, 1985, 291, pp. 695–9.
'To cope we think it imperative': ibid.
64. AIDS 'is a very serious disease': DHSS press release, 26 September 1985.
65. To allay the fears of his patients: *AIDS and the Blood: A Practical Guide*, published by the Newcastle Haemophilia Reference Centre in association with the Haemophilia Society and the Terrence Higgins Trust, February 1985.
66. Dr Jones constructed his own theory: Peter Jones, letter, 'AIDS: the African connection?', *BMJ*, 1985, 290, p. 932.
Dr Jones wrote a lengthy letter: ibid.
The letter caused some concern: E. D. Acheson, letter, 'AIDS: the African connection?', *BMJ*, 1985, 290, p. 1145.
Robert Reilly ... went on the offensive: letter, 'AIDS: the African connection?', *BMJ*, 1985, 291, p. 216.

67. Dr Jones would have none of it: letter, 'AIDS: the African connection?',
    BMJ, 1985, 291, p. 216.
68. In Koblenz, western Germany: *Independent*, 6 November 1993.
69. Most haemophiliacs in Newcastle: Jones, 'Acquired immunodeficiency
    syndrome, hepatitis, and haemophilia', op. cit.
    non-commercial British blood products: R. Cheinsong-Popov et al.,
    'Retrovirus infections among patients treated in Britain with various
    clotting factors', *BMJ*, 1986, 293, pp. 168–9.
70. 'the single biggest disaster': 'Haemophilia and AIDS: a briefing paper',
    the Haemophilia Society, October 1987.
71. over two hundred parents gathered: Dr Anthony Pinching, 'Children
    with HIV infection: Dealing with the problem', in *AIDS: A challenge in
    education*, ed. David R. Morgan (Institute of Biology/Royal Society of
    Medicine Services, 1990).
72. John Patten reaffirmed: 'Britain to be self sufficient in blood products by
    late 1986', *BMJ*, 1984, 289, p. 1545.
    the programme of heat treatment: Kenneth Clarke, *Hansard*, 5 February
    1985, 527.
    Announcing the new measures: DHSS press release, 20 February 1985.
    The question was asked by Dr Brian Mawhinney, who was later to take
    Clarke's former job at Health.
73. detained against his will: 'Court orders man to remain in hospital',
    Times, 16 September 1985.
    he had changed his mind: 'AIDS man wins in court but spurns
    freedom', *Guardian*, 25 September 1985.
    'Now he knows he can leave': ibid.
    Comprehensive testing of all blood donations: 'Two British blood tests
    launched', *Nature*, 1985, 316, p. 474; 'Date set for AIDS screening test',
    DHSS press release, 23 August 1985.
74. two notable microbiologists: 'Expert advice ignored in proposal to
    decentralize AIDS laboratory network', *Times*, 16 September 1985.
    conceded in a television interview: *This Week, Next Week*, BBC; reported
    in *Guardian*, 23 September 1985.
    wrote to all doctors in England: 'AIDS Booklet 2: Information for
    doctors concerning the introduction of the HTLV III antibody test',
    DHSS, October 1985.
75. In a written parliamentary answer: 'Extra £6.3m to combat AIDS',
    DHSS press release, 2 December 1985.
77. Expert Advisory Group on AIDS: I have relied much on the minutes of
    these meetings for the information that follows in this chapter, and for
    some of Chapters 5 and 6.
78. The minutes of the meeting: EAGA Health Education Group meeting,
    9 July 1985.

85. finally got done for rape: see Duncan Campbell, 'Doctor of Deceit', *New Statesman & Society*, 4 December 1992.

Chapter 5: Shooting Gallery
Principal interviews: Dr Ray Brettle, Dr Laurence Gruer, Joy Barlow, Paul Trainer, Hugh Dufficy.

92. Dr Donald Acheson delivered his controversial report: 'HTLV3 infection, the AIDS epidemic and the control of its spread in the UK', June 1985.
93. The first rumblings: letter, J. F. Peutherer et al., 'HTLV-III antibody in Edinburgh drug addicts', *Lancet*, 1985, 2, pp. 1129–30.
94. the situation looked even worse: 'Large numbers of intravenous drug abusers have AIDS virus', *General Practitioner*, 22 November 1985.
     They had tested stored blood samples: J. R. Robertson et al., 'Epidemic of AIDS related virus (HTLV-III/Lav) infection among intravenous drug abusers', *BMJ*, 1986, 292, pp. 527–9.
95. The history of drug use: see R. P. Brettle, 'Infection and injection drug use', *Journal of Infection*, 1992, 25, pp. 121–31.
     a system known as 'booting': ibid.
96. The Lothian and Borders Police: see *Third Report from the Social Services Committee: Problems Associated with AIDS*, HMSO, 1987. Evidence of W. G. M. Sutherland and Douglas Kerr, 12 March 1987.
     11 officers in the drug squad: ibid.
     The policemen were proud of their efforts: ibid.
97. a groundbreaking official report: *HIV infection in Scotland. Report of Scottish Committee on HIV infection and intravenous drug misuse*, Edinburgh, Scottish Home and Health Department, 1986.
     got them flustered in Westminster: 'Clean needles and syringes for drug abusers: Government reluctant to act', Commentary from Westminster, *Lancet*, 1986, 2, pp. 53–4.
     thought the idea outrageous: 'AIDS is "disease of habit"', *Hospital Doctor*, 15 May 1986.
     'a callous disregard for human misery': ibid.
     no clear party divide: 'Clean needles and syringes for drug abusers', op. cit. A letter signed by Robertson: 'Regional variations in HIV antibody seropositivity in British intravenous drug users', *Lancet*, 1986, 1, pp. 1435–6.
98. The consensus favoured needle exchanges: EAGA minutes, June and July 1986.
     'The use of a pop star': EAGA minutes, 11 September 1985.
     pilot needle exchange schemes: see 'Syringe exchanges for Scottish cities', *Pharmaceutical Journal*, 24 January 1987; A. Moss, 'AIDS and intravenous drug use: the real heterosexual epidemic', *BMJ*, 1987, 294, pp. 389–90.

101. heard evidence from Roy Robertson: *Third Report from the Social Services Committee*, op. cit., 11 March 1987.
there were 22 babies: Moss, op. cit. (These were unpublished observations from Dr Jacqueline Mok.)
At least ten partners: ibid.
102. but it was an overestimate: for general background see: L. Gruer et al., 'Distribution of HIV and acute hepatitis B infection among drug injectors in Glasgow', *International Journal of STD & AIDS*, 1991, 2, pp. 356–8; J. Emslie, 'Monitoring the spread and impact of HIV infection in Scotland, 1982–1991', *Royal Society of Medicine: The AIDS Letter*, February/March 1993.
A study of 1,786 drug injectors: Gruer et al., op. cit.
103. 'AIDS doesn't bother me': Reported 'A City at Risk', *Sunday Times Magazine*, 21 June 1987.

Chapter 6: A Plague on Both Your Houses
Principal interviews: Sir Norman Fowler, Sir Donald Acheson, Sammy Harari, Edwina Currie, Chris Smith, Professor Anthony Pinching, Baroness Jay, Peter Scott, Tony Whitehead, Zoe Schramm-Evans, Jonathan Grimshaw.

107. £100,000 would be spent: DHSS press release, 26 September 1985.
'Brave Barney has declared war on AIDS': *Doctor*, September 1985.
John Patten had also been considering: confidential DHSS/DoH source.
Norman Fowler ... was not hugely supportive: ibid.
Margaret Thatcher believed it to be a small problem: ibid.
'the Minister for Gays': ibid.
relaxed chatting to 'Bill' off camera: ibid. See also 'AIDS challenge not minister's cup of tea', *Pulse*, 16 March 1985. The headline refers to Patten's comment on *Weekend World* that he would be more than happy to drink from the same cup as a person with AIDS. According to *Pulse*, when the meeting with 'Bill' was being set up (for another Thames Television programme), 'Mr Patten ... had been very insistent that although he would come along for a chat, no tea or coffee should be on the table. The programme makers deny that they would ever have asked Mr Patten to fulfil all of his promise, but clearly the minister was taking no chances.'
'Did he really say two hundred?': confidential DHSS/DoH source.
108. 'a message from Nigel Wicks': ibid.
'a high proportion of our unanimous suggestions': *Third Report from the Social Services Committee: Problems Associated with AIDS*, HMSO, 1987
Memorandum submitted by Professor Anthony Coxon, vol. 2, p. 55.
109. 'I can remember one meeting': Dr Charles Farthing, from transcript of interview for *The Plague*, Barraclough Carey/ Channel 4.
110. the term 'anal intercourse': confidential DHSS/DoH source.

110. 'can fail to be conveyed': *Third Report from the Social Services Committee*, op. cit., vol. 1, p. XXIV, paragraph 56.
the conclusions of a survey: S. Mills et al., 'Public knowledge of AIDS and the DHSS advertisement campaign', *BMJ*, 1986, 293, pp. 1089–90.
To counteract such adverse publicity: 'Public Information Campaign on AIDS', *Lancet*, 1986, 2, p. 297.

111. 'but time is running out': 'AIDS: act now, don't pay later', *BMJ*, 1986, 293, p. 348.
The College of Health went further: 'The AIDS campaign', *Lancet*, 1986, 2, p. 353.
'I spent the quietest weekend': Sir Donald Acheson, from 'A Pale Horse In Whitehall', lecture given at St John's College, Cambridge, 6 May 1992.

112. 'have them placed by non-Governmental bodies': 'The public information campaign on AIDS', EAGA minutes, July 1986.
eight separate target groups: ibid.

113. bland language was too much for some: 'Hailsham ponders meaning of sex', *Times*, 10 July 1986.
homosexuality should be made illegal again: *Heart of the Matter* (BBC 1), 8 March 1987; quoted in Martin Durham, *Sex & Politics*, Macmillan (London, 1991), p. 125.
'a cesspool of their own making': almost all national newspapers reported this speech on 12 December 1986.

114. a problem of 'undesirable minorities': *Times*, 14 December 1988.
'my predecessors were not only not interested': the quotes in this passage come from a personal interview, but see also Edwina Currie, *Life Lines*, Sidgwick & Jackson (London, 1989), Chapter 4.

115. 'With remarkable clarity of vision': 'A Pale Horse in Whitehall', op. cit., and personal interview.
Peter Jenkins recalled a lunch with Armstrong: 'Unappetising reality of AIDS', *Sunday Times*, 9 November 1986.
Fowler was so gleeful: 'Fighting AIDS', *Lancet*, 1986, 2, p. 1291.

116. Fowler wrote in his autobiography: Norman Fowler, *Ministers Decide*, Chapmans (London, 1991), Chapter 13.
'hardly talking about AIDS': Michael Meacher in House of Commons debate on AIDS, 21 November 1986.
'AIDS: The New Holocaust': *Sunday Telegraph*, 23 November 1986.
'the greatest danger facing Britain': *Mail on Sunday*, 12 October 1986.

117. 'They look happy and healthy': *Sunday Times*, 2 November 1986.
Sir Donald Acheson left no one much the wiser: quoted in *Daily Mirror*, 21 November 1986.
broadsheets made calculations of their own: figures quoted in *Lancet*, 1987, 1, p. 175.

118. 'before *they* took any notice?': Simon Watney, 'Visual AIDS: Advertising

Ignorance', *New Socialist*, March 1987; reprinted in Simon Watney, *Practices of Freedom*, Rivers Oram Press (London, 1994), Chapter 2.

118. 'Do we know how many people *do* this sort of thing?': confidential DHSS/DoH source.

119. he 'had real problems': David Miller (Glasgow University Media Group), paper given at Seventh Conference on Social Aspects of AIDS, South Bank University, 3 July 1993.
'We used the post office for mailing': 'AIDS – are leaflets the right answer?', *Pulse*, 22 November 1986.
'human sexual behaviour in the bedroom': *Lancet*, 9 January 1988; as quoted in Zoe Schramm-Evans, unpublished thesis, p. 164.

121. two overseas trips: *Lancet*, 1987, 1, p. 234.
the Chief Rabbi ... presented Norman Fowler with a long list of misgivings: *Third Report from the Social Services Committee*, op. cit., Memorandum submitted by Sir Immanuel Jakobovits. See also Fowler, op. cit., Chapter 13.

122. 'The very least the Government could do': *Capital Gay*, 9 January 1987.
action the government should take: *Third Report from the Social Services Committee*, op. cit., Memorandum submitted by Terrence Higgins Trust, vol. 2, p. 101.

124. 'selling celibacy is like trying to market empty cans': *Sunday Telegraph*, 11 January 1987.
'the only thing that can be said in its favour': ibid.
repeated their survey nine months later: M. J. Campbell and W. E. Waters, 'Public knowledge about AIDS increasing', *BMJ*, 1987, 294, pp. 892–3.
DHSS was encouraged by the results of its own research: DHSS press release, 12 February 1987.

125. AIDS as their biggest health worry: 'Fear of AIDS second only to cancer', *Daily Telegraph*, 28 April 1987.
Football Association wrote to every professional footballer: 'Soccer AIDS War', *Daily Mirror*, 20 January 1987; 'FA's advice to players "farcical"', *Daily Telegraph*, 21 January 1987.
'Now we aim to frighten players into it': ibid.

126. 'Good Christian people': 'Afraid of AIDS? Take the wife away with you', *Daily Mail*, 13 February 1987. See also Currie, op. cit., Chapter 4.
'Beating off AIDS with the Bible': *Guardian*, 13 February 1987.
personal ads in the columns of gay newspapers: 'Infected gays seek partners', *Observer*, 1 March 1987.

127. 'The term "loose cannon"': confidential DHSS/DoH source.
a surgeon who had contracted HIV: see 'Search for 400 patients of AIDS-death doctor', *Independent*, 1 April 1988.

128. 'He came into the office with three jumpers': confidential DHSS/DoH source.
129. an independent charitable organization: DHSS press release, 5 May 1987.
a sweating Maxwell announced: 'National AIDS Trust: Mr Maxwell seeks £50 million', *Lancet*, 1987, 1, p. 1157. A private source also told me: 'Maxwell was basically just looking for his knighthood.' Sir Norman Fowler says: 'It was very difficult to stop Robert Maxwell from becoming the chairman of a [government sanctioned] national AIDS committee.'
130. two things had happened to alienate the Terrence Higgins Trust: minutes, notes and correspondence of UK AIDS Foundation.
131. 'I think we got it just about right': 'Response to AIDS about right', *Independent*, 1 April 1988.
132. 'appallingly short sighted': ibid.
the short-term predictions contained in the Cox Report: DoH press release, 30 November 1988.
a London conference on the global impact of AIDS: 'Official AIDS toll "too low"', *Guardian*, 1 March 1988.

Chapter 7: Suitable Treatment
Principal Interviews: Dr Jerome Horwitz, John Lauritsen, Professor Trevor Jones, Professor Ian Weller, Michael Cottrell, Karl Burge, Derek Jarman, Christopher Spence, Sheila Dutch, Professor Anthony Pinching, Dr Jane Cope, Dr Alan Stone.

134. obtained a 20-page document: 'Federally unapproved medications for treatment of AIDS and AIDS related conditions', Version 3.1, December 1986.
136. Norman Fowler granted a product licence: DHSS press release, 4 March 1987.
'sufficient promise to be taken forward': quoted in *Scrip*, 7 October 1985.
a conference in Minneapolis: ibid.
ribavirin was being tested by ICN: these new drug developments described in *Scrip*, 14 August 1985, 9 October 1985, 13 October 1986, 15 October 1986.
137. Jerome Horwitz was working in his laboratory: personal interview. See also Bruce Nussbaum, *Good Intentions*, Penguin (New York, 1991), Chapters 1 and 7, an exemplary account of the relationship between the worlds of science and big business.
The Wellcome group was founded in London: Wellcome Foundation Ltd's own account of its history in Press Information package.
138. another account of the development of AZT: Nussbaum, op. cit.,

Chapters 1 and 7. See also 'Who developed AZT?', *Lancet*, 14 October 1989, p. 913.

139. 'I went to one prestigious company': ibid.

140. The early clinical tests were in two phases: Robert Yarchoan et al., 'Administration of 3'-Azido-3'-Deoxythymidine, an inhibitor of HTLVIII/LAV replication, to patients with AIDS or AIDS-related complex', *Lancet*, 1986, 1, pp. 575–80. See also 'Wellcome's BW-A509U in AIDS', *Scrip*, 24 March 1986; 'Promising results halt trial of anti-AIDS Drug', *Science*, 1986, 234, pp. 15–16.

had been a considerable success: ibid.

additional plants were announced: 'Wellcome gears up production of AIDS drug', *Nature*, 12 February 1987.

stock market analysts reckoned: 'Wellcome's AZT: $12–15 million sales per year?', *Scrip*, 15 October 1986.

United States sales alone: 'Wellcome's proposed price for Retrovir', *Scrip*, 20 February 1987.

141. 'difficult to think of an achievement': reported in 'Retrovir approved in US', *Scrip*, 21 March 1987.

'Some doctors are so concerned about infection': EAGA minutes, April 1988.

'the staff at Wellcome can tell our children': Dr David Barry, *Wellcome World*, March/April 1992.

'Of all the unsolicited material': 'Promoting Retrovir', *New England Journal of Medicine*, 317, no. 18.

A Wellcome person replied: ibid.

142. many rules had been broken: 'AZT on Trial', *New York Native*, 19 October 1987. See also John Lauritsen, *Poison by Prescription*, Asklepios (New York, 1990), Chapters 1 and 2.

143. refusing to supply AZT: 'Burroughs Wellcome role in Retrovir US CTs questioned', *Scrip*, 29 April 1987.

Dr David Barry responded: ibid.

144. punctuated by bleeps: I am grateful to Adam Mars-Jones for this information.

145. the frequent use of AZT: Christine Costello et al., 'The Blood Transfusion service and zidovudine treatment for AIDS', *BMJ*, 1987, 295, p. 1486.

done extremely well out of AZT: these figures are from 'Wellcome on a high', *Independent*, 14 February 1987; 'Retrovir helps Wellcome to lift profits to £283m', *Financial Times*, 17 November 1989.

146. 'increase the total bill to the NHS dramatically': EAGA minutes, April 1988. David Barry found it 'very distressing': *Wellcome World*, March/April 1992.

148. began life in 1913 to tackle tuberculosis: from the MRC's own historical account.

148. By June 1986, it had funded 12 projects: MRC Working Party on AIDS minutes, July 1986. Much of what follows is based on documentation from these meetings.
149. 'there was an argument from government': confidential source at MRC. 'an increase in their grant in aid of £1 million': for this and subsequent grants see 'AIDS research and risks', *IMLS Gazette*, February 1987; 'Boost for MRC research', *BMJ*, 1987, 294, p. 520; 'Extra MRC funds earmarked for AIDS research in Britain', *Nature*, 5 March 1987.
150. The amount was piteously small: *Third Report from the Social Services Committee: Problems Associated with AIDS*, HMSO, 1987. Memorandum submitted by Dr Jonathan Weber, vol. 2, p. 51.
'There is no "plan" for research': ibid.
claims it took four years: *Third Report from the Social Services Committee*, op. cit., Memorandum submitted by Professor Anthony Coxon, vol. 2, p. 55.
151. a massive injection of funds was now needed: 'Directed Research on AIDS: The MRC's plans', *Lancet*, 1987, 1, pp. 578–9. See also *Third Report from the Social Services Committee*, op. cit., Evidence of the Earl Jellicoe, Sir James Gowans, Dr J. W. G. Smith, 11 February 1987.
152. The new policy had two prongs: MRC Directed programme of AIDS research programme Plan, MRC document, October 1987.
The 'market' for a vaccine: 'Progress with AIDS vaccines', *Scrip*, 27 March 1987; 'AIDS vaccine trials to start in UK', *Scrip*, May 1987; 'MRC programme for research into AIDS', *Lancet*, 1987 (19 September), p. 698.
a team led by Professor William Jarrett: 'MRC programme for research into AIDS', op. cit.
154. almost everything it had asked for: 'MRC gets £14.5 m for AIDS', *BMJ*, 1987, 294, p. 651; 'Directed Research on AIDS: The MRC's plans', op. cit.

Additional Note: In October 1987, Deirdre Cunningham and S. F. Griffiths from St Mary's Hospital constructed a detailed breakdown of the average annual treatment cost of a person with AIDS. Treatment was split between hospital and care in the community. Their work provides a useful guide not only to the financial burden, but also to the complexity and number of the services required. The breakdown was:

1) One month's inpatient care: £5,600
2) Four months' day-care treatment, including meals, one and a half hours' nursing and transport costs £3,325
3) Seven months' management by the acute district nursing service: £3,900
4) Six outpatient visits plus transport: £185
5) Home help provision: three hours per day (seven days a week) for six months, plus one hour per day (seven days a week) for four months: £2,750

6) Night sitting by nurse auxiliary: ten hours per night for
   three weeks: £1,150
7) Hospice at home: three weeks' 24-hour staff nurse: £3,630
8) Equipment: mattresses/urinals etc: £195
9) Four visits by occupational therapist: £35
10) Two visits by senior clinical psychologist: £35
    Total cost: £20,805

This total does not include the additional costs of AZT and the requisite resultant transfusions. To include this, add £5,200 for the cost of the drug and £1,050 for the costs of four transfusions, including overnight hospital stays.

Total cost including AZT treatment: £27,055
Source: *BMJ*, 10 October 1987.

Chapter 8: The Church Has AIDS
Principal interviews: Reverend Malcolm Johnson, Father John White.

160. 'The fear of disease': quoted in David Black, 'The Plague Years', *Rolling Stone*, 25 April 1985.
163. the General Synod debate: 'General Synod Report on AIDS', 10 November 1987, pp. 829–60. Compare this with the prodeedings of an inter-faith conference on AIDS and sexual health held in March 1994. George Carey, the Archbishop of Canterbury, suggested that the Church may have been partly responsible for the stigma surrounding AIDS, and may have stopped those most in need coming forward for help. 'We become part of the problem when we give the impression that the high ideals and moral standards we seek to promote are like walls surrounding a forbidding fortresss ... We may inadvertently obstruct the prevention of disease through alienating people from sources of advice and help' (quoted in 'Church fuels AIDS stigma', *Guardian*, 24 March 1994).
was the first to point the finger: ibid.
20 gay clergymen with AIDS: 'Vicars "dying from AIDS"', *Daily Express*, 9 July 1987.
Malcolm Johnson rose to his feet: ibid. See also Malcolm Johnson's General Synod briefing paper, 'The Church, homosexuals and AIDS', LGCM Theological Commission, October 1987.
issued guidelines on AIDS and pastoral care: for instance, 'AIDS: some guidelines for pastoral care', Church House Publishing, November 1986; 'AIDS and the Church', World Council of Churches, Geneva, 1987 ; 'AIDS: a challenge to the churches', British Council of Churches/Free Church Federal Council, 1989; 'The churches and AIDS', Oxford Regional Health Authority HIV and AIDS Education Programme, December 1991.

164. 'Churches are your great institutions': quoted in *Woman's Own*, 27 October 1987. In 1989 Mrs Thatcher paid a visit to the Mildmay Mission Hospital, the independent Christian hospital in London's East End. She spoke to two people with AIDS in their private rooms, but according to *Capital Gay* (11 August 1989), 'Downing Street stressed that Mrs Thatcher visited the Mildmay primarily to see a model of how she felt the health service should be, rather than to take an interest in AIDS'.
'Chris would not get closer to me than six yards': 'I'd shoot my son if he had AIDS, says vicar!', *Sun*, 14 October 1985.
were urged not to drink from the chalice: 'Curb on chalice over AIDS', *Daily Telegraph*, 25 January 1987. See also 'AIDS and the chalice', *Church Times*, 13 February 1987 and 1 May 1987.
all brides and grooms should take an HIV test: 'Check all brides for AIDS, says top priest', *Daily Mail*, 15 January 1987.
'we are witnessing the end of the era': 'Youth at risk', *Church Times*, 28 November 1986.
165. 'the black cloud of this scourge': revised transcript of Chief Rabbi's address to Union of Jewish Students, Hillel House, London, 1987; reprinted in 'AIDS: Jewish perspectives', Office of the Chief Rabbi, 1987. No issue divided the community like condoms: this continues to be the case. In April 1994 the Jewish magazine *New Moon* asked several rabbis if they would encourage people to use condoms to reduce the risk of AIDS. Rabbi Elizabeth Sarah, of Buckhurst Hill Reform Synagogue, replied: 'Of course they should wear condoms. It's simple. I don't even see that as a controversial issue.' Rabbi Nisson Shulman, of St John's Wood Orthodox Synagogue, said: 'you stop AIDS by stopping promiscuity and homosexuality. I see harm in condoning things which would normally be forbidden by Jewish law'. But Reverend Norman Gale, another orthodox rabbi from Hampstead Synagogue, believed: 'If young people feel they cannot abstain and they must have sex, then they should use a condom.'
'when the moment of temptation comes': Address to Union of Jewish Students, op. cit.
It was 'moral disorder' that led to AIDS: 'Bishops say condom use could help spread AIDS', *Independent*, 14 January 1987.

Chapter 9: Protest
Principal interviews: Jimmy Somerville, Ivan Massow, Tim Clark, Simon Watney, Ben Croall.

172. a spot of bother with the sex discrimination act: 'Formal Investigation Report: Dan Air', Equal Opportunities Commission, January 1987.
173. applicants for aircraft jobs with British Airways: 'Fighting the virus of fear in the workplace', *Independent on Sunday*, 18 November 1990. SmithKline Beecham has also defended its HIV test: ibid.

174. 'how many days off sick he would demand': 'HIV carrier sues firm in employment law test case', *Observer*, 15 April 1990.

her job with the Torbay Health Authority: 'My husband died of AIDS; but my bosses wrecked my life', *Independent*, 19 February 1990.

dealt with harshly by a tribunal: 'Employers could face claims from AIDS victims', *Independent*, 25 November 1986; 'AIDS victims "must not be sacked"', *Daily Telegraph*, 25 November 1986; 'AIDS and Employment', Department of Employment, 1986. For other guidelines see also 'AIDS and Employment Law', Financial Training Publication, 1987; 'AIDS and Human Rights: A UK Perspective', British Medical Association, 1989. In February 1994, the issue of employment protection surfaced publicly again when a worker in the Harrods food hall claimed he was sacked for failing to take an HIV test. A hundred and thirty staff were tested for HIV after an outbreak of salmonella and three refused testing. Christopher Gough, who worked on the cold meats counter, was sacked shortly after his refusal, but a Harrods spokesman claimed this was because of his 'poor interpersonal skills'. Some staff claimed that they had been tested without their consent and without counselling, which Harrods denied. The spokesman added: 'We believe it is necessary to test people involved in food preparation for HIV, because there is a likelihood of people getting cut.' Vanessa Hardy of Companies Act, the business charter on HIV and AIDS organized by the National AIDS Trust, thought it ridiculous that people working with food should be tested, suggesting that if blood got on to food, the food should always be thrown away. 'The Harrods story is an example of the misinformation about AIDS still influencing management practice.' (Source: 'Harrods workers' fury over illegal HIV tests', *Observer*, 17 April 1994; 'Harrods sparks HIV testing row', *Pink Paper*, 3 June 1994.)

Many large companies behaved creditably: 'Fighting the virus of fear in the workplace', op. cit.

specific HIV/AIDS provisions into the new Employment Act: 'Lords turn down call for ban on AIDS bias at work', *Independent*, 17 October 1989. See also the entry for 29 November 1993 in Part II.

175. wrote to all domestic port medical inspectors: 'Acquired Immune Deficiency Syndrome (AIDS) in passengers seeking to enter the UK', DHSS, 21 January 1988.

policies restricting those who were HIV positive: *WorldAIDS*, Panos Institute, March 1991. See also 'A checklist of AIDS-related visa restrictions', *Guardian*, 11 May 1988; *WorldAIDS*, July 1989; 'Have AIDS can't travel', *Sunday Correspondent*, 22 October 1989; *WorldAIDS Datafile*, May 1993.

'I know exactly how HIV is transmitted': 'Have AIDS can't travel', op. cit.

176. 'an extremely serious matter': *WorldAIDS*, November 1991. Two years earlier, Dr Mann drew a comparison between US policies and those of Britain. He said: 'Britain has been one of the leading countries in respecting human rights and the dignity of the individual with AIDS or HIV' (quoted in 'Charities threaten boycott over travel bars', *Times*, 23 December 1989). The mood improved a little in the United States with the election of Bill Clinton, yet, as with his pledge to lift the ban on gays in the military, he promised more than he delivered. There was one small breakthrough: for the 1994 Gay Games, Attorney General Janet Reno did allow all participants into the country (for a week), even if they were HIV positive.

    10.5 million life insurance policies: 'AIDS and insurance', Association of British Insurers Factfile, January 1988. This noted: 'Life insurance companies have to be prudent in the management of funds built up in this way, so that policyholders' expectations on death, maturity or retirement can be met. They must invest soundly on behalf of their policy holders, and must select carefully those lives they insure.'

    fear of close scrutiny by insurance companies: these issues explored by EAGA. Minutes of meetings, November 1987 and September 1988.

177. addressed the issue with almost boastful candour: 'AIDS quiz on mortgages', *Today*, 2 November 1986.

    'I am on dangerous ground': 'Leaked report has harsh words for insurers', *Capital Gay*, 17 February 1989.

    'all bets are off': 'Insurers' £1bn cover for AIDS', *Times*, 11 April 1988.

178. any policy worth more than £50,000: 'Blood test and sex questions for insurance applicants', *Sunday Telegraph*, 22 November 1987.

    applying for policies worth over £150,000: 'Insurers pry into AIDS risk activity', *Doctor*, 11 August 1988.

    testing for much lower amounts: ibid.

    'The future looks bleak': 'Firms censured for exploiting AIDS', *Guardian*, 16 March 1988.

    a new clause in its permanent health insurance policies: 'Insurers will cancel cover in HIV cases', *Independent*, 8 September 1990.

    cash benefits from £25,000 to £75,000 on *proof* of infection: 'Doubts over "AIDS insurance"', *Independent*, 30 June 1989.

    commissioned a survey on AIDS and life insurance: *AIDS and Life Insurance*, HMSO (London, 1991). When Minister for Health Virginia Bottomley sent a copy of the report to Chris Smith, who had expressed concern about the issue in the Commons and as vice-chair of the All-Party Parliamentary Group on AIDS, she concluded: 'The Report suggests it is likely that thousands or tens of thousands of people are dissuaded from seeking a test and these could be the people we would most like to encourage to come forward for testing.'

179. Ivan Massow says things have hardly improved: see also Ivan Massow's *Gay Finance Guide*, Fourth Estate (London, 1994).

180. A chaotic meeting: Act-Up minutes. See also 'In on the act', *20/20* magazine, March 1989.
'dedicated to improving public debate': ibid.
'If what you're hearing doesn't rouse you to anger': quoted in 'AIDS, activisim and the politics of health', *New England Journal of Medicine*, 9 January 1992.

181. the gay movement had protested widely: for a general round-up of non-AIDS related gay politics before and since, see 'Age of Consent', *Independent on Sunday Review*, 10 November 1991.
'a gathering of AIDS profiteers': 'Act-Up London!', *Capital Gay*, 20 January 1989.
'an annual Act-Up hit': 'Wellcome meeting will face protests from AIDS activists', *Financial Times*, 16 January 1990.
involved helium-filled condoms: 'In on the act', op. cit.

182. 'Pentonville Prisoners' Pricks Deserve Attention': 'Act-Up protest at Hogg's hard line', *Capital Gay*, 4 August 1989.
chained themselves to the turnstiles: 'Protest siege at newspaper HQ', *Capital Gay*, 11 August 1989.
'active homosexuals are potentially murderers': 'AIDS: Straight talk is the way to save lives', *Daily Mail*, 21 July 1989.
More grief at *Melody Maker*: 'Act Up zaps "Misery Maker" over taunts', *Capital Gay*, 31 August 1990; 'Music mag to apologise this week', *Capital Gay*, 7 September 1990.
carried away from Australia House: 'Singer held at HIV demo', *Capital Gay*, 27 October 1989; 'Five found "guilty" in new Act Up trial', *Capital Gay*, 1 December 1989.

183. Whitehall brought to a standstill: 'Dying for money', *Pink Paper*, 21 October 1989.
Westminster Bridge blocked: 'Act Up takes Westminster Bridge', *Capital Gay*, 8 December 1989.
Virgin Megastore in Oxford Street picketed: 'Act-Up zaps Virgin', *Capital Gay*, June 1989.
Middlesex Hospital picketed: 'Delays hit drug trial', *Capital Gay*, 20 April 1990.
Texaco headquarters picketed every week: 'Act Up recruits for petrol boycott', *Capital Gay*, 26 October 1990; 'Texaco job hunters must take HIV test', *Independent*, 23 January 1988.

183. other members had forged too many links: 'Why we left Act-Up', *Capital Gay*, 26 May 1990.

184. convicted of nine counts of theft: 'Act Up treasurer guilty of theft', *Capital Gay*, 21 September 1990.

Chapter 10: Really at Risk?
Principal interviews: David Mellor, Hugh Dufficy, Simon Taylor, Dr Peter
Jones, Adam Sampson, Jimmy Glass, John Campbell, Edwina Currie, Sir
Norman Fowler.

185. by 9.34 a.m. they were ready: this and the course of the debate that
follows from *Hansard*, vol. 144, no. 27, 13 January 1989, and from
personal interviews.

186. inaugural lunch of the National AIDS Trust: 'Control of HIV infection
still Government's top public health priority', DoH press release, 3
October 1988.

189. when Margaret Thatcher heard of it: 'Doubt over £500,000 sex survey',
Independent, 13 September 1989; 'Charity set to fund sex survey vetoed
by PM', *Independent*, 13 October 1989 (see also entry for 24 January 1994
in Part II).
chairman of the AIDS cabinet committee: this was disbanded by Mrs
Thatcher in September 1989.
'"Give me the facts, not the fantasy"': private source.
'something you could make a lot of headway with': private DoH source.

190. speeches she delivered as the opening and closing addresses: 'HIV &
AIDS: An assessment of current and future spread in the UK', UK
Health Departments, 24 November 1989.
heterosexual transmission in the UK: ibid. See also A. M. Johnson,
M. Laga, 'Heterosexual transmission of HIV', *AIDS*, 1988, 2, pp. 49–56.

191. Dr Johnson prepared a similar paper: 'HIV/AIDS: Is the heterosexual
population at risk?', All-Party Parliamentary Group Occasional Paper 1,
1990.
talk of such a study for over two years: this study was recommended in
the Cox Report, op. cit. See also 'Government announces new steps to
monitor the spread of HIV infection', DoH press release, 23 November
1988.
the investment in public education campaigns was justified: 'Virginia
Bottomley announces first results of anonymised HIV testing', DoH
press release, 17 May 1991.

192. 'Straight sex cannot give you AIDS – Official': quoted in '"AIDS is a
myth" say moral crusaders', *Sunday Correspondent*, 21 January 1990.
'Phony face of the war on AIDS': cited in 'The truth about AIDS',
Daily Mail, 17 November 1989.

192. 'Eton and Oxford educated Lord Kilbracken': 'Normal sex is safe row',
Daily Express, 17 November 1989.

193. 'so much to represent the AIDS situation': ibid.
his views were 'unhelpful and misleading': 'The truth about AIDS', op. cit.
'the disease is at one of its most dangerous phases': 'Normal sex is safe
row', op. cit.

193. distributed its own video: '"AIDS is a myth" say moral crusaders', op. cit.
194. withdrew a new condom campaign: 'Thatcher halts AIDS TV ads', *Campaign*, 10 November 1989; 'The politics and profits of doom', *Sunday Correspondent*, 21 January 1990.
advantage in knowing if one was HIV positive or not: 'Greater benefits now in having HIV tests, says Chief Medical Officer', DoH press release, 30 November 1990.
National AIDS Helpline reported an increase in callers: 'CMO's statement on HIV antibody testing', EAGA document, March 1991.
195. a 'dramatic' or 'marked' increase: ibid.
results would not emerge until 1993: see entry for 10 February 1994 in Part II.
little evidence of advances that may soon be of use to sick patients: this and following reports by T. Jones and G. Schild, 'All-Party Parliamentary Group on AIDS, Parliamentary AIDS Digest', Spring 1991.
196. Virginia Bottomley received a worrying report: 'HIV and AIDS Related Health Services', National Audit Office Report by the Comptroller and Auditor General, HMSO, October 1991.
197. 'some health authorities have used underspends': and figures that follow, ibid. It is noteworthy that four authorities overspent their budgets: South East Thames (£2 million), North Western (£1.5 million), Mersey (£600,000) and Yorkshire (£400,000).
198. abolished special payments to people with disabilities: 'We're dying for money', *Capital Gay*, 16 March 1990.
great discrepancies in the basic cost of health care: 'HIV and AIDS Related Health Services', op. cit.
200. how to deal with HIV and AIDS in prisons: for useful background see 'HIV, AIDS and Prisons', Prison Reform Trust, 1988 and its update March 1991. See also T. W. Harding, 'AIDS in Prison', *Lancet*, 28 November 1987; 'HIV in prisons', *BMJ*, 1988, 297, pp. 873–4; Di Robertson, 'HIV prevention in custodial settings', a discussion paper for the Health Education Authority, June 1993.
the Commons debate on AIDS: and the quotes/figures that follow, *Hansard*, vol. 144, op. cit.
202. about 50 cases of HIV identified in prisons: 'Politicians take over AIDS', *BMJ*, 1986, 293, p. 1383.
166 prisoners with HIV had passed through the system: 'HIV, AIDS and Prisons', op. cit.
the powerful Viral Infectivity Restrictions: 'Viral Infectivity Restrictions', Circular instruction from Director of Prison Medical Services, Annex D, October 1991.
203. At Wandsworth a policy of segregation: Open letter to Adam Sampson from Rosemary Wool, director Prison Medical Service, 28 March 1991.

This letter challenged many points made by the Prison Reform Trust in its updated booklet 'HIV, AIDS and Prisons'.

203. Lord Justice Woolf's report: cited in Open letter to Adam Sampson, op. cit.
a staff training video: 'HIV/AIDS: Organisation and procedures at establishment level' (and Annex A), Circular instruction from Director of Prison Medical Services. See also Open letter to Adam Sampson, op. cit. and Robertson, op. cit.

204. *AIDS Inside and Out*: ibid.
contained more people with HIV than any other prison: *Sunday Correspondent Magazine*, 18 March 1990.

205. new guidelines from the Prison Medical Services: 'HIV/AIDS: Organisation and procedures at establishment level', op. cit.
'Ministers … have not been convinced': Open letter to Adam Sampson, op. cit.

206. acknowledged the existence of illicit drug use: 'Throughcare of drug misusers', Circular instruction from Director of Prison Medical Services, 1991.
2,800 males imprisoned for drug offences: and subsequent use/confiscation figures, Robertson, op. cit.

207. creating a climate in which users would identify themselves and seek help: clearly, this is not having an effect on all inmates. In April 1994 *Our View*, a gay and lesbian magazine, received a letter from 'Michael', a British prisoner: 'As I'm sure every officer inside prison knows … sex goes on all the time, and they will never stop it. I really think the Home Office should be taken to court to say why they deny me the right to protect myself from infection and death.
'What is the use of spending thousands of pounds on officers' AIDS awareness courses when they can do nothing about the spreading of HIV, as we're not allowed to have protection. I am still as yet waiting to see the so called Home Office *AIDS: Inside and Out* video. I've heard from officers about this video, but not one person will show me it'.
somehow the drugs always get through: 'Coming clean', *ES Magazine*, September 1993.
they'd quote the findings of the 1978 Royal Commission: 'Haemophilia, AIDS and no fault compensation', *BMJ*, 17 October 1987; see also *Third Report from the Social Services Committee: Problems Associated with AIDS*, HMSO, 1987.

208. 'blood products may be used which contain viruses': quoted in 'Haemophilia, AIDS and no fault compensation', ibid.
And so a campaign got underway: 'AIDS and compensation', Haemophilia Society monthly newsletters ('The Bulletin' and 'Haemofact') and campaign updates from March 1987 to 1991; 'Haemophiliacs seek redress for HIV infection', *New Scientist*, 15 October 1987.

209. a figure of £40–£50: ibid. See also 'Plight of families trapped in AIDS stranglehold', *Guardian*, 12 October 1987.
'I see my patients become sick': 'AIDS blood victims claim £30m from NHS', *Guardian*, 14 October 1987.
but came away empty handed: 'Help for haemophiliacs', *Independent*, 11 November 1987.
suffering the unforeseen side effects: *Third Report from the Social Services Committee*, op. cit., vol. 3, 13 May 1987.
210. a change of heart: '£10m for haemophilia victims of AIDS', *Observer*, 15 November 1987; '£10m to set up AIDS trust', *Times*, 17 November 1987; Haemophilia Society monthly newsletters, op. cit.
'short-changing' the haemophiliacs: '£10m to set up AIDS trust', op. cit.
211. unsure whether the sum would be enough: report summarized in Haemophilia Society's 'The Bulletin', 1988, no. 2.
the trust had made 1,700 single hardship grants: Haemophilia Society's 'The Bulletin', 1989, no. 4.
'While some people point accusing fingers': 'The AIDS innocents', *Daily Express*, 15 October 1987.
Mr Justice Ognall heard preliminary hearings: 'Haemophiliac AIDS victims urged to seek compensation', *Daily Telegraph*, 20 July 1989.
212. 962 haemophiliacs and their families: 'Judge's pressure over HIV victims', *Times*, 1 October 1990.
Margaret Thatcher received a delegation: 'Thatcher hears haemophiliacs' plea', *Sunday Times*, 19 November 1989. The campaign by the *Sunday Times* to gain compensation was a key factor in the haemophiliacs' final success.
'She is seeing us because she cares': ibid.
more money for the Macfarlane Trust: and following quote, DoH press release, 23 November 1989 with full text of parliamentary written answer to Robert Key. See also '£19m for victims of HIV blood', *Independent*, 24 November 1989; '£100m needed for HIV compensation', *Independent*, 30 November 1989.
the possibility of settling out of court: 'Clarke may settle with HIV victims to stop court action', *Sunday Times*, 28 October 1990. See also 'Judge's pressure over HIV victims', op. cit.
large-scale advertisements in the national press: 'Paper shuns AIDS ad', *Campaign*, 5 October 1990.
213. 'those plaintiffs will die uncertain as to the outcome': 'Judge's pressure over HIV victims', op. cit.
'Our NHS is greatly threatened': 'A tragedy of nobody's making', *Sunday Times*, 28 October 1990.
'not asking the Government to admit legal liability': 'MPs in all-party cash call for AIDS victims', *Times*, 22 November 1990. See also 'MPs bill

raises hopes of earlier pay-out for haemophiliac', *Sunday Times*, 25 November 1990.

214. an out-of-court settlement in December 1990: 'Major pledges another £42m for haemophiliacs', *Times*, 12 December 1990.
'they are resigned to it': 'Haemophiliacs accept HIV virus settlement', *Independent*, 30 January 1991.
Virginia Bottomley ruled out the possibility of compensation: 'The NHS cleared this man of leukaemia, but the blood he was given was HIV-infected. The Government says it will not help him', *Observer*, 26 January 1992 (part of the *Observer*'s campaign: 'AIDS victims of the NHS').

Chapter 11: Safer Sex, Risky Sex
Principal interviews: 'Steve', Edward King, Peter Scott, Jonathan Grimshaw, Kate Grieves, Lindsay Neil, Baroness Cumberlege.

225. a letter of resignation: much of the documentation in this section comes from private sources. See also Health Education Authority's summary 'Mass media activity 1986–1993 ; HEA 'Annual Report 1992–93'. Edward King's book, *Safety in Numbers*, Cassell (London, 1993), provides a thorough, and thoroughly convincing account of gay men's health education during the epidemic. See also Simon Watney, *Practices of Freedom*, Rivers Oram Press (London, 1994), pp. 153–6, 199–203, 243–57. Back issues of *Campaign* also provided a useful general survey.
226. HEA spent £9.3 million on HIV campaigns: ibid; 'AIDS: a crisis of confidence', *Capital Gay*, 22 May 1992.
'Things have gone so wrong': ibid.
The lack of specific services: Edward King, Michael Rooney, Peter Scott, 'HIV Prevention for Gay Men: A survey of initiatives in the UK', North West Thames Regional Health Authority, July 1992.
227. 'We've no homosexual community here': ibid.
No one could take offence: see note 1 above.
228. there were some real disasters: 'The seven deadly sins of the HEA: An open letter to the All-Party Parliamentary Group on AIDS' from Edward King (reprinted in *Pink Paper*, 14 June 1992); 'AIDS: a crisis of confidence', *Capital Gay*, 22 May 1992.
230. the most widely known HIV prevention materials: Ford Hickson et al., 'Tales of gay sex: An evaluation of safer sex materials for gay men on the commercial scene', Project SIGMA Working Paper 39, April 1994.
231. a new group announced itself: 'AIDS: a crisis of confidence', *Capital Gay*, 22 May 1992.
the bulk of the campaign was confusing: confidential source. See also 'AIDS campaign falls victim to "back to basics"', *Independent*, 29 January 1994; 'Tory right halt sex education campaigns', *Independent on Sunday*, 17 April 1994.

232. conducting an investigation into condom production: 'Supply of contraceptive sheaths in the UK referred to Monopolies and Mergers Commission', Office of Fair Trading press release, 1 March 1993.

233. pretesting showed them to be well received: Margaret Sheehan, 'Pretesting of safer sex advice advertisements', printed March 1994. Obtained from HEA.

234. The relationship between the HEA and the DoH: for background see 'BMP threat as Govt orders AIDS rethink', *Campaign*, 2 April 1993; 'BMP starts anti-AIDS blitz', *Campaign*, 15 October 1993.
another agency had beaten the HEA's agency: 'Govt awards AIDS work to start-up Lane Earl and Cox', *Campaign*, 7 May 1993.
HEA pulled its own travel-safe posters: 'HEA delays BMP AIDS push after airline complaints', *Campaign*, 2 July 1993.

Chapter 12: Stars and Red Ribbons
Principal interviews: Holly Johnson, Stephen Fry, Jimmy Somerville, Simon Watney, Tim Bussell, Lyndall Stein, Patrick O'Connell, Andrew Butterfield, Ceri Hutton.

236. I hope you don't mind me ringing you at home: the text of this conversation taken from the script of THT Financial Emergency Appeal conducted by Facter Fox, 28 November 1991.

238. 'just have a look at that list': 'Charity Trends 1993', 16th Edition, Charities Aid Foundation, Tonbridge, 1993.

240. the response from the art world was slow: for a general discussion of AIDS' impact on the arts see 'Tragedy', *Independent on Sunday Review*, 1 December 1991; 'Day of the locust', *Premiere*, February 1992; 'Rudi, art and the matter of life and death', Derek Jarman, *Independent*, 8 January 1993; 'A Lost Generation', *Newsweek*, 18 January 1993.
people would assume he was HIV positive: 'Tragedy', op. cit.
'like walking into an Equity meeting': 'Actor's Death from AIDS highlights "obsession"', *Independent*, 13 January 1990.

242. sold his record collection: 'Elton John sale raises AIDS funds', *Guardian*, 30 July 1993. See also Elton John interview in *10 Percent magazine*, Summer 1993.
lucky to be alive: 'Elton: I take an AIDS test every 6 months', *Daily Mirror*, 29 July 1993.

255. Jeremy Irons explained: (and details that follow) from conversation with Patrick O'Connell. Other background information on red ribbon from Red Ribbon International's presentation to the World Health Organization, August 1993; 'Wear a ribbon, win an Oscar', *Independent*, 30 March 1993.

257. Andy Butterfield first became interested: this history drawn from conversations with Butterfield, O'Connell and confidential sources. The

correspondence that concludes this section obtained from confidential
source.

PART II
Journal of a Plague Year

270. the launch of National Condom Week: as reported by Press Association.
'My lover has been really ill': quotes from South London Press/Press
Association.
271. metaphors for the more extensive branding: Benetton press release at
launch, 15 September 1993.
272. 'There's only one pullover': 'AIDS charity hits back at Benetton with
condom ad', *Campaign*, April 1992.
280. 'We heard a lot about the Princess wearing gloves': 'Di's hand of hope',
Evening Standard, 9 April 1987.
'You can't get away anyway': 'AIDS sufferers are reassured by Princess',
Daily Telegraph, 14 September 1988.
'I never read the *Sun*': 'My hamsters eat the Sun, says Diana', *Evening
Standard*, 13 September 1988.
'I'm as thick as a plank': 'A princess positive about AIDS', *Independent*,
30 November 1991.
'Princess Ann doesn't pick up babies': 'Di gets real', *Vanity Fair*,
December 1989.
281. 'a classic own-goal': 'AIDS is own-goal by human race, says Princess',
Daily Telegraph, 27 January 1988.
'the exact spot on my workbench': 'AIDS pioneer praises Princess's
gesture', *Times*, 9 November 1988.
283. her close friend Adrian Ward-Jackson: for a full account of how Diana
nursed Ward-Jackson see Andrew Morton, *Diana: Her True Story*,
Michael O'Mara Books (London, 1992).
284. 'I wish to help her': 'A princess positive about AIDS', op. cit.
'how she feels about the [negative] reaction': ibid.
'I reached a depth inside': Morton, op. cit.
287. a new set of predictions: 'The incidence and prevalence of AIDS and
other severe HIV disease in England and Wales for 1992–97: projections
using data to the end of June 1992', PHLS, June 1993.
288. one other big stat at the World AIDS Day launch: 'HIV & AIDS: It's
time to Act', Health Education Authority press release, 24 November
1993.
290. 'past the time when money was needed for pump priming': *The World
This Weekend* (BBC Radio 4), 16 May 1993.
292. The plan was to roam Europe in search of images: (and subsequent
history) from Network/THT minutes of meetings, 1990–93.

293. 'Each of the photographs ... is a *memento mori*': Stephen Mayes and Lyndall Stein (eds), *Positive Lives: Responses to HIV – a Photodocumentary*, Cassell (London, 1993).

295. established a basecamp in the corner of Jack Straw's Castle car park: this was repeated in 1994.

303. the survey of sexual behaviour in Britain: Kaye Wellings et al., *Sexual Behaviour in Britain*, Penguin/ Blackwell Scientific Publications (London, 1994). This precis of some of the findings taken from 'The facts of homosexual life', *Independent on Sunday Review*, 23 January 1994.

305. Gays Against Genocide haven't gathered to protest this afternoon: see journal entry for 10 February 1994.

307. In June 1991, Frontliners ... was forced to cease trading: see 'Managing and Funding AIDS Organisations: Experience from the closure of Frontliners', Department of Health, 1992.
    partly he blames the *Sunday Times*: see journal entry for 14 June 1994.

311. we all already really know the results: (and subsequent figures) 'Preliminary analysis of the Concorde trial', *Lancet*, 1993, 341, pp. 889–90. See also 'AIDS Treatment Update' (*National AIDS Manual*), Issue 6, April 1993; and (pre-Concorde) Ian V. D. Weller, 'The treatment of asymptomatic HIV infection: lessons from the zidovudine experience', *AIDS*, 1989, 3, pp. 215–20.

312. 'I tolerated AZT fairly easily': Arthur Ashe, *Days of Grace*, Heinemann (London, 1993).
    it could delay the progression of the disease: P. A. Volberding et al., 'Zidovudine in asymptomatic human immunodeficiency virus infection: a controlled trial in persons with fewer than 500 CD-4 positive cells per cubic millimeter', *New England Journal of Medicine*, 1990, 332, pp. 941–9 (trial known as ACTG 019). See also 'Shares soar after AIDS breakthrough', *Times*, 19 August 1989; 'Success stops trial of AIDS drug', *New Scientist*, 26 August 1989; 'Concorde remains aloft', *Lancet*, 28 October 1989, pp. 1017–18.
    AZT had caused cancer in rodents: 'Setback for anti-AIDS drug', *Financial Times*, 6 December 1989.

313. The company's share price was hammered: 'AZT: Wellcome's bitter pill', *Observer*, 4 April 1993.
    unhappy with the way the results were released: 'Wellcome hits back over AIDS drug results', *New Scientist*, 17 April 1993. In July 1994 Professor Jones announced he was leaving Wellcome to become director general of the Association of the British Pharmaceutical Industry. His departure had been expected for some time, ever since David Barry, his counterpart in the United States, also took on the role of director of research and development in the UK.

315. An emotional climax of sorts: 'HIV in the work place', speech by J. A.

Breitman at Positive Action, 22 June 1992. I am grateful to Neil
McKenna for informing me of this.

315. the alternative self-help group Positively Healthy: in the late 1980s
Positively Healthy had been involved in a libel dispute with Duncan
Campbell, the *New Statesman* journalist who had done much valuable
work in exposing quack AIDS doctors and their bogus drugs. The
dispute with PH's Cass Mann centred on the relative benefits of
conventional treatments, including AZT, and the alternative, sometimes
ineffectual, compounds and therapies offered by Mann. See also 'Health
and Safety', *Observer*, Uncensored supplement, 17 April 1994; 'Dirty
Tricksters', *Time Out*, 23 February 1994.

316. 'a naïve hope that Holland and Barrett will produce a herbal tea': (and
subsequent information in this entry) 'The rise and fall of AZT',
Independent on Sunday Review, 2 May 1993.
it had all turned rather sour: High Court writ, 11 June 1993; 'Gay
activists picket AIDS charity after pair jailed', *Independent*, 20 July 1993.

317. believed that HIV was not the cause of AIDS: see entry for 14 June 1994.
granted legal aid to pursue a similar case: 'Woman gets legal aid to sue
over AZT AIDS drug', *Guardian*, 31 August 1993.

319. this morning came some bad news: see also 'Police hunt AIDS charity's
missing £500,000', *Independent*, 15 February 1994; 'Police launch
investigation into AIDS group', *Pink Paper*, 18 February 1994.

322. Jarman wrote an eloquent letter: 'Why shutting Bart's would be a crime',
Independent, 5 May 1993.

323. anal sex has been on the agenda: for example, during a discussion of the
age of consent at a meeting of Preston Council in mid-February,
councillor Ken Hudson said there was 'no money in the budget for
shirtlifters'. Hudson later apologized, and abstained when the council
supported lowering the age to 16. (Source: *Pink Paper*, 18 February
1994.)
'The present laws prevent us': 'Young gay men being exposed to risk of
AIDS', *Independent*, 29 January 1994.

324. 'party political broadcast for the Buggers' Party': quoted in *Pink Paper*,
25 February 1994.
Paul Muldownie began with a knife: 'AIDS robber terrified victim with
syringe', *Times*, 1 March 1994; 'AIDS raider used syringe to terrify',
Guardian, 1 March 1994.

326. MRC co-ordinated a European study in 1991: 'European collaborative
study. Children born to women with HIV-1 infection: natural history
and risk of transmission', *Lancet*, 1991, 337, pp. 253–60.
prevent a pregnant HIV positive woman infecting her baby: 'AZT tests
yield new hope for babies of women with HIV', *Guardian*, 22 February
1994.

326. transmission normally occurs about 15 per cent of the time: see A. E. Ades et al., 'Vertically transmitted HIV infection in the British Isles', *BMJ*, 1993, 306, pp. 1296–9. The vertical transmission rate in the British Isles was found to be 13.7 per cent (23 cases out of 168), and 23 per cent of infected children developed AIDS in the first year of life.
a new MRC programme to develop vaginal virucides: for this and other ongoing research mentioned here see *Report on MRC AIDS research 1993*, MRC (London, 1993).

327. a report on AIDS and the over-fifties: *A Crisis of Silence: HIV, AIDS and Older People* (Age Concern Greater London, 1993).

332. pioneering same-day test: see S. B. Squire et al., 'Open access clinic providing HIV-1 antibody result on day of testing: the first twelve months', *BMJ*, 1991, 302, pp. 1383–6.

334. *Your Pocket Guide to Sex*: an extract: 'All I did was hold his cock in the palm of my hand. It was stiff as a board and I could feel it throbbing. I looked him in the eyes and said: "You know there's only two things in the world that I want right now – your cock deep inside me, and your cock inside a condom."'

335. Condoms were moving out of Chingford, Essex: 'LIG's plant closures to cost 1,000 British jobs', *Independent*, 20 April 1994.
some contrast to 1987: 'Soaring demand for condoms help LIG advance by 13%', *Financial Times*, 19 June 1987. See also 'The condom market', *Lancet*, 21 November 1987.
an important meeting was taking place: based on confidential minutes.

336. blowing up 17,000 condoms: 'Condom brands fail to satisfy standards test', *Guardian*, 10 August 1993; Press Association, 9 August 1993. Despite some poor results, the magazine concluded, 'Thankfully, poor quality condoms are few and far between'.
The BSI revises its guidelines on condoms: details of revisions from BSI Text of new edition of BS 3704, 22 April 1994.

337. condoms be made available for use by prisoners: 'Prison health adviser backs free condoms', *Guardian*, 17 May 1994.

339. Roy Cornes … died today: 'Husband accused of spreading AIDS dies', *Daily Telegraph*, 7 June 1994. See also 'AIDS: from them to us', *Independent on Sunday*, 28 June 1992; 'When AIDS struck home', *Sunday Telegraph*, 28 June 1992; 'The fear and the fury of wisdom after the event', *Daily Telegraph*, 14 December 1993.

344. the potential for its heterosexual growth was only too visible: 'AIDS epidemic shows signs of decline as new cases peak', *Sunday Times*, 13 August 1989.
a *Dispatches* programme for Channel 4: 'The AIDS Catch', Channel 4, 13 June 1990. The 1987 programme was called 'AIDS – The Unheard Voices'.

345. Duesberg liked to quote Lewis Carroll: 'AIDS acquired by drug consumption and other noncontagious risk factors', *Pharmacology and Therapeutics*, 1992, 55, pp. 201–277.
a fondness for Sherlock Holmes: ibid.
Duesberg claimed that HIV was a harmless retrovirus: for concise summaries of the Duesberg theories see 'A challenge to the AIDS establishment', *Bio/Technology*, vol. 5, November 1987; 'AIDS and the "innocent" virus', *New Scientist*, 28 April 1988 (and the response from Jonathan Weber, 'AIDS and the "guilty" virus', *New Scientist*, 5 May 1988). For a good round-up of Duesberg and supporters, 'Does this man know something we don't?', *Telegraph Magazine*, 20 November 1993.

346. 'a kind of conspiracy beginning to develop': 'Unlikely saviour of the gay community?', *Continuum*, October/November 1993. See also Neil's letter, 'AIDS and the *Sunday Times*', *Guardian*, 17 December 1993.
run almost in its entirety: 'AIDS: Can we be positive?', *Sunday Times*, 26 April 1992.

347. The campaign then took off: 'AIDS: Why we won't be silenced', *Sunday Times*, 12 December 1993, provides a summary of past articles and main arguments. For a response to some points raised see 'HIV: beyond reasonable doubt', *New Scientist*, 15 January 1994.

348. 'one of the greatest peace-time scandals of the 20th century': 'Unlikely saviour of the gay community?', op. cit.
HIV may not be the sole cause of AIDS: they believe that HIV is still necessary for AIDS, but there may also be 'co-factors', other unsepecified elements which determine progression to AIDS.

349. 60 times more likely to die within two years: see 'Africa study showsHIV victims 60 times likelier to die in 2 years'. *Guardian*, 22 April 1994.

350. a forceful opponent of Duesberg and his supporters: see in particular 'The truth about growing menace of heterosexual AIDS', *Independent on Sunday*, 21 May 1993.
three Nobel prize-winners working at Cambridge University: 'Nobel scientists reaffirm HIV link with AIDS', *Independent*, 20 May 1992.
a doctor working in Nairobi: 'Paper accused of AIDS "distortion"', *Independent*, 9 January 1994.

351. 'closer comparison would be with the Hitler diaries': 'HIV, AIDS, and the anatomy of dissent', *Independent*, 6 December 1993.

352. arrested and charged with 11 joint offences: according to *Pink Paper*, 15 July 1994, Michael Cottrell has called off GAG's campaign from his prison cell.

353. an editorial she has just completed: 'Non-progression in HIV infection', *AIDS*, 1994, vol. 8, no. 8.
Additional note: Two significant small-scale studies appeared at the end of 1994. Researchers at the Royal Free Hospital, London, reported that

one in four people may not develop AIDS for up to 20 years after infection. The projection was based on studies of the CD4 counts of 111 haemophiliacs. Another study, based at Turin University, looked at 18 lesbian couples in long-term sexually active relationships; one member of each couple was HIV positive (usually through intravenous drug use), and the other was negative. The couples engaged in theoretically high-risk activity without protective barriers, but there was no viral transmission. The researchers concluded that the risk of transmission was 'non-existent'.

Index